Methods in Neurosciences

Volume 8

Neurotoxins

Methods in Neurosciences

Edited by

P. Michael Conn

Department of Pharmacology
The University of Iowa
College of Medicine
Iowa City, Iowa

Volume 8

Neurotoxins

ACADEMIC PRESS, INC.
Harcourt Brace Jovanovich, Publishers
San Diego   New York   Boston
London   Sydney   Tokyo   Toronto

Front Cover illustration (paperback edition only): Most neurotoxins are naturally derived products and owe their specificity and potency to millions of years of evolution. The cover image is the editor's rendering of the wood scorpion (*Androctonus aeneus)* noted for its potent neurotoxin.

This book is printed on acid-free paper. ∞

Academic Press, Inc.
1250 Sixth Avenue, San Diego, California 92101

United Kingdom Edition published by
Academic Press Limited
24–28 Oval Road, London NW1 7DX

International Standard Serial Number: 1043-9471

International Standard Book Number: 0-12-185265-2 (Hardcover)

International Standard Book Number: 0-12-185266-0 (Paperback)

PRINTED IN THE UNITED STATES OF AMERICA
92 93 94 95 96 97   EB   9 8 7 6 5 4 3 2 1

Table of Contents

Contributors to Volume 8

Article numbers are in parentheses following the names of contributors. Affiliations listed are current.

FRANCES C. G. ALEXANDER (12), Protein Toxins Group, Division of Biologics, PHLS Centre for Applied Microbiology and Research, Salisbury, Wiltshire SP4 OJG, England

A. J. ANDERSON (29), Department of Physiology and Pharmacology, Strathclyde Institute for Drug Research, University of Strathclyde, Glasgow G1 1XW, Scotland

M. ARITA (22), Department of Pharmacology, University of Occupational and Environmental Health, School of Medicine, Yahatanishiku, Kitakyushu 807, Japan

JOHANNA BALVINSDOTTIR (7), Department of Biological Sciences, The Royal Danish School of Pharmacy, 2100 Ø Copenhagen, Denmark

EVELYNE BENOIT (11), Laboratoire de Physiologie Comparée, Unité Associée du Centre de la Recherche Scientifique, Université de Paris XI, 91405 Orsay, France

ROLAND BENZ (1), Lehrstuhl für Biotechnologie, Universität Würzburg, D-8700 Würzburg, Germany

MORDECAI BLAUSTEIN (16), Department of Physiology and Medicine, School of Medicine, University of Maryland, Baltimore, Maryland 21201

PETER M. BLUMBERG (27), Laboratory of Cellular Carcinogenesis and Tumor Promotion, National Institutes of Health, National Cancer Institute, Bethesda, Maryland 20892

JEAN-PHILIPPE BREITTMAYER (17, 25), Faculté de Médecine, Université de Nice, 06034 Nice, France

BARRY S. BREWSTER (2), Jerry Lewis Muscle Research Center, Department of Pediatrics and Neonatal Medicine, Royal Postgraduate Medical School, Hammersmith Hospital, London W12 ONN, England

CARLOS CERVEÑANSKY (18), Division of Neurochemistry, Instituto de Investigaciones Biológicas Clemente Estable, 11600 Montevideo, Uruguay

Trinad Chakraborty (1), Lehrstuhl für Mikrobiologie, Universität Würzburg, D-8700 Würzburg, Germany

Jens Dencker Christensen (7), Department of Biological Sciences, The Royal Danish School of Pharmacy, 2100 Ø Copenhagen, Denmark

F. Clementi (6), CNR Center of Cytopharmacology, Department of Medical Pharmacology, University of Milan, 20129 Milan, Italy

Joan X. Comella (11), Facultat de Medicina, Estudi General de Lleida, Universitat de Barcelona, Lleida E-25006, Spain

Cyrus R. Creveling (3), Laboratory of Bioorganic Chemistry, National Institute of Diabetes and Digestive and Kidney Diseases, National Institutes of Health, Bethesda, Maryland 20892

Federico Dajas (18), Division of Neurochemistry, Instituto de Investigaciones Biológicas Clemente Estable, 11600 Montevideo, Uruguay

John W. Daly (3), Laboratory of Bioorganic Chemistry, National Institute of Diabetes, Digestive, and Kidney Diseases, National Institutes of Health, Bethesda, Maryland 20892

Thu T. Dinh (9), Department of Veterinary and Comparative Anatomy, Pharmacology, and Physiology, Washington State University, Pullman, Washington 99164

A. Esparis-Ogando (6), CNR Center of Cytopharmacology, Department of Medical Pharmacology, University of Milan, 20129 Milan, Italy

Bjarne Fjalland (7), Department of Biological Sciences, The Royal Danish School of Pharmacy, 2100 Ø Copenhagen, Denmark

Christian Frelin (17, 25), Institut de Pharmacologie Moléculaire et Cellulaire, Centre National de la Recherche Scientifique, Sophia Antipolis, 06560 Valbonne, France

Maria L. Garcia (10), Department of Membrane Biochemistry and Biophysics, Merck Institute for Therapeutic Research, Rahway, New Jersey 07065

Margarita Garcia-Calvo (10), Department of Membrane Biochemistry and Biophysics, Merck Institute for Therapeutic Research, Rahway, New Jersey 07065

C. Gotti (6), CNR Center of Cytopharmacology, Department of Medical Pharmacology, University of Milan, 20129 Milan, Italy

Claude Granier (28), Laboratoire de Biochemie, Centre National de la Recherche Scientifique, Faculté de Médecine, 13326 Marseille Cedex 15, France

JOHN B. HARRIS (21), Division of Neurobiology, School of Neurosciences, University of Newcastle upon Tyne, Medical School, Newcastle upon Tyne, NEZ 4AB, England

A. L. HARVEY (29), Department of Physiology and Pharmacology, Strathclyde Institute for Drug Research, University of Strathclyde, Glasgow G1 1XW, Scotland

N. H. HIMMELREICH (20), Department of Neurochemistry, A. V. Palladin Institute of Biochemistry, Ukrainian Academy of Sciences, 252030 Kiev, U.S.S.R.

F. IZUMI (22), Department of Pharmacology, University of Occupational and Environmental Health, School of Medicine, Yahatanishiku, Kitakyushu 807, Japan

ANNETTE JØRGENSEN (7), Department of Biological Sciences, The Royal Danish School of Pharmacy, 2100 Ø Copenhagen, Denmark

GREGORY J. KACZOROWSKI (10), Department of Membrane Biochemistry and Biophysics, Merck Institute for Therapeutic Research, Rahway, New Jersey 07065

H. KOBAYASHI (22), Department of Pharmacology, University of Occupational and Environmental Health, School of Medicine, Yahatanishiku, Kitakyushu 807, Japan

SUSAN F. LAW (26), Department of Pharmacology, University of Pennsylvania, School of Medicine, Philadelphia, Pennsylvania 19104

ANNE-MARIE LEGRAND (11), Institut Territorial de Recherches Médicales Louis Malardé, Associé à l'Institute Pasteur, Papeete, Tahiti, Polynésie, Francaise

IDA J. LLEWELLYN-SMITH (13), Center for Neuroscience and Department of Medicine, Flinders University School of Medicine, Bedford Park, South Australia 5042, Australia

KARSTEN LOLLIKE (7), Institute of Medical Physiology and Biotechnology, Center for Signal Peptide Research, The Panum Institute, University of Copenhagen, 2200 N Copenhagen, Denmark

ERWANN P. LORET (28), Department of Biochemistry and Biophysics, Oregon State University, Corvallis, Oregon 97331

JANE B. MINSON (13), Center for Neuroscience and Department of Medicine, Flinders University School of Medicine, Bedford Park, South Australia 5042, Australia

FRANÇIS MIRANDA (28), Laboratoire de Biochemie, Centre National de la Recherche Scientifique, Faculté de Médecine, 13326 Marseille Cedex 15, France

JORDI MOLGO (4, 11), Laboratoire de Neurobiologie Cellulaire et Moléculaire, Centre National de la Recherche Scientifique, 91198 Gif-sur-Yvette, France

M. MORETTI (6), CNR Center of Cytopharmacology, Department of Medical Pharmacology, University of Milan, 20129 Milan, Italy

HIDESHI NAKAMURA (19), Department of Chemistry, Faculty of Medicine, Hokkaido University, Sapporo 060, Japan

JEAN J. NORDMANN (14), Centre de Neurochimie du Centre National de la Recherche Scientifique, 67084 Strasbourg, France

YASUSHI OHIZUMI (19), Pharmacological Institute, Tohoku University, Sendai 980, Japan

PAUL M. PILOWSKY (13), Center for Neuroscience and Department of Medicine, Flinders University School of Medicine, Bedford Park, SA 5042, Australia

BERNARD POULAIN (4), Laboratoire de Neurobiologie Cellulaire et Moléculaire, Centre National de la Recherche Scientific, 91198 Gif-sur-Yvette, France

TERRY REISINE (26), Department of Pharmacology, University of Pennsylvania, School of Medicine, Philadelphia, Pennsylvania 19104

SUE RITTER (9), Department of Veterinary and Comparative Anatomy, Pharmacology, and Physiology, Washington State University, Pullman, Washington 99164

HERVÉ ROCHAT (28), Laboratoire de Biochemie, Centre National de la Recherche Scientifique, Faculté de Médecine, 13326 Marseille Cedex 15, France

E. G. ROWAN (29), Department of Physiology and Pharmacology, Strathclyde Institute for Drug Research, University of Strathclyde, Glasgow G1 1XW, Scotland

FRANÇOIS SAMPIERI (28), Laboratoire de Biochemie, Centre National de la Recherche Scientifique, Faculté de Médecine, 13326 Marseille, France

KAZUKI SATO (19), Mitsubishi Kasei Institute of Life Sciences, Machida, Tokyo 194, Japan

MARTIN-PIERRE SAUVIAT (24), Laboratoire de Physiologie Comparée, Université de Paris-SUD, 91405 Orsay, France

CLIFFORD C. SHONE (12), Protein Toxins Group, Division of Biologics, PHLS Centre for Applied Microbiology and Research, Salisbury, Wiltshire SP4 0JG, England

RODOLFO SILVEIRA (18), Division of Neurochemistry, Instituto de Investigaciones Biológicas Clemente Estable, 11600 Montevideo, Uruguay

LANCE L. SIMPSON (5), Department of Medicine, Division of Environmental Medicine and Toxicology, Jefferson Medical College, Philadelphia, Pennsylvania 19107

YU. V. SOKOLOV (20), Department of Neurochemistry, A. A. Bogomoletez Institute of Physiology, Ukrainian Academy of Sciences, 252030 Kiev, U.S.S.R.

ROGER G. SORENSEN (16), Department of Medicine, Division of Environmental Medicine and Toxicology, Thomas Jefferson University, Philadelphia, Pennsylvania 19107

PETER N. STRONG (2), Jerry Lewis Muscle Research Center, Department of Pediatrics and Neonatal Medicine, Royal Postgraduate Medical School, Hammersmith Hospital, London W12 ONN, England

ARPAD SZALLASI (27), Laboratory of Cellular Carcinogenesis and Tumor Promotion, National Cancer Institute, National Institutes of Health, Bethesda, Maryland 20892

KEN TAKEDA (14), Laboratoire de Pharmacologie Cellulaire et Moléculaire, Université Louis Pasteur de Strasbourg, Centre National de la Recherche Scientifique, 67401 Illkirch, France

MOTOHIKO TAKEMURA (15), Department of Pharmacology II, Faculty of Medicine, Osaka University, Suita, Osaka 565, Japan

YA. T. TERLETSKAYA (20), Department of Neurochemistry, A. V. Palladin Institute of Biochemistry, Ukrainian Academy of Sciences, 252030 Kiev, U.S.S.R.

HOWARD S. TRANTER (12), Small Scale Production Group, Division of Biologics, PHLS Centre for Applied Microbiology and Research, Salisbury, Wiltshire SP4 0JG, England

MAREK TREIMAN (7), Institute of Medical Physiology and Biotechnology, Center for Signal Peptide Research, The Panum Institute, University of Copenhagen, 2200 N Copenhagen, Denmark

K. TSUJI (22), Department of Medicinal Chemistry of Natural Products, University of Shizuoka, School of Pharmaceutical Sciences, Shizuoka 422, Japan

Y. UEZONO (22), Department of Pharmacology, University of Occupational and Environmental Health, School of Medicine, Yahatanishiku, Kitakyushu 807, Japan

JESUS VAZQUEZ (10), Department of Membrane Biochemistry and Biophysics, Merck Institute for Therapeutic Research, Rahway, New Jersey 07065

A. WADA (22), Department of Pharmacology, University of Occupational and Environmental Health, School of Medicine, Yahatanishiku, Kitakyushu 807, Japan

I. WESSLER (8), Department of Pharmacology, University of Mainz, D-6500 Mainz, Germany

N. YANAGIHARA (22), Department of Pharmacology, University of Occupational and Environmental Health, School of Medicine, Yahatanishiku, Kitakyushu 807, Japan

FRANK ZUFALL (23), Physiologisches Institut der Technischen Universität München, D-8000 München 40, Germany

Preface

The exquisite specificity and potency of toxins have made them valuable probes of neural systems. These compounds have been extremely helpful in probing second messenger molecules, ion channels, G proteins, and in electrophysiological studies. Because of the impact of this methodology on the development of and progress in the neurosciences, it was felt that a volume containing representative methodology in this area should be included among the first ten volumes in this series. Every effort has been made to provide representative examples of the useful techniques that have made this area a productive component of the neurosciences.

In this volume, techniques are described for the preparation, handling, and, particularly, for the use of neurotoxins. Model systems are presented in which these neurotoxins have been extremely valuable in developing an understanding of the cellular and molecular basis of secretion and electro-physiological events leading to altered cell function.

The goal of this volume, as well as of those to follow, is to provide in one source a view of the contemporary techniques significant to a particular branch of neurosciences, information which will prove invaluable not only to the experienced researcher but to the student as well. Of necessity some archival material will be included, but the authors have been encouraged to present information that has not yet been published, to compare (in a way not found in other publications) different approaches to similar problems, and to provide tables that direct the reader, in a systematic fashion, to earlier literature and as an efficient means to summarize data. Flow diagrams and summary charts will guide the reader through the processes described.

The nature of this series permits the presentation of methods in fine detail, revealing "tricks" and short cuts that frequently do not appear in the literature owing to space limitations. Lengthy operating instructions for common equipment will not be included except in cases of unusual application. The contributors have been given wide latitude in nomenclature and usage since they are best able to make judgments consistent with current changes.

I wish to express my appreciation to Mrs. Sue Birely for assisting in the organization and maintenance of records and especially to the staff of Academic Press for their energetic enthusiasm and efficient coordination of production. Appreciation is also expressed to the contributors, particularly for meeting their deadlines for the prompt and timely publication of the volume.

P. MICHAEL CONN

Methods in Neurosciences
Edited by P. Michael Conn

[1] Comparison of α-Toxin of *Staphylococcus aureus* and Aerolysin for Formation of Ion-Permeable Channels

Roland Benz and Trinad Chakraborty

Introduction

Mammalian cells are surrounded by a fluid mosaic membrane that is composed of lipids, proteins, and carbohydrates (1). The lipids are amphiphilic molecules with a hydrophilic head and a hydrocarbon side chain. They are arranged in a fluid bilayer structure. Pure lipid bilayer membranes have a very small permeability for hydrophilic and charged solutes (2). Integral proteins are responsible for the specific permeability properties of biological membranes. These proteins act either as channels, carriers, or pumps. As a result of the action of ion pumps, such as the Na^+,K^+-ATPase, cell membranes have on both sides different concentrations of potassium and sodium ions. The interior of mammalian cells is enriched in potassium, whereas the external media contain high concentrations of sodium. The asymmetric distribution of ions and the function of the cell membrane as a barrier are essential for cell function. The loss of the barrier function of cell membranes for any length of time leads to cell death.

Many bacteria of pathogenic origin synthesize toxins that are capable of lysing mammalian cells. The frequent correlation of hemolytic activity with pathogenic bacteria has led to the suggestion that these "cytotoxins" or "pore-forming toxins" are virulence factors (3, 4). With the availability of purified toxins, it has been shown that many toxins indeed form ion-permeable channels of different ionic specificity.

Synthesis of cytotoxins has been reported through a broad spectrum of gram-negative and gram-positive bacteria (3). They are frequently found in the supernatant of cultures of pathogenic cells. Cytotoxins are exoproteins, and are exported out of the cells in a water-soluble form. In the presence of membranes, they completely change their structure and act as membrane channels, which have hydrophobic exteriors. The insertion of these channels into the cytoplasmic membrane results in permeability changes. Subsequently the osmotic balance across the cytoplasmic membrane is disturbed and the cells swell and lyse if components responsible for the active transport of ions cannot balance the permeability increase. The *in vivo* action of cytotoxins ultimately causes physical damage to a variety of eukaryotic cells. In this chapter we discuss the molecular properties of two of these cytotoxins and the nature of the ion-permeable channels they form in lipid bilayer membranes.

Species of the gram-negative bacterial genus *Aeromonas* elaborate the potent cytotoxin aerolysin (5, 6). Aerolysin is a single polypeptide with a molecular mass of 54 kDa and is secreted as a proenzyme (7, 8). There exist two precursor forms of aerolysin. The first, preproaerolysin, contains the typical signal sequence of 23 amino acids that is cotranslationally removed as the protein crosses the inner bacterial membrane. Active toxin is produced by proteolytic cleavage of the protoxin at its carboxy-terminal end (9). The biological properties include lethality to mice, enterotoxicity in rabbit ileal segments, and cytotoxicity in a large variety of cell lines *in vitro*. Independent cloning and sequencing of the aerolysin gene have been reported (7, 10). This has now opened the way for a molecular analysis of the various properties reported for the toxin.

α-Toxin of *Staphylococcus aureus* is a proteinaceous exotoxin, the hemolytic, dermonecrotic, and lethal properties of which have been known for a long time (11–13). The toxin is produced as a water-soluble polypeptide with a molecular mass of 34 kDa (14). It binds to cell membranes with a cell type-specific affinity (12). In the presence of lipids, α-toxin forms hexamers that can be detected in electron microscopic analysis of target membranes and liposomes (15). The toxin has been shown to act as a membrane-permeabilizing compound (14). Molecular cloning of its gene has been reported (16), and its involvement in staphylococcal infections demonstrated by the use of site-directed insertion mutants within the gene (17).

Isolation and Purification of Aerolysin and α-Toxin

Aerolysin of *Aeromonas* species and α-toxin of *S. aureus* are found in the supernatant of cell cultures. Culture supernatants are obtained by centrifugation. The supernatant fluid of the *Aeromonas* culture is concentrated 50-fold by ultrafiltration using an Amicon (Danvers, MA) "hollow fiber" filter (cutoff molecular mass approximately 10 kDa). Aerolysin is precipitated from the concentrated supernatant by adjustment to pH 4.5 after addition of a yeast tRNA solution to a final concentration of 0.3 mg/ml (18). The pellet is dissolved in buffer containing 50 mM Tris-HCl and 1 M urea and loaded onto an anion-exchange column. Elution is performed using a salt gradient and hemolytic activity elutes as a sharp peak between 0.22 and 0.25 M NaCl. Fractions containing electrophoretically pure aerolysin are concentrated by dialysis against the urea–Tris-HCl buffer containing 150 mM NaCl and 20%

polyethylene glycol (PEG) 20,000 and stored at $-70°C$ in 50 mM Tris-HCl, 4 M urea, and 20% glycerol.

α-Toxin is precipitated from the supernatant by the addition of solid ammonium sulfate to 75% saturation. The precipitated crude toxin is dialyzed against 20 mM NaCl, 10 mM sodium acetate, pH 5, and loaded onto a cation-exchange column. Elution is performed with a linear salt gradient of 200 mM NaCl, 10 mM sodium acetate, pH 5. The fractions exhibiting toxin activity are concentrated and loaded onto a Superose gel filtration column. Elution with 10 mM NaCl, 10 mM sodium phosphate buffer, pH 7, yields electrophoretically pure toxin (14).

Methodology of Lipid Bilayer Membranes

It is possible to study the action of toxins in patch-clamp experiments with cell membranes (19). However, many more studies have been performed using the lipid bilayer technique (20–23). Two basically different methods have successfully been used for formation of lipid bilayer membranes and for the study of channels in *in vitro* systems. The first method was proposed by Mueller *et al.* (24), and has been described in a number of different publications (2, 22–26). The cell used for membrane formation consists of a Teflon chamber with a thin wall separating two aqueous compartments. The Teflon divider has small circular holes with an area of either 1 or 2 mm^2 (for macroscopic conductance measurements) or 0.1 mm^2 (for single-channel experiments). For membrane formation, the lipid is dissolved mainly in *n*-decane in a concentration of 1 of to 2% (w/v). However, other organic solvents, such as *n*-hexadecane, squalene, or triolein, have successfully been used for membrane formation. The basic difference between them is the amount of residual solvent in the membrane after it is in the "black" state, i.e., the solvents influence the membrane thickness (27, 28). In particular, this type of solvent has no influence on the properties of reconstituted channels. The lipid solution is painted over the holes to form a lamella. The membrane experiments start after the lamella thins out and turns optically black in reflected light, which suggests that the membrane is much thinner than the wavelength of the light (28). The addition of small amounts of *n*-butanol (10%, v/v) to the membrane-forming solutions stabilizes the membranes.

A second method is the formation of "solvent-free" or "solvent-depleted" lipid bilayer membranes according to the method of Montal and Mueller (29). The cell for membrane formation is basically the same as described above for the formation of solvent-containing membranes, with the exception that the holes in the Teflon divider are extremely small (diameter 10 to 50 μm).

The surfaces of the aqueous phases on both sides of the hole are adjusted below it. Lipid dissolved in hexane is now added to both surfaces to form monolayers (in fact, the lipid must be sufficient for many monolayers). Then the aqueous phases are raised over the hole and a lipid bilayer membrane may be formed. It should be noted that the hole must be pretreated with small amounts of petroleum jelly, hexadecane, or other organic solvents for successful formation of membranes (27). Solvent-depleted membranes cannot be controlled optically because of their small surface area. The control of successful membrane formation (as opposed to the possibility that the hole is simply plugged with lipid) is possible only on the basis of the measurement of the membrane capacitance (27, 29). This method has the advantage that reconstituted vesicles can be used for the formation of the lipid bilayer membranes. In this case, the reconstituted vesicles are spread on the surfaces on both sides of the Teflon divider to form monolayers. It is believed that the membrane formed by these monolayers contains protein reconstituted into the vesicles (30).

The lipid bilayer technique allows the sensitive detection of current through the membrane. It is, however, not very well suited for the study of fluxes of uncharged solutes. For sensitive electrical measurements, the membrane cell must be surrounded by a Faraday cage to avoid the 50- or 60-cycle noise of the line and other pertubations caused by electric fields. It is also necessary to insulate the membrane cell against mechanical oscillations. Two Ag/AgCl or calomel electrodes are inserted into the aqueous phases on both sides of the membrane. Electrodes with salt bridges must be used in case of salt gradients across the membrane or if the aqueous phase does not contain a sufficient concentration of chloride. The electrodes are switched in series with a voltage source (output voltage 5 to 250 mV) and an electrometer (Keithley 602 or 616; Cleveland, OH). In the case of the single-channel recordings the electrometer is replaced by a current amplifier (Keithley 427 or a current-to-voltage converter based on an operational amplifier). The amplified signal is monitored with a storage oscilloscope and recorded with a tape or a strip chart recorder.

The sensitivity of the method is of the order of 0.1 pA (which corresponds to a flux of about 5×10^5 ions/sec) or a few picosiemens (pS; 10^{-12} A/V). The lipid bilayer technique allows good access from both sides of the membrane. This means that with this technique the ionic composition on both sides of the membrane can be controlled. It is possible to establish salt gradients across the membrane by the addition of concentrated salt solution to one side of the membrane. Zero-current membrane potential measurements allow the measurement of the ionic selectivity of channels if the membrane contains a sufficient number of channels (26).

Toxins in Lipid Bilayer Membranes

The study of the toxin is performed as follows (21, 22). Purified toxin is added in small concentration (10 ng/ml to 1 μg/ml) with stirring. This allows equilibration to the aqueous phase bathing a black lipid bilayer membrane, formed by either of the two different methods described above. After a short lag time of about 2 min the membrane current starts to increase, reaching many orders of magnitude within 15 to 20 min (21). This process is similar for aerolysin and α-toxin. It indicates the insertion of membrane-active, ion-permeable material into the membrane. After about 30 min, the membrane conductance (i.e., the current per unit voltage) increases at a much slower rate. This slow conductance increase continues usually until the lipid bilayer membranes are mechanically disrupted. When the rate of conductance increase is relatively slow (as compared to the initial one) it is possible to study the membrane conductance as a function of the protein concentration. Interestingly, the specific conductance is steeper than the toxin concentration. This result indicates that more than one toxin molecule is involved in channel formation. In fact, both toxins form sodium dodecyl sulfate (SDS)-stable oligomers (possibly hexamers) in the presence of lipids (11, 21, 31). These oligomers have been detected in electron microscope studies of membranes in the presence of α-toxin (15).

Single-Channel Analysis and Pore Diameter

The addition of smaller amounts of both toxins to lipid bilayer membranes allows the resolution of step increases in conductance as shown in Fig. 1. This means that the membrane activity described above is caused by the formation of ion-permeable channels in the membranes. One step reflects the insertion of one conductive unit (i.e., of one channel into the membrane). These conductance steps are specific to the presence of the toxins. They are not observed when only concentrated supernatants of cells lacking the toxins are added to the aqueous phase. This means that the channels are not formed by porins of *Aeromonas sobria*. *Staphylococcus aureus* does not contain porins. Figure 1 shows that the conductance steps observed in the presence of both toxins are almost exclusively directed upward. Closing events are only rarely observed at small transmembrane potentials of about 20 mV. The most frequent value for the single-channel conductance of aerolysin in 1 M KCl (the conditions of Fig. 1) was about 0.65 nS. The single-channel conductance of the α-toxin channel is, with 0.82 nS, about 20% higher under the same conditions. Only a limited number of larger steps are observed for

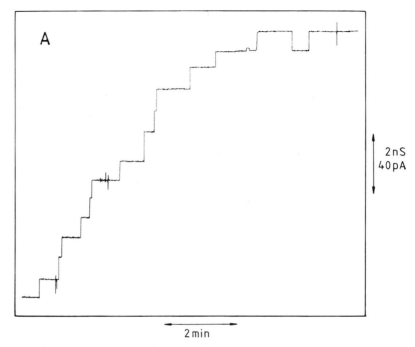

FIG. 1   Single-channel recordings of diphytanoylphosphatidylcholine membranes after the addition of 5 ng/ml aerolysin of *Aeromonas sobria* (A) or 10 ng/ml α-toxin of *Staphylococcus aureus* (B) to the aqueous phase. The aqueous phase contained 1 *M* KCl, pH 6. The applied potential was 20 mV; 25°C.

both toxins (see Fig. 2 for a histogram of the conductance fluctuations observed with both toxins in 1 *M* KCl). These larger conductance fluctuations are probably caused by the formation of two channels at the same time.

At voltages up to 50 mV the closing events represent only a minor fraction of the total number of current fluctuations. However, at membrane potentials higher than 50 mV the closing events are more frequent. Figure 3 shows a single-channel recording of a membrane in the presence of aerolysin at 100 mV. The "on" steps have a mean single-channel conductance of 0.65 nS (similar as at 20 mV), but the mean of the "off" steps is only about 0.50 nS. This result indicates that the aerolysin channels do not close completely but switch to a substate of small permeability as a consequence of the high membrane potential. In the multichannel system the decay of the membrane current following a voltage step can be described by a single exponential

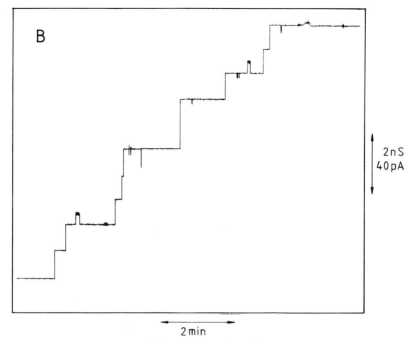

2 nS
40 pA

2 min

Fig. 1   (*continued*)

decay. The time constant of this exponential decay is about 10 sec at 100 mV. Higher membrane potentials cause faster decays of membrane current.

A comparison of the macroscopic conductance data derived from multi-channel experiments shows that a channel density of more than 10^6 channels/cm^2 can be obtained in reconstitution experiments. This suggests that the formation of toxin channels is not a rare event and is definitely not an artifact.

The lipid bilayer technique allows excellent access to both sides of the membrane. As a consequence, it is possible to perform single-channel experiments in different salts and concentrations (see Table I). A large variety of different ions are permeable through the toxin channels. Furthermore, the single-channel conductance of aerolysin and α-toxin is a linear function of the specific conductance σ of the bulk aqueous phase. Obviously, both aerolysin and α-toxin form water-filled channels since the ions move inside the channels with a similar mobility sequence as in the aqueous phase. This means that despite a large variation of the average single-channel conductance as a function of the bulk aqueous conductivity the ratio G/σ varies only little.

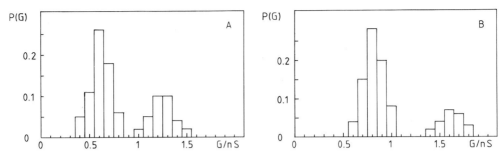

FIG. 2 Histograms of conductance fluctuations observed with membranes from diphytanoylphosphatidylcholine/*n*-decane in the presence of aerolysin (A) and α-toxin (B). The aqueous phase contained 1 *M* KCl. The applied voltage was 20 mV. The average single-channel conductance was 0.68 nS for 253 steps in the case of aerolysin and 0.85 nS for 186 single events in the case of α-toxin; 25°C.

The single-channel conductance, G, of the toxins can be used to calculate the effective diameter of the channels according to an established procedure (26). Assuming that the pores are filled with a solution of the same specific conductivity, σ, as the bulk aqueous solution and assuming a cylindrical pore with a length l of 6 nm (corresponding to the approximate thickness of a lipid bilayer membrane), the effective pore diameter d ($= 2r$) can be calculated according to Eq. (1).

$$G = \sigma\pi r^2/l \tag{1}$$

Using the single-channel conductances in 1 *M* KCl ($= 110$ mS/cm), the effective diameter d ($= 2r$) of both toxins can be estimated to be approximately 0.8 nm. The diameter of the channel formed by α-toxin of *S. aureus* has also been studied by electron microscopy of toxin-containing liposomes (15) and by permeability measurements of erythrocyte membranes (3). Both methods suggest a diameter of about 2 nm. This could mean that our estimate must be considered as a lower limit since the channel interior may not be perfectly shielded from the low dielectric of the hydrocarbon core as it is in the case of the porins (32).

Ion Selectivity of Aerolysin and α-Toxin

Ions move through the channels formed by aerolysin and α-toxin in a manner similar to the way they move in the bulk aqueous phase. Nevertheless, the channels exhibit a certain specificity for charged solutes, because the single-

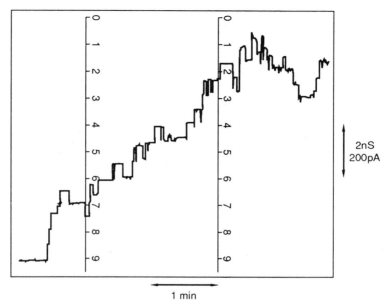

FIG. 3   Single-channel recording of a diphytanoylphosphatidylcholine membrane after the addition of 10 ng/ml aerolysin of *Aeromonas sobria* to the aqueous phase. The aqueous phase contained 1 *M* KCl, pH 6. The applied membrane potential was 100 mV; 25°C. Note that the "on" steps are approximately 600 pS, while "off" steps are about 500 pS.

channel conductance is larger in LiCl than it is in potassium acetate. Both salts have the same specific conductivity in the aqueous phase, which suggests that the channels have a limited selectivity for anions (21–23). The lipid bilayer assay allows the evaluation of the ionic selectivity by measuring the membrane potential under zero-current conditions. From the measured V_m as a consequence of the externally applied concentration gradient, c''/c', across the membrane, the ratio P_a/P_c of the permeabilities (P_a for anions and P_c of cations) can be calculated using the Goldman–Hodgkin–Katz equation (26). Table II shows the zero-current membrane potentials and the permeability ratios for the two toxins in potassium chloride, potassium acetate, and lithium chloride. It is obvious from the data in Table II that the asymmetry potential and the ion selectivity of the toxins are dependent on the combination of different anions and cations. The channel is moderately anion selective for the equally mobile potassium and chloride ions. For the combination of the less mobile lithium ion [because of the larger hydration shell (33)] with chloride, the anion selectivity increases. The selectivity decreases for po-

TABLE I   Average Single-Channel Conductance of
Aerolysin of *Aeromonas sobria* and α-Toxin of
Staphylococcus aureus[a]

| Salt | c (M) | Concentration, conductance, G (nS) | |
		Aerolysin from *A. sobria*	α-Toxin from *S. aureus*
KCl	0.01	0.008	0.010
	0.03	0.024	nm
	0.1	0.072	0.089
	0.3	0.22	0.28
	1	0.65	0.82
	3	1.7	2.5
CsCl	1	0.67	nm
NaCl	1	0.60	nm
LiCl	1	0.50	0.58
CH$_3$ COOK	1	0.28	0.38
K$_2$SO$_4$	0.5	0.34	0.42
MgCl$_2$	0.5	0.55	0.62

[a] In different salt solutions of concentration c. The aqueous salt solutions contained about 20 ng/ml of the toxins; the pH was between 6.0 and 7.0. The membranes were made from diphytanoylphosphatidylcholine/n-decane; 25°C; V_m = 20 mV. G was determined by recording at least 100 conductance steps and averaging over the distribution of the values. nm, Not measured. (From Ref. 21 by permission.)

tassium acetate, presumably because of the smaller mobility of acetate as compared with chloride. Again, the ions move inside the channels in a similar mobility sequence as in the aqueous phase.

Discussion

The single-channel experiments with artificial lipid bilayer membranes suggest that the channels formed by aerolysin and α-toxin behave as general diffusion channels. This means that the single-channel conductance is a linear function of the bulk aqueous conductance and does not show any saturation, which would be needed for the existence of an ion-binding site inside the channel. Our results for aerolysin and α-toxin are in agreement with the published literature (22, 23). Both channels are anionically selective. This may be explained by the presence of an excess of positively charged groups, possibly lysines (32), in or near the pore. However, the permeability ratio is

TABLE II   Zero-Current Membrane Potentials
of Membranes from
Diphytanoylphosphatidylcholine/n-Decane in
the Presence of Aerolysin and α-Toxin

Toxin salt	Membrane potential, V_m (mV)	P_a/P_c
Aerolysin		
KCl (pH 6)	−31	4.8
LiCl (pH 6)	−38	7.7
Potassium acetate (pH 7)	−17	2.2
α-Toxin		
KCl (pH 6)	−28	4.0
LiCl (pH 6)	−35	6.3
Potassium acetate (pH 7)	−13	1.9

[a] Measured over a 10-fold gradient of different salts. V_m is defined as the potential of the dilute side (10 mM) relative to that of the concentrated side (100 mM); the temperature was 25°C. P_a/P_c was calculated from the Goldman–Hodgkin–Katz Eq. (26) from at least four individual experiments. (From Ref. 21 by permission.)

a function of the aqueous mobility of the different ions (see Table II). This result is also consistent with the assumption of general diffusion channels, since the selectivity of highly selective channels is not dependent on the mobility of anions and cations in the aqueous phase (32).

The toxin channels described here appear to be very similar to those that have been observed in the presence of a variety of different bacterial porins (32). The toxins form channels that are long lasting and have a lifetime of at least 5 min. This is not, however, a general feature of all toxins. Hemolysin of *Escherichia coli* forms transient channels with a short lifetime of only a few seconds (20) and cannot be detected by electron microscopic analysis as are the α-toxin oligomers of *S. aureus* (3). On the other hand, the structural analogy between porin and the toxins studied here is striking. Both primary and secondary structural features of aerolysin and α-toxin are reminiscent of those found in bacterial porins (32). Indeed, the toxins are devoid of α-helical structures and their amino acid sequences are extremely hydrophilic and most likely form pleated sheet structures as do the porins (8, 32, 34, 35). Spectroscopic analysis and preliminary X-ray crystallographic data suggest that aerolysin consists entirely of β-structure (36), analogous to the porin proteins from which it may have evolved. This has also been seen with circular dichroism spectroscopy analysis of the α-toxin of *S. aureus* (37).

Recent studies using site-directed mutagenesis of the cloned aerolysin gene have revealed further insight into the nature of residues involved in oligomerization and binding of the toxin (36). Mutational changes of His-107 and His-132, located at the N-terminal end of the molecule, demonstrated that both residues are required for oligomerization of the toxin before entry into the lipid bilayer. These residues appear to be located within the aqueous channel lumen. Mutation of the C-terminal His-332 residue resulted in lower binding affinity of the mutated toxin to erythrocyte membranes, suggesting that it may be in or close to a receptor-binding site. All mutations described lead to lowered hemolytic activity, underlining their contribution to the toxicity of this protein. We have in addition found that the mutation at residue His-132 results in abrogation of the enterotoxic properties of this protein (T. Chakraborty, unpublished observations, 1990).

Many of the biological properties of aerolysin and α-toxin can be attributed to the insertion of the toxin molecule into the membrane of the target cell to form channels. Channel formation is dissectable into two steps. Toxin monomers bind to lipid bilayers without generating bilayer leakiness (13, 21, 23, 36, 38, 39). Membrane-bound monomers then laterally diffuse to form noncovalently bonded oligomers that then generate the pores, allowing flux of ions and small molecules across the bilayer membrane. In cells such as erythrocytes, which are devoid of membrane turnover, cytolysis will occur. When toxin pores form in the membrane of nucleated cells, repair of a limited number of lesions will occur. Nevertheless, transiently formed ion fluxes may trigger secondary responses, such as the release of inflammatory mediators from target cells (3, 4), which are of pathophysiological relevance to the infected host.

Acknowledgments

This work was supported by the Deutsche Forschungsgemeinschaft (SFB 176) and the Fonds der Chemischen Industrie.

References

1. S. Singer and G. Nicolsen, *Science* **175,** 720 (1972).
2. O. S. Andersen, *in* "Renal Function" (G. H. Giebisch and E. F. Purcell, eds.), p. 71. Independent Publishers Group, Port Washington, New York, (1978).
3. S. Bhakdi and J. Tranum-Jensen, *Rev. Physiol. Biochem. Pharmacol.* **107,** 147 (1987).
4. O. P. Daily, S. W. Josepf, J. C. Coolbaugh, R. I. Walker, B. R. Merell, D. M. Rollins, R. J. Seidler, R. R. Colwell, and C. R. Lissner, *J. Clin. Microbiol.* **13,** 769 (1981).

5. V. Burke, J. Robinson, H. M. Atkinson, and M. Gracey, *J. Clin. Microbiol.* **15,** 48 (1982).
6. S. P. Howard and J. T. Buckley, *Biochemistry* **21,** 1662 (1985).
7. S. P. Howard, W. J. Garland, M. J. Greene, and J. T. Buckley, *J. Bacteriol.* **169,** 2869 (1987).
8. V. Husslein, B. Huhle, T. Jarchau, R. Kurz, W. Goebel, and T. Chakraborty, *Mol. Microbiol.* **2,** 507 (1988).
9. S. P. Howard and J. T. Buckley, *J. Bacteriol.* **163,** 336 (1985).
10. T. Chakraborty, B. Huhle, H. Bergbauer, and W. Goebel, *J. Bacteriol.* **167,** 368 (1986).
11. I. P. Arbuthnott, I. H. Freer, and B. Bileliffe, *J. Gen. Microbiol.* **75,** 309 (1973).
12. I. H. Freer, I. P. Arbuthnott, and W. Bernheimer, *J. Bacteriol.* **95,** 1153 (1968).
13. M. Rogolski, *Microbiol. Rev.* **43,** 320 (1979).
14. I. Lind, G. Ahnert-Hilger, G. Fuchs, and M. Gratzl, *Anal. Biochem.* **164,** 84 (1987).
15. S. Bhakdi and J. Tranum-Jensen, *Philos. Trans. R. Soc. London, B* **306,** 311 (1984).
16. M. Kehoe, J. Duncan, T. Foster, W. Fairweather, and W. Douglas, *Infect. Immun.* **41,** 1105 (1983).
17. M. O'Reilly, J. C. S. de Azavedo, S. Kennedy, and T. J. Foster, *Microb. Pathog.* **1,** 125 (1986).
18. T. Asao, Y. Kinoshita, S. Kozaki, T. Uemura, and G. Sakaguchi, *Infect. Immun.* **46,** 228 (1984).
19. F. Dreyer, K. Maric, and F. Lutz, *Zentralbl. Bakteriol., Suppl.* **19,** 227 (1990).
20. R. Benz, A. Schmid, W. Wagner, and W. Goebel, *Infect. Immun.* **57,** 887 (1989).
21. T. Chakraborty, A. Schmid, S. Notermans, and R. Benz, *Infect. Immun.* **58,** 2127 (1990).
22. G. Menestrina, *J. Membr. Biol.* **90,** 177 (1986).
23. H. U. Wilmsen, F. Pattus, and J. T. Buckley, *J. Membr. Biol.* **115,** 71 (1990).
24. P. Mueller, D. O. Rudin, H. T. Tien, and W. C. Wescott, *Nature (London)* **194,** 979 (1962).
25. R. Benz, K. Janko, W. Boos, and P. Läuger, *Biochim. Biophys. Acta* **511,** 305 (1978).
26. R. Benz, K. Janko, and P. Läuger, *Biochem. Biophys. Acta* **551,** 238 (1979).
27. R. Benz, O. Fröhlich, P. Läuger, and M. Montal, *Biochim. Biophys. Acta* **394,** 323 (1975).
28. J. P. Dilger and R. Benz, *J. Membr. Biol.* **85,** 181 (1985).
29. M. Montal and P. Mueller, *Proc. Natl. Acad. Sci. U.S.A.* **69,** 3561 (1972).
30. J. H. Lakey and F. Pattus, *Eur. J. Biochem.* **186,** 303 (1978).
31. H. Ikigai and T. Nakae, *Biochem. Biophys. Res. Commun.* **130,** 175 (1985).
32. R. Benz, *Annu. Rev. Microbiol.* **42,** 359 (1988).
33. G. W. Castellan, "Physical Chemistry." Addison-Wesley, Reading, Massachusetts, 1983.
34. T. Chakraborty, H. Bergbauer, V. Husslein, and R. Benz, *Zentralbl. Bakteriol., Suppl.* **19,** 325 (1990).

35. T. Chakraborty, B. Huhle, H. Hof, H. Bergbauer, and W. Goebel, *Infect. Immun.* **55,** 2274 (1987).
36. M. J. Green and T. J. Buckley, *Biochemistry* **29,** 2177 (1990).
37. N. Tobkes, B. A. Wallace, and H. Bayley, *Biochemistry* **24,** 1915 (1985).
38. F. Hugo, A. Sinner, J. Reichwein, and S. Bhakdi, *Infect. Immun.* **55,** 2922 (1987).
39. J. Reichwein, F. Hugo, M. Roth, A. Sinner, and S. Bhakdi, *Infect. Immun.* **55,** 2940 (1987).

[2] Apamin: A Probe for Small-Conductance, Calcium-Activated Potassium Channels

Peter N. Strong and Barry S. Brewster

Introduction

Small-conductance calcium-activated potassium channels (SK channels) can be operationally defined as those having single-channel conductances of less than 20 pS. These channels are found in a wide range of excitable and nonexcitable cells. In nerve and muscle, the ionic currents that flow through these channels are responsible for maintaining the slow after-hyperpolarizing potential (AHP) that follows bursts of action potentials. In nonexcitable cells (e.g., hepatocytes and adipocytes), channel activity is stimulated by hormones and receptor agonists, the channel thereby providing a means for metabolic activity (as reflected in alterations in cytoplasmic calcium levels) to regulate the plasma membrane potential of the cell.

Two venom toxins have been characterized to date that appear to interact specifically with SK channels: apamin and leiurotoxin (1–3). Apamin, a neurotoxin isolated from the venom of the European honey bee *Apis mellifera,* was the first potassium channel toxin to be isolated and characterized, although for a long time its precise site of action was unknown, and it was simply described as a centrally acting neurotoxin. Apamin is a highly basic peptide with a molecular weight of 2000. It has been used as a pharmacological tool to characterize ionic currents flowing through SK channels as well as for the quantification of apamin-binding sites and the identification of putative SK channel polypeptides. Apamin-binding assays have been used to monitor the solubilization and purification of SK channel proteins. The toxin has also been used to provide evidence of a regulatory role for SK channels in cell metabolism. Leiurotoxin is a more recently identified toxin, isolated from the venom of the Israeli scorpion *Leiurus quinquestriatus hebraeus*. It was discovered by screening scorpion venoms for toxins that possessed apamin-like pharmacological activity. Leiurotoxin has a molecular weight of 3400 and is immunologically and structurally unrelated to apamin (3).

Purification of Apamin

Although apamin is available from several sources (Sigma, St. Louis, MO; Serva, Westbury, NY; Bachem Bubendorf, Switzerland; Research Biochemicals, Inc., Natick, MA), the quality of commercial samples is variable. The main problems are contamination with mellitin and the removal of traces of other extremely basic venom peptides of very similar molecular weight [e.g., mast cell degranulating (MCD) peptide].

Method

Crude bee venom (25 g) is dissolved in 200 ml formic acid (0.1 M) and dialyzed (Visking tubing, M_r cutoff 12,000) against four changes of the same buffer for 48 hr at 4°C. The dialysate is lyophilized and 5 g of lyophilized powder is dissolved in 10 ml ammonium phosphate (0.5 M) adjusted to pH 7.4. This solution is applied to a column (100 × 5 cm in diameter) of Sephadex G-50 (Pharmacia, Piscataway, NJ) equilibrated in the same buffer at room temperature. The column is eluted with 0.5 M ammonium phosphate, pH 7.4 (3 liters) and the eluate is monitored at 229 or 254 nm. Fractions are run on cellulose thin-layer chromatography (TLC) plates (Merck, Poole, UK) and the chromatogram is developed in a solvent of butanol; pyridine : acetic acid : water (3 : 3 : 1 : 3, v/v). Peptide spots are detected using ninhydrin; apamin has an R_f value of 0.30 in this system. Apamin-rich fractions are combined before desalting on a Sephadex G-10 column, which is eluted with 2% (v/v) acetic acid. Column fractions are monitored as above. The eluate is lyophilized and can be stored at −20°C indefinitely.

Five milligrams of the lyophilized, apamin-rich fraction dissolved in 3 ml of sodium phosphate buffer (10 mM, pH 6.8) is applied to a column (12 × 0.9 cm diameter) of heparin-Sepharose CL-6B (Pharmacia) equilibrated in the same buffer. The column is then eluted with a linear salt gradient (0.02–1.5 M NaCl, total volume 600 ml) in the same buffer. Apamin is eluted at a salt concentration of 0.1 M NaCl. The purified toxin is desalted on a 1-ml C_{18} reversed-phase column (Bond-Elut; Analytichem, Harbor City, CA), eluting with methanol : acetonitrile : water (3 : 1 : 30, v/v) containing 1% (v/v) phosphoric acid. Apamin can then be lyophilized and stored desiccated at −20°C for at least 5 years.

The purity of the apamin preparation can be checked by reversed-phase chromatography on a Synchropak RP-C_{18} column (250 × 4 mm diameter). The column is eluted under isocratic conditions with a buffer of 2% 2-propanol, 3 mM methylsulfonic acid, 10 mM triethylamine phosphate, pH 2.5, at 1 ml/min. Protein peaks are monitored spectrophotometrically at 229 nm. Mellitin contamination of apamin preparations can be checked fluorimetrically. The tryptophan fluorescence of suspected samples (295-nm excitation; 354-nm emission) can be measured and compared with a standard linear calibration curve of synthetic mellitin (Bachem) in the range 0.1–50 μM.

Notes

1. This procedure, currently used by the authors, is one that they acknowledge as being refined and adapted from original published methods (4–6).

2. Mellitin is an amphipathic, extremely hydrophobic peptide, comprising 50% of the dry weight of crude bee venom (cf. apamin, comprising 2%). The hydrophobic properties of monomeric mellitin cause it to bind tightly to both the column matrices and other peptides.

3. Crude bee venom can be obtained from Sigma but it is most reliably obtained from a specialist supplier of venoms (6a).

4. WARNING—Lyophilized bee venom can cause severe respiratory allergies. It is recommended that a face mask be worn at all times.

5. Mellitin (2800 Da) associates as a stable tetramer in 0.5 M phosphate buffer; it can be more easily separated from apamin on gel-permeation columns run in high salt solution because of its higher apparent molecular weight (ca 12,000) and its decreased hydrophobicity.

6. Heparin-Sepharose provides an excellent affinity support for separating apamin from its major contaminants, MCD peptide and mellitin. The latter two peptides bind extremely tightly to this matrix and are eluted only at high salt concentrations (0.3 M NaCl or greater), whereas apamin is eluted at 0.1 M NaCl. This technique can be easily scaled down to purify commercial samples of apamin where necessary.

7. Ion-pair reagents are essential for the resolution of apamin and other closely related, extremely basic peptides (e.g., MCD peptide, secapin) that are found in bee venom. Radial compression C_{18} columns provide sufficient resolution for preparative uses.

8. Contamination of apamin preparations with mellitin is a serious problem. The detergent-like properties of mellitin rapidly cause cell lysis; even 1% levels of contamination can compromise the use of apamin as a pharmacological and biochemical probe.

9. Apamin has negligible absorbance at 280 nm due to the complete absence of any aromatic amino acids and is therefore conveniently monitored in column eluates at either 254 or 229 nm. The absence of tryptophan residues in apamin itself facilitates the use of a simple and sensitive fluorimetric assay for detecting contamination of apamin samples with tryptophan-containing peptides (such as mellitin). Mellitin contamination of 0.1% can easily be detected by this method.

10. Apamin has also been synthesized using solid-state methods and the synthetic peptide folds correctly to exhibit native biological activity and circular dichroic (CD) structure (7, 8).

Identification of Calcium-Activated Potassium Permeabilities Inhibited by Apamin

Apamin blocks calcium-activated potassium permeabilities that result from receptor activation. For example, a variety of α-adrenergic agonists and hormones have been shown to affect apamin-sensitive potassium fluxes from hepatocytes; the toxin can therefore be used to provide evidence of a regulatory role for SK channels in cell metabolism. Another means of activating potassium ion flow through the same channel is to induce efflux artificially by the application of calcium ionophores such as A23187 or ionomycin (Calbiochem, La Jolla, CA). In both these cases, apamin-sensitive potassium fluxes can be measured with potassium ion-sensitive electrodes or by using ^{42}K or ^{86}Rb (Amersham, Arlington Heights, IL) as radioactive tracers (Table I).

Identification of Apamin-Sensitive After-Hyperpolarization Currents

The slow after-hyperpolarization (AHP) in many cells, which follows bursts of action potentials, often results from the activation of calcium-dependent potassium currents flowing through SK channels. Apamin has been shown

TABLE I   Potassium Permeabilities Blocked by Apamin

Preparation	Agonist	Assay	Apamin (nM)	Ref.
Guinea pig hepatocytes	Noradrenaline ATP A23187 ionophore	K electrode	1–10	a
	Angiotensin II		1 (EC$_{50}$)	b
Guinea pig taenia caeci	Adrenaline	^{42}K flux	100	c
	Noradrenaline	^{86}Rb flux	100	d
Hamster brown adipocytes	A23187 ionophore		2 (EC$_{50}$)	e
Rat embryonic neurons			0.3 (EC$_{50}$)	f
Pheochromocytoma (PC12)			0.2 (EC$_{50}$)	g

[a] G. M. Burgess, M. Claret, and D. H. Jenkinson, *J. Physiol. (London)* **317,** 67 (1981).
[b] N. S. Cook and D. G. Haylett, *J. Physiol (London)* **358,** 373 (1985).
[c] A. J. J. Maas, A. den Hertog, R. Ras, and J. van den Akker, *Eur. J. Pharmacol.* **67,** 265 (1980).
[d] S. S. Weir and A. H. Weston, *Br. J. Pharmacol.* **88,** 113 (1986).
[e] E. Nanberg, E. Connolly, and J. Nedergaard, *Biochim. Biophys. Acta* **844,** 42 (1985).
[f] M. J. Seagar, C. Granier, and F. Couraud, *J. Biol. Chem.* **259,** 1491 (1984).
[g] Schmid-Antomarchi, M. Hugues, and M. Lazdunski, *J. Biol. Chem.* **261,** 8633 (1986).

to reduce the amplitude of many AHP currents, without affecting their decay rate (Table II). Although the effects of apamin are rapid, blockade is often incomplete and washout times of 1 hr are usually required for full recovery.

In contrast to high-conductance calcium-activated potassium channels, it has not proved easy to measure single-channel SK conductances due to the problems of filtering out extraneous signal noise. The identification of unitary SK channels in isolated patches of either rat myotubes or guinea pig hepatocytes has been crucially supported by the pharmacological observations that these channels can be blocked by apamin. Single-channel conductance values range from 12 to 20 pS in symmetrical (ca. 140 mM) potassium solutions (9, 10).

Use of Mono[125I]iodoapamin for Identification of Toxin-Binding Sites

Mono[125I]iodoapamin can be used to identify toxin-binding molecules (putative components of SK channel proteins) and to monitor the solubilization and purification of these proteins. Although toxin-binding sites have been

TABLE II   Apamin-Sensitive After-Hyperpolarization

Preparation	Apamin (nM)	Ref.
Rat embryonic myotubes	10	a
Rat skeletal muscle (denervated)	10	b
Frog skeletal muscle	20	c
Frog sympathetic ganglia	2.5–25	d
Rat sympathetic ganglia	15 (IC$_{50}$)	e
Neuroblastoma (N1E115)	100	f
Neuroblastoma/glioma hybrids	100–400	g
Cat spinal motoneurons	25	h
Rat supraoptic neurosecretory neurons	1.3 (IC$_{50}$)	i

[a] M. Hugues, H. Schmid, G. Romey, D. Duval, C. Frelin, and M. Lazdunski, *EMBO J.* **1**, 1039 (1981).

[b] H. Schmid-Antomarchi, J.-F. Renaud, G. Romey, M. Hugues, and M. Lazdunski, *Proc. Natl. Acad. Sci. U.S.A.* **82**, 2188 (1985).

[c] C. Cognard, F. Traore, D. Potreau, and G. Raymond, *Pfluegers Arch.* **402**, 222 (1984).

[d] P. Pennefather, B. Lancaster, P. Adams, and R. A. Nicoll, *Proc. Natl. Acad. Sci. U.S.A.* **82**, 3040 (1985).

[e] T. Kawai and M. N. Watanabe, *Br. J. Pharmacol.* **87**, 225 (1986).

[f] M. Hugues, G. Romey, D. Duval, J. P. Vincent, and M. Lazdunski, *Proc. Natl. Acad. Sci. U.S.A.* **79**, 1308 (1981).

[g] D. A. Brown and H. Higashida, *J. Physiol. (London)* **397**, 149 (1988).

[h] L. Zhang and K. Krnjevic, *Neurosci. Lett.* **74**, 58 (1987).

[i] C. W. Bourque and D. A. Brown, *Neurosci. Lett.* **82**, 185 (1987).

characterized in many tissues (Table III) and toxin-binding polypeptides identified, purification of the solubilized toxin-binding macromolecules has proved an elusive task at the present time (11, 12).

Preparation of Monoiodoapamin

Apamin can be conveniently iodinated using the Iodogen procedure. Ten milligrams of Iodogen (Pierce, Rockford, IL) is dissolved in dichloromethane (25 ml) and an 80-μl aliquot is dispensed to a flat-bottomed tube and evapo-

TABLE III   Apamin-Binding Constants

Buffer and tissue[a]	K_D (pM)	B_{max} (fmol/mg)	Assay	Ref.
Low ionic strength buffer				
Synaptosomes	15–25	12.5	Filtration	d
Cerebral cortex				e
Postsynaptic density	24	30.2		
Synaptic membrane	33	17.3		
Neuroblastoma	15–22	12		f
Smooth muscle				
Colon	36	30		g
Ileum	67	42		h
Embryonic skeletal muscle	30–60	3.5		i
Liver	13	4.2		j
	15	43		h
Heart	59	24		
Physiological buffer				
Hepatocytes	350–390	1.1[b]	Centrifugation	k
Primary cardiac cells	69	2.8	Plate wash[c]	h
Embryonic neurons	60–120	3–8		l

[a] All assays performed at 4°C except with hepatocytes (37°C).

[b] Femtomoles per milligram dry weight of cells.

[c] Cells grown as monolayers and incubated/washed *in situ*.

[d] M. Hugues, D. Duval, P. Kitabgi, M. Lazdunski, and J. P. Vincent, *J. Biol. Chem.* **257**, 2762 (1982).

[e] C. F. Wu, R. Carlin, I. Sachs, and P. Siekewitz, *Brain Res.* **360**, 183 (1985).

[f] M. Hugues, G. Romey, D. Duval, J. P. Vincent, and M. Lazdunski, *Proc. Natl. Acad. Sci. U.S.A.* **79**, 1308 (1981).

[g] M. Hugues, D. Duval, H. Schmid, P. Kitabgi, M. Lazdunski, and J. P. Vincent, *Life Sci.* **31**, 437 (1981).

[h] B. Marqueze, M. Seagar, and F. Couraud, *Eur. J. Biochem.* **169**, 295 (1987).

[i] M. Hugues, H. Schmid, G. Romey, D. Duval, C. Frelin, and M. Lazdunski, *EMBO J.* **1**, 1039 (1981).

[j] P. N. Strong and W. H. Evans, *Eur. J. Biochem.* **163**, 267 (1987).

[k] N. S. Cook, D. G. Haylett, and P. N. Strong, *FEBS Lett.* **152**, 265 (1983).

[l] M. J. Seagar, C. Granier, and F. Couraud, *J. Biol. Chem.* **259**, 1491 (1984).

rated to dryness under a gentle stream of nitrogen at 4°C. To one of these Iodogen tubes (containing 75 nmol Iodogen) is added (1) 100 μg apamin (50 nmol) dissolved in 80 μl Tris-HCl buffer (10 mM, pH 8.6), (2) 2 mCi Na^{125}I (Amersham), and (3) an aliquot of 10 mM Tris-HCl buffer to bring the final reaction volume to 160 μl. The Iodogen tube is incubated at room temperature for 20 min, shaking intermittently, and then the contents decanted into a clean plastic vial for 10 min. The reaction mixture is then applied to an S-Sepharose (Pharmacia) column (14 × 0.9 cm) equilibrated in 160 mM NaCl/ 50 mM sodium phosphate buffer, pH 6.0 and eluted with the same buffer (1-ml fractions, ~8 ml/hr). Two peaks of radioactivity are obtained, the first being unincorporated Na^{125}I, the second being mono[^{125}I]iodoapamin. After approximately six column volumes of the equilibration buffer, the unlabeled apamin is eluted with three column volumes of a high-salt buffer (300 mM NaCl/50 mM sodium phosphate, pH 6.0). Mono[^{125}I]iodoapamin is stored at 4°C in the presence of bovine serum albumin (2 mg/ml) and retains full binding activity for at least 2 months.

Notes

1. This procedure is a refinement of previously published work (13–15). It produces homogeneous mono[^{125}I]iodoapamin, free from unlabeled apamin, at a specific activity of 2200Ci/mmol. Approximately 50% of iodinated material loaded on to the column is recovered as mono[^{125}I]iodoapamin.

2. Iodogen tubes can be stored in a vacuum desiccator at 4°C for 1 month.

3. The reaction mixture is decanted from the reaction tube and allowed to sit for 10 min in order to permit unincorporated ^{125}I$^+$ to revert to molecular iodine. This greatly reduces nonspecific labelling of the gel bed and permits the same column to be used many times.

4. Subtle differences in ion-exchange properties between S-Sepharose (this method) and SP-Sephadex C-25 (13–15) simplify the separation of mono[^{125}I]iodoapamin from unlabeled apamin.

5. Although this method avoids contaminating a high-performance liquid chromatography (HPLC) apparatus or having a dedicated apparatus for use with radioactive samples, mono[^{125}I]iodoapamin can be separated and purified on a C_{18} reversed-phase column as described for the preparation of apamin.

6. A minor radioactive peak, sometimes occurring between free iodine and mono[^{125}I]iodoapamin, is due to di[^{125}I]$_2$iodoapamin and should be discarded.

7. Unlabeled apamin can be detected in the high salt eluate by HPLC (see above) or by radioimmunoassay with anti-apamin antibodies (16).

Apamin-Binding Assays

Mono[^{125}I]iodoapamin binding to isolated membranes can be conveniently measured using a filtration binding assay (13, 15). Additionally, the measurement of apamin-binding sites under physiological conditions, using cells in suspension (e.g., hepatocytes), may be measured using a rapid centrifugation assay (14). The incubation conditions in these two assays described below (or close variants of them) have been used to characterize apamin-binding proteins in a variety of preparations (Table III).

Filtration Assay

Membranes (100 μg) are incubated with mono[^{125}I]iodoapamin (0.9–50 pM) in a final volume of 1 ml, all dilutions being made in incubation buffer (5.4 mM KCl, 0.1% bovine serum albumin, 10 mM Tris/HEPES, pH 7.4). Samples are incubated in triplicate for 90 min at 0–4°C with gentle shaking. At the end of the incubation period, samples are filtered through cellulose acetate filters (0.45 μm; Sartorius 11106, Bohemia, NY) that have been soaked in incubation buffer for at least 1 hr at 0°C and then rinsed with a 5-ml aliquot of ice-cold buffer immediately prior to application of the membrane sample. After filtration of the membranes, the filter is washed rapidly (<25 sec) with two further 5-ml aliquots of ice-cold buffer. Wet filters can be counted directly in a calibrated gamma counter. Noninhibitable binding is determined with unlabeled apamin (100 nM). Binding data is analyzed using a nonlinear least-squares curve-fitting procedure, available in a variety of commercial software packages (e.g., Fig P; Biosoft, Cambridge, England).

Notes

1. Whatman (Clifton, NJ) glass fiber GF/B filters [presoaked in aqueous polyethyleneimine (0.5%, v/v) for 2 hr at 4°] can be used equally satisfactorily as cellulose acetate filters and have the advantage of being considerably cheaper.

2. Binding site density is extremely low on most membranes (on the order of femtomoles per milligram protein, see Table III); the use of purified mono[^{125}I]iodoapamin, specific activity 2200 Ci/mmol, is vital for reliable and accurate quantitation.

Centrifugation Assay

A suspension (8×10^6 cells/ml) of isolated hepatocytes (17) is incubated at 37°C in Eagle's minimum essential medium (MEM, Wellcome) supplemented with 10% (v/v) newborn calf serum and 2% (v/v) bovine serum albumin. An aliquot (0.3 ml) of this suspension is layered above 0.25 ml di-*n*-butyl phthalate (oil layer) in a 1.5-ml plastic centrifuge tube. Then 0.2 ml of mono[^{125}I]iodoapamin

(20–1000 pM), diluted in the same hepatocyte incubation medium, is added and the cells incubated with labeled toxin for 2 min at 37°C. Incubations are performed in quadruplicate and at the end of the incubation period the cells are rapidly centrifuged (15 sec, 6000 g) through the oil layer to separate bound from unbound toxin. After removing the aqueous layer (top) and the oil layer by careful aspiration, the bottom of the tubes, containing the cell pellets, are cut off with a guillotine. Noninhibitable binding is measured in the presence of unlabeled apamin (1 μM). Pellets are counted in a calibrated gamma counter.

Notes

1. [^{3}H]Inulin can be used to determine the amount of extracellular fluid carried through with the cells after centrifugation. This carryover is the predominant contributor to noninhibitable binding.

2. Attainment of equilibrium is extremely rapid, approaching the diffusion-limited rate. Dissociation is equally fast [half-time for dissociation at 37°C is 40 sec (18)] and therefore demands crucial attention to the speed at which labeled cells are separated.

3. Inorganic cations inhibit apamin binding ($K_{0.5}$ for Na$^+$ is 35 mM); therefore the affinity of apamin for its binding protein is considerably reduced in physiological saline as compared with the low ionic strength buffer used for all membrane assays.

Acknowledgments

The contributions of Professors D. H. Jenkinson and B. E. C. Banks, and Drs. D. G. Haylett, N. S. Cook, and N. A. Castle to the work described here are gratefully acknowledged. We thank the Muscular Dystrophy Group of Great Britain and the Wellcome Trust for financial support.

References

1. E. Moczydlowski, K. Lucchesi, and A. Ravindran, *J. Membr. Biol.* **105,** 95 (1988).
2. N. A. Castle, D. G. Haylett, and D. H. Jenkinson, *Trends Pharmacol. Sci.* **12,** 59 (1989).
3. P. N. Strong, *Pharmacol. Ther.* **46,** 137 (1990).
4. J. Gauldie, J. M. Hanson, R. A. Shipolini, and C. A. Vernon, *Eur. J. Biochem.* **83,** 40 (1976).
5. B. E. C. Banks, C. E. Dempsey, F. L.Pearce, C. A. Vernon, and T. E. Wholley, *Anal. Biochem.* **116,** 48 (1981).

6. E. M. Dotimas, R. C. Hider, U. Ragnarsson, and A. S. Tatham, *Proc. Eur. Pept. Symp., 18th* p. 141 (1984).

6a. Details of suppliers can be found in any current *Newsletter of the International Society of Toxicology.* (For more information contact the society treasurer: Dr. D. Mebs, Zentrum für Rechtsmedizin, Universität Frankfurt, Kennedyalle 104, D6000 Frankfurt 70, Germany.)

7. W. L. Cosland and R. B. Merrifield, *Proc. Natl. Acad. Sci. U.S.A.* **74,** 2771 (1977).

8. C. Granier, E. P. Muller, and J. Van Rietschoten, *Eur. J. Biochem.* **82,** 293 (1978).

9. A. L. Blatz and K. L. Magleby, *Nature (London)* **323,** 718 (1986).

10. T. Capiod and D. C. Ogden, *J. Physiol (London)* **409,** 285 (1989).

11. P. Auguste, M. Hugues, and M. Lazdunski, *FEBS Lett.* **248,** 150 (1989).

12. M. J. Seagar, B. Marqueze, and F. Couraud, *J. Neurosci.* **7,** 565 (1987).

13. M. Hugues, D. Duval, P. Kitabgi, M. Lazdunski, and J. P. Vincent, *J. Biol. Chem.* **257,** 2762 (1982).

14. N. S. Cook, D. G. Haylett, and P. N. Strong, *FEBS Lett.* **152,** 265 (1983).

15. P. N. Strong and W. H. Evans, *Eur. J. Biochem.* **163,** 267 (1987).

16. H. Schweitz and M. Lazdunski, *Toxicon* **22,** 985 (1984).

17. N. C. Cook and D. G. Haylett, *J. Physiol. (London)* **358,** 373 (1985).

18. N. A. Castle, Ph.D. thesis. Univ. of London, London, 1987.

[3] Batrachotoxinin A [³H]Benzoate Binding to Sodium Channels

Cyrus R. Creveling and John W. Daly

Introduction

Voltage-dependent Na⁺ channels are responsible for a selective increase in Na⁺ permeability that underlies the generation of action potentials in excitable membranes of nerve and muscle. The major subunit of the Na⁺ channel is a large (260 kDa) glycoprotein: Smaller (30–40 kDa) β-subunits are associated with Na⁺ channels of brain (1, 2). An initial threshold depolarization of nerve and muscle activates the voltage-dependent Na⁺ channel and induces a series of conformational changes, leading to a transient open or conducting state. This is followed by a voltage-dependent conversion to an inactive nonconductive state, from which state the channel then returns to the resting state. There appear to be several different subtypes of Na⁺ channels, but all are likely to be similar in structure and functional attributes. The primary structures of Na⁺ channels from eel and rat have been deduced and models proposed in which four homologous units, each with six transmembrane sections, are organized to form a central pore (2).

Several classes of neurotoxins bind specifically to sites associated with the Na⁺ channel and affect the conformational changes that underlie the function of the channel. The site and mechanism of action of each of these classes of neurotoxins have led to better understanding of this functionally important protein. Radioligands for the different sites have been developed and a system of nomenclature introduced (1). Site 1 is at the external ion pore and binds the guanidinium toxins, tetrodotoxin and saxitoxin. This is also the site that binds μ-conotoxin, a polypeptide from marine gastropods. Binding of toxins to site 1 blocks Na⁺ flux through the channel. Site 2 appears to be associated with a voltage-sensitive "gate" of the channel. A number of lipid-soluble toxins, including the alkaloids batrachotoxin (BTX), veratridine, and aconitine, and the diterpene grayanotoxin, interact with site 2. Batrachotoxin is the most potent of the ligands for this site and binding results in the stabilization of the channel in an open conformation. A BTX analog has been developed as a radioligand for study of site 2 on the Na⁺ channel (3). Site 3, one of two polypeptide-binding sites, is on the external face of the Na⁺ channel. It binds polypeptide neurotoxins from Old World scorpions, the scorpion α-toxins,

Batrachotoxinin A   (BTX-A)   R =   ——H

Batrachotoxinin-A Benzoate   (BTX-B)   R =

Batrachotoxin   (BTX)   R =

Homobatrachotoxin   (HomoBTX)   R =

and polypeptide neurotoxins from sea anemones, the anemone toxins. Binding of toxins to site 3 is voltage dependent and results in a slowing of the inactivation of the channel. Binding of polypeptide toxins at site 3 enhances binding of a BTX analog (3) and other toxins to site 2 and converts partial activators at site 2, such as veratridine and aconitine, to full activators. Site 4 is also on the external face and binds another class of polypeptide toxins, the scorpion β-toxins from New World scorpions. The location of site 4 is different from that of the scorpion α-toxin-binding site and, instead of slowing inactivation, binding of a scorpion β-toxin enhances activation of the channel by shifting the voltage dependence of the channel to more negative membrane potentials. Site 5 appears to be associated with the voltage-sensing region of the channel, since ligands for the site, namely brevetoxin and ciquatoxin, which are polyether toxins from marine dinoflagellates, enhance the binding of a BTX analog (4–6) and other toxins at site 2, a site known to be associated with the voltage-sensitive gate. Brevetoxin, however, does not affect binding of the scorpion α-toxins to site 3, but instead enhances binding of scorpion β-toxins to site 4. Binding of the marine polyether toxins results in repetitive firing and slows inactivation of the channel. Another lipophilic alkaloid, pumiliotoxin B, has similar effects on channel function to those of the brevetoxins. The site of action of pumiliotoxin B is not yet clear. Unlike brevetoxins, there is no effect of pumiliotoxin B on binding of a BTX analog to site 2 (7, 8). There is a cooperative augmentation of effects of pumiliotoxin B by brevetoxin, acting at site 5, and by scorpion toxins, acting at site 3 or 4. It now appears likely that pumiliotoxin B interacts with a subdomain of site 2 shared with aconitine, but not with BTX (9). Finally, there are several other classes of agents that allosterically affect function of Na⁺ channels. These include local anesthetics, which antagonize the binding of a BTX analog to site 2 (10, 11), and the action of BTX and other site 2 toxins, and pyrethroids, which cause repetitive firing and delay inactivation, and can enhance binding of a BTX analog to site 2 (12, 13). Recent reviews focused on the interactions of toxins with the Na⁺ channel are available (1, 14).

The remarkable allosteric interactions of various classes of neurotoxins at Na⁺ channels would have been difficult to define without specific radioligands for each site. In 1981 a synthetic, radioactive analog of BTX, which retains full biological activity, was prepared (15). This derivative, batrachotoxinin

---

FIG. 1   Structures of batrachotoxin and the major congeners, homobatrachotoxin and batrachotoxinin A, from the poison-dart frogs (*Phyllobates* species), and the structure of batrachotoxinin A 20α-benzoate (BTX-B). Isotopically labeled BTX-B has been prepared as the 4-tritio- and 2,5-ditritiobenzoates.

A 20 α-[benzoyl-4-^{3}H]benzoate ([^{3}H]BTX-B) binds specifically to site 2 on Na$^+$ channels and has been used extensively in investigations of the properties of the Na$^+$ channel. The present chapter details the procedures for measurement of the specific binding of [^{3}H]BTX-B and documents effects of the various Na$^+$ channel toxins and other agents on such binding. The structures of the important naturally occurring batrachotoxin alkaloids and the partially synthetic [^{3}H]BTX-B are shown in Fig. 1.

Measurement of Specific Binding of [^{3}H]BTX-B

Most procedures for the measurement of the specific binding of [^{3}H]BTX-B to brain preparations represent minor modifications of the initial procedure reported for rat synaptosomes (3). Specific binding has been measured most successfully in vesicular preparations from rodent brain. The vesicular brain preparations that have been used for [^{3}H]BTX-B binding include the following: synaptosomes, synaptoneurosomes, and synaptosomal fractions from brain or specific brain regions of guinea pig, mouse, and rat (3, 6, 10, 11, 16). Scorpion α-toxin, anemone toxin, or scorpion venom (*Leiurus quinquestriatus*) have been used to enhance high-affinity binding. A relatively low-affinity binding for [^{3}H]BTX-B was reported for a rat brain "microsomal" fraction (13). The affinity was enhanced more than twofold by anemone toxin. Specific binding of high concentrations (0.1–1 μM) of [^{3}H]BTX-B to rat atrial membrane preparations and rat brain synaptoneurosomes has been reported in the absence of scorpion toxin (17, 18). Muscarinic agonists caused a marked increase in specific binding. High-affinity binding of [^{3}H]BTX-B has been reported in a particulate fraction from house fly heads (19) and in a particulate fraction from eel electroplax (20). [^{3}H]BTX-B, in conjunction with scorpion venom or anemone toxin to enhance binding, has been used for autoradiographic localization of binding sites in sections of rat brain (13, 21). High-affinity binding of [^{3}H]BTX-B occurs on intact rat ventricular myocytes in the presence of anemone toxin (22). A comparison of high-affinity [^{3}H]BTX-B binding to rat brain and rat heart membrane preparations has been reported (23, 24).

An essential requirement for [^{3}H]BTX-B binding is the retention of membrane potential, since the high-affinity binding is minimal except in the presence of a scorpion α-toxin or anemone toxin, and the action of these polypeptide toxins is dependent on a membrane potential. The earliest studies on the specific binding of [^{3}H]BTX-B were attempted with a particulate fraction from homogenates of mouse cerebral cortex (15). These early studies were performed in the absence of scorpion venom in normal Ringer's solution at 0–5°C with a sedimentation method. There was only 10% specific binding as defined by the presence of veratridine. Addition of scorpion venom, anemone toxin, or tetrodotoxin had no effect on specific binding at 0°C. The pH dependency of specific binding suggested the involvement of a histidine residue (25). The substitution of choline chloride for NaCl in the reaction medium and an increase in the incubation temperature to 36°C resulted in a high level of specific binding (70–80%) in the presence, but not in the absence, of scorpion α-toxin (3).

Binding assays with [³H]BTX-B are initiated by the addition of vesicular preparations from brain to a defined Na$^+$-free medium in which Na$^+$ salts have been replaced by choline chloride at pH 7.4 in the presence of anemone toxin, scorpion α-toxin, or scorpion venom (L. quinquestriatus), tetrodotoxin, glucose, and 2–35 nM [³H]BTX-B. After an incubation for 30–60 min at 36 or 37°C, the reaction is terminated by dilution with cold medium containing Ca^{2+}, in addition to other components, followed by vacuum-assisted filtration through glass fiber filters. Total binding determined by scintillation spectroscopy represents the [³H]BTX-B retained on the glass fibers. Nonspecific binding is defined by the binding that remains in the presence of veratridine, aconitine, or unlabeled BTX-B. Results are expressed as femtomoles of [³H]BTX-B bound per milligram of vesicular protein.

Procedure for Measurement of Specific Binding of [³H]BTX-B to Na$^+$ Channels in Synaptoneurosomal Preparation from Guinea Pig Cerebral Cortex

A vesicular preparation from guinea pig cerebral cortical tissue has been referred to as synaptoneurosomes (26). The major components of this preparation appear to be resealed postsynaptic membranes with attached resealed presynaptic elements. The preparation is as follows: slices of gray matter are cut manually with a chilled razor blade from the cerebral cortex of guinea pig (male Hartley, 200–250 g). The slices, approximately 1 g wet weight, are homogenized in 4 ml of binding medium, containing the following: 130 mM choline chloride, 50 mM HEPES/Tris buffer, pH 7.4, 5.5 mM glucose, 0.8 mM MgSO$_4$, and 5.4 mM KCl. Homogenization is with 10–12 strokes of a glass–glass conical homogenizer. The final volume is adjusted to 10 ml and centrifuged at 1000 g at 4°C for 15 min. The pellet is washed once with 10 ml of buffer and resuspended in the same volume of buffer to yield the vesicular preparation. Incubations are carried out in a final volume of 250 μl of binding buffer containing 1 μM tetrodotoxin, 0.03 mg scorpion venom (L. quinquestriatus), and 2 to 20 nM [³H]BTX-B (batrachotoxinin A 20α-[benzoyl-

2,5-³H]benzoate, specific activity 40 Ci/mmol; New England Nuclear, Boston, MA). The binding assay is initiated by the addition of 100 μl of the vesicular preparation, containing approximately 400 μg of protein. Maximal specific binding is achieved after incubation for 45 min at 37°C. The reaction is terminated by dilution with 3 ml of ice-cold wash buffer and collection of the vesicles under vacuum on glass fiber filters (GF/C filters; Whatman, Clifton, NJ). The filters are washed three times with 3 ml of cold wash buffer. Filtration of sets of 24 samples can be accomplished with a Brandel cell harvester (Gaithersburg, MD). The wash buffer contains the following: 163 mM choline chloride, 5 mM HEPES/Tris buffer, pH 7.4, 1.8 mM CaCl$_2$, and 0.8 mM MgSO$_4$. Radioactivity, retained on the filters, is measured in a scintillation counter using 10 ml of Hydroflor (National Diagnostics, Manville, NJ) with a counting efficiency for tritium of 43%. Specific binding is obtained by subtracting the nonspecific binding obtained in parallel reactions, containing 300 μM veratridine or 500 μM aconitine from the total binding. Specific binding ranges from 77 to 86% of total binding. Protein concentrations in the vesicular preparation can be determined by the method of either Peterson (27) or Lowry *et al.* (28). In the latter case, the vesicular preparation must be centrifuged and washed with phosphate-buffered saline (PBS) in order to remove the HEPES/Tris.

A stock solution of HEPES/Tris buffer is prepared by titration of a 1 M stock solution of HEPES acid (N-2-hydroxyethylpiperazine-N'-2-ethanesulfonic acid, Ultrol HEPES; Calbiochem, La Jolla, CA) with a 1 M stock solution of Tris base [tris(hydroxymethyl)aminomethane; Ultrol Tris, Calbiochem] to pH 7.4. Stock solutions of the other components of the binding buffer are prepared as follows: 1.3 M choline chloride (Calbiochem), 80 mM magnesium sulfate heptahydrate, 540 mM potassium chloride, and for the wash buffer, 180 mM calcium chloride. To prepare the binding buffer 50 ml HEPES/Tris, 100 ml choline chloride, 10 ml MgSO$_4$, and 10 ml KCl of the stock solutions are diluted to 1 liter with water. Glucose, 1 g/liter, is added as a solid. To prepare the wash buffer the same stock solutions are used (omitting KCl and adding CaCl$_2$) by diluting 25 ml HEPES/Tris, 627 ml choline chloride, 50 ml MgSO$_4$, and 50 ml CaCl$_2$ to 5 liters with water. Veratridine (16.9 mg/ml) or aconitine (16.2 mg/ml) is prepared as a 25 mM stock solution in 50 mM H$_2$SO$_4$ (both from Sigma Chemical Co., St. Louis, MO). Tetrodotoxin (Calbiochem) is prepared as a 12.5 mM stock solution (4 mg/ml) in water and diluted 1:100 to give a 125 μM working solution. Scorpion venom (*L. quinquestriatus*) (Sigma) is prepared as an aqueous solution (10 mg/ml) and stored as 0.5-ml aliquots at -70°C. In practice it has been necessary to titrate each lot of scorpion venom against the specific binding of [³H]BTX-B to determine the concentration of scorpion venom needed to achieve optimum enhancement (approximately 25-fold) of binding.

The optimum concentration has ranged from a final concentration of 20 to 120 μg/ml with five separate lots of venom. Alternatively, venom can be replaced with 1 μM scorpion α-toxin, purified by ion-exchange chromatography according to Catterall (29). Anemone toxin (100 μM) (Ferring GmbH, Keil, Germany) also has been used (13). The commercial radioligand, [³H]BTX-B, is stored as received in an ethanol solution at −20°C. This ethanol solution is stable for at least 6 months. To prepare a working solution, an aliquot of 10 μl is removed as needed and diluted 1 : 100 in water to provide sufficient ligand, when used at 10 μl per assay tube, to give approximately 0.1 μCi at a final concentration of approximately 10 nM [³H]BTX-B. The working solution of [³H]BTX-B is stable for 3–4 days at −20°C.

Supplemental Notes

[³H]BTX-B binding is readily measured in synaptosomes or synaptosomal preparations (3, 11, 23, 30–32) as well as the above synaptoneurosome preparation. Preparation of synaptosomes are described in the above references. [³H]BTX-B binding also has been measured with a similar protocol in a particulate preparation from heart (23, 24).

It is important that the temperature of the incubation with brain vesicular preparations be maintained at 37°C, since occupancy of site 1 by either tetrodotoxin or saxitoxin can inhibit [³H]BTX-B binding at lower temperatures (16): at 37°C this inhibition is negligible, while at 18 to 25°C both tetrodotoxin and saxitoxin inhibit [³H]BTX-B binding to mouse synaptoneurosomes in a concentration-dependent manner. However, the effects of tetrodotoxin and saxitoxin may require further study. Thus, Garritsen et al. (31) reported that with rat brain synaptosomes, 1 μM tetrodotoxin can inhibit the binding of [³H]BTX-B by about 50% at *both* 25 and 37°C. Garritsen et al. (31) also reported that in HEPES/Tris buffer alone, compared to buffer containing choline chloride, MgCl₂, KCl, etc., there was a twofold increase in specific binding of [³H]BTX-B. There was less inhibition of [³H]BTX-B binding by tetrodotoxin in the presence of magnesium. The MgCl₂ (0.8 mM) in the standard buffer appeared to be responsible for about a 50% inhibition of [³H]BTX-B binding. Choline chloride and KCl of the standard buffer had minimal effects on binding. While binding of [³H]BTX-B is enhanced in magnesium-free HEPES/Tris buffer (31), almost all studies to date have been with buffers similar to or identical with that reported in the present procedure for assay of [³H]BTX-B binding.

Toxins that interact with site 3, such as scorpion α-toxin and anemone toxin, markedly enhance binding of [³H]BTX-B (3). Indeed, high-affinity binding of [³H]BTX-B has not been measured effectively except in the presence of a site 3 toxin. The scorpion β-toxins, which bind to site 4, should not affect the binding of [^{3}H]BTX-B. Marine polyether toxins, such as brevetoxin and ciquatoxin, bind to site 5, and allosterically enhance the binding of [^{3}H]BTX-B to site 2 even in the presence of scorpion α-toxin (4–6).

Other agents affect voltage-dependent channels and enhance binding of [^{3}H]BTX-B. These include the pyrethroids, which can cause repetitive firing and activation of Na$^+$ channels. Type II pyrethroids enhance the binding of [^{3}H]BTX-B (12, 13). Type I pyrethroids inhibit the effect of type II pyrethroid (12). Pumiliotoxin B, one of a series of congeneric alkaloids from tropical frogs, enhances Na$^+$ flux and, like pyrethroids, causes repetitive firing and activation of Na$^+$ channels (33). Pumiliotoxin B does not directly affect [^{3}H]BTX-B binding (7, 8), but it does reduce the inhibition of [^{3}H]BTX-B binding by aconitine in a concentration-dependent manner, suggesting that pumiliotoxin B interacts with a subdomain of site 2 shared by aconitine, but not by BTX (9, 34). Striatoxin, a polypeptide from a marine gastropod, slightly increases [^{3}H]BTX-B binding, apparently through interaction with yet another site on Na$^+$ channels (35). In the presence of scorpion α-toxin, striatoxin has no effect.

A summary of the affinity constants for binding of [^{3}H]BTX-B is presented in Table I (3, 4, 10–13, 16, 19, 20, 22–24, 26, 36–44). Scatchard analyses have in many cases been conducted at a fixed concentration of [^{3}H]BTX-B and increasing concentrations of BTX-B. A range of K_D values from 27 to 194 nM has been reported in rodent brain vesicular preparation with either scorpion venom (*L. quinquestriatus*) or scorpion α-toxin. Brevetoxin and pyrethroids can elicit further increases in the affinity of [^{3}H]BTX-B. In one study, with rat heart membrane fractions, a K_D value of 44 nM was determined in the presence of scorpion venom (23, 24).

A wide range of compounds inhibit binding of [^{3}H]BTX-B. These are summarized in Table II (10, 11, 21, 23, 24, 30, 32, 36–57) and represent local anesthetics, and compounds with local anesthetic activity, including antiarrhythmics and anticonvulsants. The inhibition of [^{3}H]BTX-B binding by local anesthetics appears to occur in a competitive manner (10). However, the apparent competitive inhibition actually results from an allosteric coupling between the binding of local anesthetics and related compounds and the binding of [^{3}H]BTX-B at site 2. This results in a concentration-dependent increase in the dissociation rate of [^{3}H]BTX-B from site 2 (11). An increase in the dissociation rate of [^{3}H]BTX-B (off rate) has been reported in several studies (11, 30, 38, 40, 48, 57). Local anesthetics also can decrease the association rate for binding of [^{3}H]BTX-B (57). Yohimbine has no effect on the dissociation rate, leading to the proposal that it is a direct competitive antagonist against [^{3}H]BTX-B binding (41, 43). An *N*-alkylamide insecticide reduces the association rate, but has no effect on the off rate for [^{3}H]BTX-

TABLE I   Affinity (K_D) and Maximum Binding Capacity (B_{max}) of [³H]BTX-B in Na^+ Channel Preparations

Preparation	$K_D{}^a$ (nM)	$B_{max}{}^a$ (pmol/mg vesicular protein)	Additions	Refs.
Rat brain synaptosomes (Sprague-Dawley)	82	2.1 ± 0.2	Scorpion α-toxin	3
	65 ± 9 (3)	1.3 ± 0.17 (3)	Scorpion α-toxin	11
	116	0.32	Scorpion α-toxin	4
	270	0.31	Brevetoxin	
	68	0.33	Scorpion α-toxin + brevetoxin	
Rat brain synaptosomes (Wistar)	38 ± 3 (4)	1.24 ± 0.02 (4)	Scorpion venom	36
	83 ± 13 (5)	1.8 ± 0.1 (5)	Scorpion venom	23, 24
	194 ± 30 (3)	6 ± 0.7 (3)	Scorpion venom	44
	343 ± 21 (3)	15 ± 1.1 (3)	Scorpion venom + amiloride	
Rat cerebrocortical synaptoneurosomes (Sprague-Dawley)	95	2.2	Scorpion venom	12
	35	2.4	Scorpion venom + deltamethrin	
Rat brain microsomal fraction	460	2.2	None	13
	200	2.2	Anemone toxin	
	15	2.2	Pyrethroid (RU39568)	
	70	2.2	Anemone toxin + brevetoxin	
	12	2.2	Anemone toxin + brevetoxin + deltamethrin	
	2.9	2.2	Anemone toxin + brevetoxin + RU39568	
Guinea pig cerebrocortical synaptoneurosomes (Hartley)	35 ± 5 (10)^b	1.5 ± 0.1 (9)	Scorpion venom	10
	134 ± 46 (7)^c	3.6 ± 0.7 (7)	Scorpion venom	
	118	2.1	Scorpion venom	38
	29 ± 1 (6)	2.0 ± 0.3 (6)	Scorpion venom	37
	48	2.1	Scorpion venom	39
	137 ± 13 (5)^d	4.0 ± 0.5 (5)	Scorpion venom	26
	164 ± 14 (3)^e	3.6 ± 14 (3)	Scorpion venom	
Mouse brain synaptosomes (BALB/cBy)	62	—	Scorpion α-toxin	40
Mouse brain synaptoneurosomes (Swiss Webster)	30	1.0	Scorpion venom	10
	65^f	—	Scorpion venom	16
	180^f	—	Scorpion venom + tetrodotoxin	
Mouse brain synaptoneurosomes (BALB/cBy)	62	—	Scorpion α-toxin	40
	50 ± 5 (3)	3.5 ± 0.5 (3)	Scorpion venom	43
	33 ± 6.3 (3)^g	2.5 ± 0.3 (3)	Scorpion venom	41
Mouse brain synaptoneurosomes (ICR)	50	7.4	Scorpion venom	42
Rat cardiac myocytes	35.3 ± 3.5 (4)	(0.033 ± 0.01 per 6 × 10⁻⁵ cells)	Anemone toxin	22
Rat heart membrane fraction (Wistar)	44 ± 8 (5)	0.5 ± 0.006 (5)	Scorpion venom	23, 24
Eel electroplax membrane fraction (*Electrophorus electricus*)	138	3.3	Scorpion venom	20
House fly head preparation (*Musca domestica L.*)	140	1.3	None	19
	80	1.5	Scorpion venom	

^{a} Values in parentheses indicate the number of separate binding assays.
^{b} Value from Scatchard analysis using a constant concentration of [³H]BTX-B and increasing concentrations of cold BTX-B.
^{c} Value from Scatchard analysis using increasing concentrations of [³H]BTX-B.
^{d} Synaptoneurosomes filtered through a 10-μm filter (LCWP-047; Millipore, Bedford, MA).
^{e} Unfiltered synaptoneurosomes.
^{f} Assay at 25°C.
^{g} At a higher concentration of scorpion venom a more complex binding curve was cited to be indicative of "more binding sites" (41).

TABLE II   Inhibition of [^{3}H]BTX-B Binding by Local Anesthetics and Other Agents

Preparation	Agent	Refs.
Brain vesicular	Local anesthetics	10, 11, 23, 24, 32, 38, 39, 40, 47, 49, 52
	Anticonvulsants	21, 30, 47, 51, 52, 55
	Antiarrhythmics	32
	Antidepressants	47
	Analgesics	32, 47, 49
	Cardiotonics	37
	Calcium antagonists	23, 32, 47, 54
	Adrenergic antagonists	23, 47, 53, 54
	Dopaminergic antagonists	32, 47, 54
	Histaminergic antagonists	32, 47
	Serotinergic antagonists	32, 47
	Amiloride	44
	Cocaine	32, 40, 47
	Yohimbine	41, 43, 47
	Ethanol	36, 45, 46
	Phencyclidine	48, 49, 50
	Histrionicotoxins	48
	Insecticides	42
Heart vesicular	Local anesthetics	23, 24
	Calcium antagonists	23, 24
Heart myocytes	Local anesthetics	57
	Antiarrhythmics	56, 57

B (42). Amiloride decreases the K_D for [^{3}H]BTX-B, but remarkably appears to increase the B_{max} (44). There have been excellent correlations between local anesthetic activity and inhibition of [^{3}H]BTX-B binding (10, 11, 32, 47, 52, 58). The inhibition potencies of calcium channel antagonists, adrenergic blockers, and tetracaine versus [^{3}H]BTX-B were compared for rat brain and rat heart vesicular preparations (23, 24). It should be noted that ethanol has an inhibitory effect on [^{3}H]BTX-B binding (36, 45, 46). Like local anesthetics, ethanol increases the dissociation rate for [^{3}H]BTX-B. The inhibitory effect of alcohols is of practical importance when methanol or ethanol is used as a solvent for agents examined as inhibitors of [^{3}H]BTX-B. The IC_{50} values for methanol and ethanol are 1.0 and 0.60 M, respectively, or expressed in microliters per tube (total volume = 250 μl) are 11 and 9 μl (unpublished observations, 1990). A procaine isothiocyanate and a proparacaine isothiocyanate cause irreversible inhibition of [^{3}H]BTX-B binding (38, 39), presumably through reaction with sulfhydryl or amino groups at local anesthetic-binding sites. The former markedly increases the dissociation rate of [^{3}H]BTX-B (38). Although the site of interaction of [^{3}H]BTX-B with voltage-dependent channels remains unknown, efforts to develop irreversible radiolabeled analogs are in progress. Radiation–inactivation analysis of the binding of [³H]BTX-B in rat synaptosomes indicated two target sites of ~290 and 50 kDa (59).

References

1. W. A. Catterall, *ISI Atlas Sci.: Pharmacol.* **2,** 190 (1988).
2. M. Noda and S. Numa, *J. Recept. Res.* **7,** 467 (1987).
3. W. A. Catterall, C. S. Morrow, J. W. Daly, and G. B. Brown, *J. Biol. Chem.* **256,** 9822 (1981).
4. R. G. Sharkey, E. Jover, F. Couraud, D. G. Baden, and W. A. Catterall, *Mol. Pharmacol.* **31,** 273 (1987).
5. W. A. Catterall and M. Gainer, *Toxicon* **23,** 497 (1985).
6. A. Lombet, J.-N. Bidard, and M. Lazdunski, *FEBS Lett.* **219,** 355 (1987).
7. F. Gusovsky, D. P. Rossignol, E. T. McNeal, and J. W. Daly, *Proc. Natl. Acad. Sci. U.S.A.* **85,** 1272 (1988).
8. J. W. Daly, F. Gusovsky, E. T. McNeal, S. Secunda, M. Bell, C. R. Creveling, Y. Nishizawa, L. E. Overman, M. J. Sharp, and D. P. Rossignol, *Biochem. Pharmacol.* **40,** 315 (1990).
9. F. Gusovsky, W. Padgett, and J. W. Daly, *Soc. Neurosci. Abstr.* **16,** 182 (1990).
10. C. R. Creveling, E. T. McNeal, J. W. Daly, and G. B. Brown, *Mol. Pharmacol.* **23,** 350 (1983).
11. S. W. Postma and W. A. Catterall, *Mol. Pharmacol.* **25,** 219 (1984).
12. G. B. Brown, J. E. Gaupp, and R. W. Olsen, *Mol. Pharmacol.* **34,** 54 (1988).
13. A. Lombet, C. Mourre, and M. Lazdunski, *Brain Res.* **459,** 44 (1988).
14. G. Strichartz, T. Rando, and G. K. Wang, *Annu. Rev. Neurosci.* **10,** 237 (1987).
15. G. B. Brown, S. C. Tieszen, J. W. Daly, J. E. Warnick, and E. X. Albuquerque, *Cell. Mol. Neurobiol.* **1,** 19 (1981).
16. G. B. Brown, *J. Neurosci.* **6,** 2064 (1986).
17. M. Cohen-Armon, H. Garty, and M. Sokolovsky, *Biochemistry* **27,** 368 (1988).
18. M. Cohen-Armon and M. Sokolovsky, *J. Biol. Chem.* **261,** 12498 (1986).
19. D. M. Soderlund, R. E. Grubs, and P. M. Adams, *Comp. Biochem. Physiol. C* **94C,** 255 (1989).
20. E. T. McNeal and J. W. Daly, *Neurochem. Int.* **9,** 487 (1986).
21. P. F. Worley and J. M. Baraban, *Proc. Natl. Acad. Sci. U.S.A.* **84,** 3051 (1987).
22. R. S. Sheldon, N. J. Cannon, and H. J. Duff, *Mol. Pharmacol.* **30,** 617 (1986).
23. J. Velly, M. Grima, G. Marciniak, M. O. Spach, and J. Schwartz, *Naunyn-Schmiedeberg's Arch. Pharmacol.* **355,** 176 (1987).
24. M. Grima, J. Schwartz, M. O. Spach, and J. Velly, *Br. J. Pharmacol.* **89,** 641 (1985).
25. G. B. Brown and J. W. Daly, *Cell. Mol. Neurobiol.* **1,** 361 (1981).
26. E. B. Hollingsworth, E. T. McNeal, J. L. Burton, R. J. Williams, J. W. Daly, and C. R. Creveling, *J. Neurosci.* **5,** 2240 (1985).

27. G. L. Peterson, *Anal. Biochem.* **83,** 346 (1977).
28. O. H. Lowry, N. J. Rosebrough, A. L. Farr, and R. J. Randall, *J. Biol. Chem.* **193,** 265 (1951).
29. W. A. Catterall, *J. Biol. Chem.* **252,** 8669 (1977).
30. M. Willow and W. A. Catterall, *Mol. Pharmacol.* **22,** 627 (1982).
31. A. Garritsen, A. P. Ijzerman, and W. Soudijn, *Eur. J. Pharmacol.* **145,** 261 (1988).
32. P. J. Pauwels, J. E. Leysen, and P. M. Laduron, *Eur. J. Pharmacol.* **124,** 291 (1986).
33. K. S. Rao, J. E. Warnick, J. W. Daly, and E. X. Albuquerque, *J. Pharmacol. Exp. Ther.* **243,** 775 (1987).
34. F. Gusovsky, W. L. Padgett, C. R. Creveling, and J. W. Daly, *Mol. Pharmacol.* (submitted) (1991).
35. T. Gonoi, Y. Ohizumi, J. Kobayashi, H. Nahamura, and W. A. Catterall, *Mol. Pharmacol.* **32,** 691 (1987).
36. M. J. Mullin and W. A. Hunt, *J. Pharmacol. Exp. Ther.* **242,** 536 (1987).
37. G. Romey, I. Quast, D. Pauron, C. Frelin, J. F. Renaud, and M. Lazdunski, *Proc. Natl. Acad. Sci. U.S.A.* **84,** 896 (1987).
38. C. R. Creveling, M. E. Bell, T. R. Burke, E. Chang, G. A. Lewandowski-Lovenberg, C.-H. Kim, K. C. Rice, and J. W. Daly, *Neurochem. Res.* **15,** 441 (1990).
39. F. Gusovsky, Y. Nishizawa, W. Padgett, E. T. McNeal, K. Rice, C.-H. Kim, C. R. Creveling, and J. W. Daly, *Brain Res.* **518,** 101 (1990).
40. M. E. A. Reith, S. S. Kim, and A. Lajtha, *J. Biol. Chem.* **261,** 7300 (1986).
41. I. Zimanyi, A. Lajtha, E. S. Vizi, and M. E. A. Reith, *Biochem. Pharmacol.* **37,** 641 (1988).
42. J. A. Ottea, G. T. Payne, J. R. Bloomquist, and D. M. Soderlund, *Mol. Pharmacol.* **36,** 280 (1989).
43. I. Zimanyi, A. Lajtha, E. S. Vizi, E. Wang, and M. E. A. Reith, *Neuropharmacology* **27,** 1205 (1986).
44. J. Velly, M. Grima, N. Decker, E. J. Cragoe, and J. Schwartz, *Eur. J. Pharmacol.* **149,** 97 (1988).
45. I. Zimanyi, A. Lajtha, and M. E. A. Reith, *Eur. J. Pharmacol.* **146,** 7 (1988).
46. M. J. Mullin, T. K. Dalton, W. A. Hunt, R. A. Harris, and E. Majchrowicz, *J. Pharmacol. Exp. Ther.* **242,** 541 (1987).
47. E. T. McNeal, G. A. Lewandowski, J. W. Daly, and C. R. Creveling, *J. Med. Chem.* **28,** 381 (1985).
48. T. Lovenberg and J. W. Daly, *Neurochem. Res.* **11,** 1609 (1986).
49. C. R. Creveling, E. T. McNeal, G. A. Lewandowski, M. Rafferty, E. H. Harrison, A. E. Jacobson, K. C. Rice, and J. W. Daly, *Neuropeptides* **5,** 353 (1985).
50. H. Allaoua and R. Chicheportiche, *Eur. J. Pharmacol.* **163,** 327 (1989).
51. J. A. Waters, E. B. Hollingworth, J. W. Daly, G. A. Lewandowski, and C. R. Creveling, *J. Med. Chem.* **29,** 1512 (1986).
52. I. Zimanyi, S. R. B. Weiss, A. Lajtha, R. M. Post, and M. E. A. Reith, *Eur. J. Pharmacol.* **167,** 419 (1989).
53. A. P. Ijzerman, A. Nagesser, and A. Garritsen, *Biochem. Pharmacol.* **36,** 4239 (1987).

54. P. J. Pauwels and P. M. Laduron, *Eur. J. Pharmacol.* **132,** 289 (1986).

55. W. J. Brouillette, G. B. Brown, T. M. DeLorey, S. S. Shirali, and G. L. Grunewald, *J. Med. Chem.* **31,** 2218 (1988).

56. R. S. Sheldon, N. J. Cannon, A. S. Nies, and H. J. Duff, *Mol. Pharmacol.* **33,** 327 (1988).

57. R. J. Hill, H. J. Duff, and R. S. Sheldon, *Mol. Pharmacol.* **36,** 150 (1989).

58. Y. Nishizawa, F. Gusovsky, and J. W. Daly, *Mol. Pharmacol.* **34,** 707 (1988).

59. K. J. Angelides, T. J. Nutter, L. W. Elmer, and E. S. Kemper, *J. Biol. Chem.* **260,** 3431 (1955).

[4] Botulinal Neurotoxins: Mode of Action on Neurotransmitter Release

Bernard Poulain and Jordi Molgo

Botulinal neurotoxins (BoNTs) are among the most potent biological agents so far known. Seven immunologically distinguishable forms of these neuroparalytic proteins, designated as types A, B, C_1, D, E, F, and G, are produced by different strains of the anaerobic, spore-forming bacterium, *Clostridium botulinum*. These neurotoxins are synthesized as single-chain proteins. Depending on the physiology of the bacterium and the conditions of the bacterial culture, they may be cleaved (nicked) to a dichain protein. The constituent heavy chain (HC) and light chain (LC) of BoNTs, of $M_r \sim 100,000$ and $\sim 50,000$, respectively (Fig. 1), are held together by disulfide and noncovalent bonds. In general, BoNTs may be isolated from the bacterial culture as a single chain (e.g., BoNT type E) or as a dichain (e.g., BoNT type A); the dichain form of the neurotoxins has a higher toxicity than the single-chain form. Despite the lack of antigenic cross-reactivity among the serologically distinct BoNTs the comparison of their amino acid composition indicates that they have similar molecular sizes and share a common subunit structure (1–4).

Studies with BoNTs have been directed toward the understanding of the toxicity and the clinical problems of botulinum intoxication, which most often result either from ingestion of the toxin in contaminated food, or in infants from colonization of the intestine by *C. botulinum* (1, 5). In recent years, these neurotoxins have been used in the treatment of neuromuscular dystonias as an alternative to surgical treatments (6).

Botulinal neurotoxins are known to act primarily on peripheral synapses that store and release acetylcholine (ACh). Like other toxic proteins, BoNTs have been suggested to act through a sequence of three steps in producing their neuroparalytic effect (7). There is an initial binding step whereby BoNTs attach to specific acceptors located on the cholinergic presynaptic membrane. Then an internalization step ensues, in which the neurotoxins are translocated across the cholinergic membrane to the cytosol of the nerve terminal, where they inhibit ACh release in a long-lasting manner. Functional recovery of poisoned terminals is believed to occur mainly by the remodeling of pre- and postsynaptic structures (8).

The purpose of the present article is to give an overview of the various experimental approaches that have been used to study the mode of action of botulinal toxins, with emphasis on electrophysiological and new experimental

Methods in Neurosciences, Volume 8

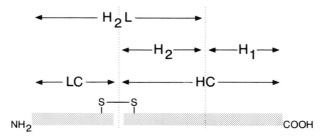

FIG. 1   Schematic representation of chains and fragments of *Clostridium botulinum* neurotoxin (BoNT).

methods that have been developed in various laboratories (for more comprehensive reviews see Refs. 7 and 9–14).

Models and Methods Used in Studying the Mode of Action of Botulinal Neurotoxins

One of the most accessible and studied peripheral cholinergic synapse is the vertebrate skeletal neuromuscular junction. Because BoNTs affect cholinergic transmission specifically, the vertebrate neuromuscular junction has been used more than any other synapse to dissect the site(s) of action of these neurotoxins. For this purpose mammalian and amphibian neuromuscular junctions have been poisoned *in vivo*. The general procedure consisted of injecting sublethal doses of the toxin into a given muscle group. The toxin requirements depend on the purity of the toxin, species of experimental animal, and site of injection. At various times after the injection, the neuromuscular preparation can be isolated from the poisoned animal and studied *in vitro*. The *in vivo* poisoning has been widely used not only to study the actions of BoNTs but also as a pharmacological tool to block neuromuscular transmission in studies of trophic influences between nerve and muscle (8). In most of these latter studies the toxin was administered subcutaneously to maximize the local toxin concentration and to reduce its systemic toxic effects. *In vitro* poisoning involves the application of BoNTs or their constituent chains to the extracellular medium bathing the isolated neuromuscular preparation.

The intracellular action of BoNTs can be addressed independently of the membrane steps (binding and/or internalization) by applying BoNTs directly to the cells. In order to introduce BoNTs or their fragments into motor nerve terminals a method was recently developed in which liposomes were loaded with BoNT, or its chains, and intracellular delivery of toxin samples was achieved by the fusion of the liposomes with the plasma membrane (15).

For assaying the effects of BoNTs, different mammalian neuromuscular preparations have been proposed as alternatives to the classic rat or mouse phrenic nerve-hemidiaphragm, extensor digitorum longus, and soleus nerve-muscle preparations. These include the mouse triangularis sterni (16, 17), the lumbrical muscles of the hind paw of the mouse (18), and the mouse levator auris longus nerve-muscle preparation (19, 20).

The techniques that have been used to quantify the effects of the toxins have been measurements of indirectly elicited muscle twitch contraction (21–24) and conventional electrophysiological methods that allow a high time resolution of presynaptic and postsynaptic events related to the release of acetylcholine (presynaptic current recordings, quantal analysis of evoked and spontaneous quantal or nonquantal ACh release) (Fig. 2a–f). Ultrastructural and autoradiographic studies of motor nerve terminals supplying vertebrate neuromuscular junctions have also been performed (20, 25–28).

Neurochemical and radioligand studies may be easily performed using synaptosomes from the electric organ of *Torpedo,* which are ontogenetically equivalent to cholinergic motor nerve terminals (29, 30).

Another convenient preparation is constituted by easily identifiable couples of neurons making cholinergic or noncholinergic synapses in isolated ganglia of the marine mollusk *Aplysia.* These offer the possibility, using micropipettes, of air pressure injections of toxins or their fragments into the presynaptic cell bodies (75- to 300-μm diameter), which are relatively close to the terminals (300–500 μm) (31–34) (Fig. 3). Visual monitoring of the injection is possible through the use of a vital dye (fast-green FCF) mixed to the toxin. Injected neurons remain alive for several days when cultured and transmitter release can be evaluated by conventional electrophysiological methods (31, 33) (Fig. 2g–i and Fig. 3).

In the vertebrate central nervous system (CNS) various experimental approaches have been developed to bypass the problems resulting from the inherent intricacy and heterogeneity of neuronal networks. Several isolated preparations from the CNS, i.e., brain slices, broken cells, brain particles, or synaptosomes, have been used to characterize the action of BoNTs. However, the different preparations remain quite heterogeneous in the type of cells they include and their active lifetime is only a few hours. Thus, the use of high toxin concentrations is required to obtain rapid and significant effects. Cultured cells [primary cell cultures from brain or spinal chord, which are also heterogeneous, chromaffin cells, or several tumor cell lines (e.g., PC-12 cells)] permit the use of low toxin concentrations since their lifetime is not limited (reviewed in Ref. 11).

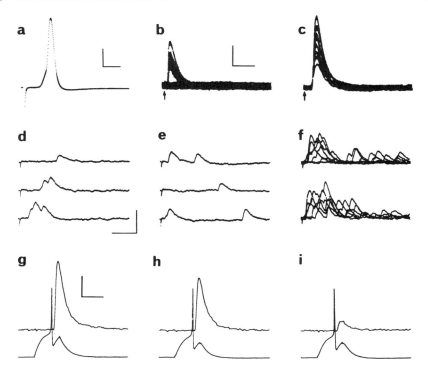

FIG. 2   Typical electrophysiological recordings performed at mouse neuromuscular junctions (a–f) and at a cholinergic synapse of *Aplysia* buccal ganglion (g–i) during the action of BoNT types A (b, c), D (d–f), and B (g–i). (a) Synaptically evoked muscle action potential elicited by nerve stimulation at a single unpoisoned junction. (b) and (c): Superimposed end-plate potentials (EPPs) recorded in a junction previously poisoned with BoNT-A. In (b), note the many failures of release and the low amplitude of the EPPs on nerve stimulation at 1 Hz. (c) Synchronized EPPs elicited at 10 Hz show the absence of failures of release after the addition of 3,4-diaminopyridine (10 μM). In (b) and (c), the medium contained 8 mM Ca^{2+}; arrows indicate stimulus artifact. Traces in (d–f) were obtained from a junction previously poisoned with BoNT type D during 1-Hz (d, e) and 5-Hz (f) nerve stimulation in a medium containing 8 mM Ca^{2+} and 100 μM 3,4-diaminopyridine. Notice the asynchronous responses on nerve stimulation. (g–i) Presynaptic action potentials (lower trace) and elicited postsynaptic current response (upper trace) before (g) and after (h, i) the intracellular injection of BoNT type B. Note the absence of change in the presynaptic action potential at the time the postsynaptic response decreased after 30 min (h) and 120 min (i) of BoNT action. Vertical and horizontal calibration in (a) is 20 mV and 2 msec; in (b), 0.5 mV and 5 msec; in (c), 2 mV and 5 msec [calibration of (b)]; in (d–f), 1 mV and 20 msec. Calibration in (g–i), 5 nA and 20 mV, 32 msec.

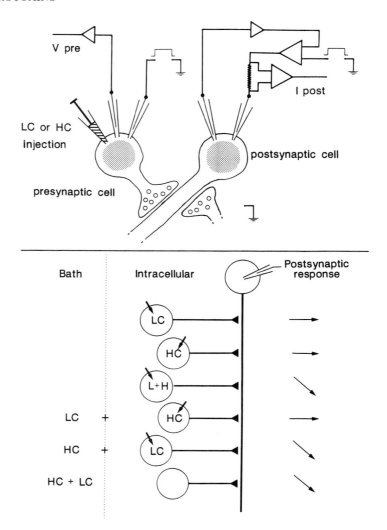

FIG. 3   Schematic representation of the experimental setup for intracellular recording and injection in *Aplysia* neurons (*top*). The role of the various chains or fragments of BoNT in their inhibition of neurotransmitter release in *Aplysia* is presented schematically (*bottom*). Chains or fragments that were administered extracellularly are denoted in the "bath" column and those injected into presynaptic neurons are in the column labeled "intracellular." Evolution of postsynaptic response is symbolized by the position of the thin arrow (horizontal, no effect; falling arrow, depression of evoked release). It can be deduced that both LC and HC are intracellularly required for inhibition of transmitter release but only the HC can enter on its own or mediate internalization of LC.

Recently, bovine adrenal chromaffin cells, which are feebly sensitive to BoNTs (35), and the PC-12 cell line were extensively used for studying the intracellular action of BoNTs. For this purpose, the BoNT was applied using a patch micropipette (36). Under these conditions, the toxin diffused into the chromaffin cell from the micropipette. However, the use of such a method does not allow the actual intracellular concentration of toxin to be known.

The permeabilization of cell membranes using digitonin (a steroid glycoside that interacts specifically with 3β-hydroxysterol) or streptolysin O has been used by several authors to introduce BoNTs or their fragments into bovine chromaffin cells (37, 38), PC12 cells (39), or neurosecretory cells releasing vasopressin (40). The use of detergents to render the plasma membrane permeable allows a precise control of the intracellular medium such as intracellular Ca^{2+} buffering and the introduction of toxins at a given concentration into the cells. However, the half-life of permeabilized preparations is relatively short.

Specificity of Action of Botulinal Neurotoxins

It is well known that BoNTs exhibit cholinergic specificity in their actions on nerve terminals. The evidence obtained at the vertebrate neuromuscular junction and in other cholinergic systems strongly supported this current view (7, 10, 11). The use of higher concentrations than those required at cholinergic terminals in noncholinergic preparations of the autonomic or CNS revealed that the cholinergic specificity of BoNTs was not absolute (7, 41). Indeed, it has been shown that BoNT type A also inhibits the release of various neurotransmitters such as noradrenaline, dopamine, serotonin, γ-aminobutyrate, glycine (42–46), and the peptide methionine-enkephalin (47). In addition, BoNTs have been shown to inhibit catecholamine secretion from bovine adrenal medullary cells (35). From these studies, it remained unclear whether the preferential action of BoNTs on ACh release resulted from differences between secretory processes and/or intracellular efficacies or to differences in membrane targeting.

Direct introduction of BoNTs into cells or neurons showed that BoNTs have *no intracellular cholinergic specificity*. Using intracellular injection of BoNTs [type A into chromaffin cells (36), types A, B, and E into cholinergic and noncholinergic identified neurons in *Aplysia* (31–33), or application of BoNT types A, B, and E to permeabilized chromaffin cells (37, 38) or PC-12 cells (39)] it was shown that bypassing the membrane-related events (binding/internalization) abolished the cholinergic selectivity of BoNTs. These studies have definitely established that the final target of BoNTs is intracellular and suggested that a toxin-sensitive component of the release process exists in several, if not all, nerve terminal types. The relative cholinergic specificity of action of BoNT can be attributed to its interaction with unique acceptors located onto the plasma membrane of cholinergic terminals.

Binding of Botulinal Neurotoxins

Due to difficulties in isolating sufficient amounts of membrane material from peripheral nerve terminals, binding studies using radiolabeled BoNTs have been performed mainly on preparations from the CNS that are, in general, less sensitive to the action of BoNTs. The easiest way to localize the binding sites of BoNTs onto nerve terminals has been the use of autoradiographic techniques with ^{125}I-labeled BoNT. It has been shown that ^{125}I-labeled BoNT type A or B interacted saturably and independently of temperature with distinct acceptors on motor nerve terminals (27, 28). The labeling was distributed uniformly on all unmyelinated areas of the terminals at densities of ~150–650 sites/μm^2. However, the number of binding sites on motor terminals by far exceeds the number of molecules needed for paralysis, suggesting that only a fraction of these binding sites is implicated in the neurotoxic action.

Radioligand studies on cerebrocortical synaptosomes have characterized the existence of saturable, temperature-independent, and high-affinity binding sites for BoNTs. Each BoNT type binds to at least two species of acceptors, one of high affinity ($K_d \sim 0.1$–0.6 nM) for type A (48), B (49), C_1 (50), D (51), and F (52), and the other of lower affinity. Cross-competition experiments revealed different acceptors for the various BoNT types (27, 28, 49, 52). However, the acceptors for type E were related to those of type A (53) and there was competitive binding between types C_1 and D (51). The physiological meaning of these radiolabeled-characterized acceptors remains to be determined, since BoNT type A has not been found to be noticeably toxic when injected into brain (48).

The binding of BoNTs causes by itself no detectable changes in the physiological parameters of neurotransmission. However, in electrophysiological experiments, it has been possible to dissociate the binding from the ensuing steps involved in toxin action and to deduce some features related to the binding. In such experiments, BoNT was applied under conditions that allowed binding but prevented internalization (see below). Then, various treatments supposed to affect the binding were performed (washing out of the toxin, addition of specific antibodies or toxin fragments, etc.). On return to physiological conditions the modified action of BoNT was evaluated. Following this experimental approach it was shown that the binding of BoNTs was irreversible, little or not affected by temperature (21, 22, 32), and still accessible to the neutralization by specific antibodies (21, 54).

Identification of Toxin Moieties Implicated in Binding

Using an autoradiographic approach, when internalization was minimized, the HC alone was found to abolish completely the binding of ^{125}I-labeled BoNT to motor nerve terminal (27, 28). Accordingly, the HC can prevent the binding of ^{125}I-labeled BoNT to rat brain membranes (48, 51, 53). At an *Aplysia* cholinergic synapse, once the internalization step was blocked, the HC fully prevented BoNT binding (32). Similarly, high concentrations of the HC delayed the action of BoNT type A and B on murine phrenic nerve-hemidiaphragm muscle preparations (23). It is worth noting that the LC was found to be unable to compete with the holoneurotoxin. These results indicate that the binding of BoNTs is mediated by the HC. However, at the murine neuromuscular junction, when competition experiments were done under the same condition as specified for autoradiographic studies, the HC did not antagonize the blocking action of BoNTs (24). These and other results, described elsewhere (24, 32, 33), suggested that only the dichain species of BoNT is able to recognize efficiently those acceptors involved in the poisoning of motor nerve terminals (24, 55).

An alternative approach to gain insight into the molecular domains of BoNT implicated in binding is the use of monoclonal antibodies directed against selected BoNT epitopes (10, 54). Results obtained under these conditions support the view that the HC of BoNT is directly implicated in the binding step.

Enzymatic removal of the C-terminal half of the HC prevented the binding of the remaining ^{125}I-labeled BoNT fragment, named H_2L, to either rat cerebrocortical synaptosomes (56) or motor nerve terminals (32). In this latter preparation, as expected, the H_2L fragment was unable to inhibit BoNT binding (32). However, when tested in *Aplysia* neurons, this nontoxic fragment was shown to antagonize the binding of BoNT (32). The discrepancy between the results obtained in vertebrates and invertebrates could be due to evolutionary divergence in the nature of BoNT acceptors.

Nature of Neuronal Acceptors for Botulinal Neurotoxins

To date, the receptors for BoNTs have not been isolated (for reviews, see Refs. 10–12, 57, and 58. By analogy with tetanus neurotoxin (TeNT), it was initially proposed that BoNTs bind to ganglioside components (GT_{1b} or GD_{1a})

of the presynaptic membrane. The digestion by neuraminidase of GD_{1a} on chromaffin cells caused the loss of BoNT ability to inhibit carbachol-induced [^{3}H]noradrenaline release. Additionally, following incorporation of a mixture of gangliosides (GM_1, GD_{1a}, GD_{1b}, GT_{1b}), the potency of BoNT type A increased (59). Botulinal toxin type A binding has been found to be neuraminidase sensitive in both cerebrocortical synaptosomes (48, 49) or cultured cells from mouse spinal cord and brain (43, 44). Also, on isolated neuromuscular preparations, gangliosides produced a loss of BoNT activity, the extent of which depended on the serotype used (60).

The involvement of a protein component(s) in the binding of BoNTs has been suggested because target tissues for BoNTs have not been found to be especially enriched with the above-mentioned gangliosides (57). This suggestion also gained support by the observation that pretreatment of rat brain synaptosome membranes with trypsin prevented specific binding (48) and because ^{125}I-labeled BoNT type A was found to bind to peptides from the presynaptic membrane of *Torpedo* electric organ (30). A model in which the HC of BoNTs binds first via its carboxy terminus to a ganglioside region and thereafter via its amino-terminal region to a proteinaceous component has been proposed (57).

Internalization of Botulinal Neurotoxins

Internalization of BoNTs has been deduced from the fact that their final target is intracellular and from autoradiographic studies showing the presence of ^{125}I-labeled BoNT inside motor nerve terminals (27, 28). Possible models for the translocation of BoNTs have been discussed (7, 10, 12, 57, 58).

The internalization of BoNT is an energy-dependent process as shown by its dependence on temperature and energy metabolism. The internalization of ^{125}I-labeled BoNT may be blocked by lowering temperature or by the addition of inhibitors of energy production, such as azide or α-dinitrophenol (28). A selective inhibition of the internalization of BoNT is obtained by reducing the temperature at murine motor nerve terminals or *Aplysia* neurons, and by reducing extracellular Ca^{2+} and increasing Mg^{2+} concentration (21, 23, 24, 32).

Autoradiographic studies have revealed that ^{125}I-labeled BoNT is associated with endocytotic structures within motor terminals (28), thereby supporting the view that the translocation of BoNT from the extra- to the intracellular medium is due to acceptor-mediated endocytosis. It is worth noting that agents that impair receptor-mediated endocytosis such as methylamine or ammonium chloride and lysomotropic agents like chloroquine delay the onset of blockade induced by BoNT types A, B, C, and E (61).

Toxin Moiety Implicated in Internalization of Botulinal Neurotoxins

The sequential application of the constituent chains of BoNT on both the phrenic nerve-hemidiaphragm muscle preparation (23) and *Aplysia* synapses (24, 33) has shown that when one chain (either the LC or the HC) is applied and washed out, subsequent addition of the complementary chain causes inhibition only when the initially applied chain is the HC. Thus, the HC is considered to mediate the internalization of the LC. Although in *Aplysia* neurons both chains of BoNT are required intracellularly to inhibit neurotransmitter release, only the HC was able to internalize on its own (31) (see Fig. 3). Recent experiments in *Aplysia* have further indicated that the N-terminal half of the HC mediates the internalization of BoNT (33).

A possible role for the N-terminal half (H$_2$) of the HC in the translocation process has been suggested on the basis of biophysical studies performed on lipid bilayer membranes. It has been found that not only the holotoxin but also the N-terminal region of the HC of BoNT forms channels at low pH (62–64). These channels seem to be large enough to ensure the passage of the LC through the membrane.

Intracellular Actions of Botulinal Neurotoxins on Neurotransmitter Release

The most striking action of BoNTs is the long-lasting blockade of neurotransmitter release from nerve terminals. Most of the information available has been obtained with electrophysiological methods at the vertebrate neuromuscular junction.

Evoked Quantal Transmitter Release

Botulinal neurotoxins reduce nerve impulse-evoked quantal transmitter release from motor endings in such a way that, in general, only a few ACh quanta are released on nerve stimulation. Even when the quantal content of end-plate potentials (EPPs) is reduced to low levels, transmitter release continues to be random and spatially dispersed all over the nerve terminal.

The low probability of transmitter release from BoNT type A-poisoned terminals can be enhanced by increasing the extra- and intracellular Ca^{2+} concentration (65) and frequency of nerve stimulation (66), and by lowering temperature (22, 67, 68). On both PC-12 cells and synaptosomes, the BoNT type A-induced blockade of K^+-evoked release may not be reversed by increasing Ca^{2+} concentration (39, 45) unless the Ca^{2+} ionophore A23187 was added (55). Drugs that enhance phasic presynaptic Ca^{2+} influx by blocking voltage-dependent K^+ channels such as 4-aminopyridine (4-AP) and 3,4-diaminopyridine (3,4-DAP) are found to be potent antagonists of the neuromuscular block produced by BoNT types A (69) and E (70). However, it should be emphasized that when evoked transmitter release is *completely* abolished by BoNT types A and E, these drugs cannot reverse the inhibition of release. No effect of 4-AP is observed on K^+-evoked release of [^{3}H]ACh or [^{3}H]noradrenaline from synaptosomes treated with BoNT type A (45).

When the effects of 4-AP or 3,4-DAP were examined at junctions poisoned with BoNT types B, D, and F, the drugs, instead of increasing the evoked synchronous release giving rise to EPPs, as seen with type A or E (20, 69, 70), induced an asynchronous quantal release recorded as an increase in miniature EPP (MEPP) frequency in response to nerve impulses (17, 20, 71, 72) (Fig. 2). Such asynchronous release prevented the buildup of EPPs so that neuromuscular transmission remained blocked. The differences in the action of aminopyridines with these serotypes were so impressive that they raised the question as to whether the BoNT types B, D, and F had a mode of action similar to that of types A and E. Other studies have also reported subtle differences in the action of the various BoNTs (38, 55).

We know little about the mechanism whereby Ca^{2+} influx following nerve impulses triggers synchronous transmitter release. The results obtained with BoNT types B, D, and F suggest that a special mechanism exists for the synchronization of quantal transmitter release and raise the possibility that this mechanism may be the target of these neurotoxins. It has been hypothesized that BoNT types B, D, and F could modify the coordinated transport of synaptic vesicles toward the presynaptic membrane (14, 17). Related to this issue, it is worth noting that destruction of actin-based cytoskeleton in brain synaptosomes with cytochalasin D or disassembly of microtubules with colchicine, nocodazole, or griseofulvin antagonizes the intracellular action of BoNT type B but not of type A (55).

Spontaneous Quantal and Nonquantal Acetylcholine Release

As recently reviewed (14, 73, 74), there is general agreement that, following *in vitro* or *in vivo* BoNT type A poisoning, spontaneous MEPP frequency is reduced by more than 99%. Contradictory results were, however, obtained when the molecular leakage of ACh was evaluated by different methods (11). Comparative studies have reported that MEPP frequency is less affected by BoNT types B, D, E, or F than by type A. The mean MEPP amplitude is decreased during the first few days of *in vivo* or *in vitro* poisoning with BoNTs (14). Following BoNT type A poisoning *in vivo*, slow-rising MEPPs of the Ca^{2+}-insensitive type increase in frequency and become particularly prominent within about 15 days (75). As the effects of the toxin subside, the frequency of these MEPPs is reduced while the number of fast-rising Ca^{2+}-sensitive MEPPs increases (73, 75).

The decreased probability of spontaneous quantal release from BoNT type A-poisoned terminals is not restored by increasing the extracellular Ca^{2+} concentration or by elevating intraterminal Ca^{2+} by the calcium ionophore A23187 (26, 65). These findings indicate that the process of transmitter release in poisoned terminals has a reduced sensitivity to intracellular Ca^{2+}. This is supported by numerous experimental findings in which intraterminal Ca^{2+} was modified by depolarizing with high extracellular K^+ (71, 75), by blockade of the Na^+,K^+-ATPase with ouabain (65, 76), or by metabolic inhibitors (71, 74). In addition, La^{3+}, Zn^{2+}, and Cd^{2+}, which induce within minutes a large increase in MEPP frequency in normal junctions, appear to be far less effective at promoting ACh release from BoNT type A-paralyzed junctions. These findings indicate that the spontaneous Ca^{2+}-dependent quantal transmitter release from BoNT-poisoned terminals seems to be resistant not only to the release-promoting action of Ca^{2+}, but also to other cations known to support transmitter release (reviewed in Ref. 74).

Identification of Intracellularly Active Moieties of Botulinal Neurotoxins

In *Aplysia* neurons the injection of a single isolated chain (either the HC or the LC of BoNT types A or B) has, by itself, no toxic action. Both the LC and the C-terminal half of the HC of BoNT have been required intracellularly to express neurotoxicity (31, 33). These results are in marked contrast to those obtained with permeabilized bovine chromaffin cells (37, 38), PC-12 cells (39), or with nerve endings releasing vasopressin (40). In those preparations it was shown that only the LC of BoNT was intracellularly active. Similar results have been obtained recently when the LC of BoNT-A was introduced into motor nerve terminals by liposome fusion (15). The reason for the discrepancy between results on molluskan neurons and secretory cells or motor nerve terminals is still controversial.

The elucidation of the primary structure of several BoNTs by molecular biotechnology (2, 3) has opened new possibilities in the study of the active chain domains of BoNTs. A novel approach to test the biological properties of the LC of clostridial toxins has been developed (34). In those studies the mRNA encoding the LC of BoNT type A was injected into an identified cholinergic neuron of *Aplysia* leading to the intracellular synthesis of the corresponding peptide within ~35 min (34). The translation of the LC of BoNT induced no effect until the complementary HC, which can enter the neuron on its own, was applied to the extracellular medium. This new methodology makes possible the identification of the protein domains directly implicated in the action of BoNTs by the study of modified LCs intraneuronally translated from mRNA encoding deletions or punctual modifications (by site-directed mutagenesis).

Intracellular Site of Action(s) of Botulinal Neurotoxins

The possibility that BoNTs could affect presynaptic Ca^{2+} entry and/or intraterminal Ca^{2+} levels has been tested. Using microelectrodes inserted in the perineurium of small preterminal nerve bundles to record electric signals related to membrane currents, it was found that BoNT type A or D poisoned endings display normal Ca^{2+} currents (16, 19, 20, 77). This is in agreement with results showing that $^{45}Ca^{2+}$ fluxes remained unaffected by BoNT type A, B, or D in chromaffin cells (35) or cholinergic synaptosomes from *Torpedo* electric organ (29). In addition, it has been shown that the presynaptic Ca^{2+}-dependent K^+ current in junctions poisoned with BoNT types A or D is indistinguishable from that observed in control conditions (19, 20). These results indicate that neither Ca^{2+} entry nor intraterminal levels of Ca^{2+} are markedly affected by BoNTs. Thus, it is possible that BoNTs may either reduce the efficacy of the release-promoting action of Ca^{2+} or affect directly the transmitter release process.

The present prevailing belief is that BoNTs once internalized may modify a substrate that governs ACh release through an enzymatic action. Botulinal toxin type D but not type A was reported to ADP-ribosylate a protein of M_r 21,000 (78) that behaves as a GTP-binding protein. This finding led to the attractive hypothesis that BoNT type D-induced ADP-ribosylation of a G protein could inhibit secretion. This was contradicted by studies showing that the ADP-ribosylation was due to a botulinum ADP-ribosyltransferase C3 present in the BoNT type D sample used (79, 80). Accordingly, no ADP-ribosylation of brain proteins has been detected under conditions where BoNT type A or B abolish transmitter release (45, 46, 80).

In pure cholinergic synaptosomes isolated from the electric organ of *Torpedo* it was found that BoNT type A inhibited depolarization-stimulated protein phosphorylation (81). Protein phosphorylation and distinct Ca^{2+}-dependent protein kinases have been implicated in the regulation of neurotransmitter release. Botulinal toxin types A and B apparently cause no detectable alteration in the phosphorylation of synaptosomal proteins or in the activity of various kinases, including those dependent on cAMP, Ca^{2+}, Ca^{2+}-calmodulin, and Ca^{2+}-phospholipid, under conditions in which inhibition of transmitter release is observed (13, 55). Further studies are required to identify the major proteins involved directly in the inhibition of neurotransmitter release caused by BoNTs.

In conclusion, in recent years there has been increasing interest in the study of the mode of action of botulinal toxins at the cellular level. This is due mainly to the unique ability of these toxins to effectively block neurotransmitter release in all types of terminals once they gain access inside the nerve terminals. During the last decade progress has been made in the identification of the functional domains of BoNTs implicated in the multiple facets of their mode of action. Deciphering their intracellular molecular actions awaits clarification and remains a challenge for future research.

Acknowledgments

This study was supported in part by Direction des Recherches Etudes et Techniques, Association Française contre les Myopathies (AFM), and by the CNRS. The authors thank Mr. Louis-Eric Trudeau for many helpful editorial comments.

References

1. H. Sugiyama, *Microbiol. Rev.* **44,** 419 (1980).
2. D. E. Thompson, J. K. Brehm, J. D. Oultram, T. J. Swinfield, C. C. Shone, T. Atkinson, J. Melling, and N. P. Minton, *Eur. J. Biochem.* **189,** 73 (1990).
3. T. Binz, H. Kurazono, M. Wille, J. Frevert, K. Wernars, and H. Niemann, *J. Biol. Chem.* **265,** 9153 (1990).
4. B. R. DasGupta, *J. Physiol. (Paris)* **84,** 220 (1990).
5. S. S. Arnon, *J. Infect. Dis.* **154,** 201 (1986).
6. J. Elston, *J. Physiol. (Paris)* **84,** 285 (1990).
7. L. L. Simpson, *Pharmacol. Rev.* **33,** 155 (1981).
8. S. Thesleff, J. Molgo, and S. Tägerud, *J. Physiol. (Paris)* **84,** 167 (1990).
9. C. B. Gundersen, *Prog. Neurobiol.* **14,** 99 (1980).
10. L. L. Simpson, *in* "Botulinum Neurotoxin and Tetanus Toxin" (L. L. Simpson, ed.), p. 153. Academic Press, San Diego, California, 1989.
11. E. Habermann and F. Dreyer, *Curr. Top. Microbiol. Immunol.* **129,** 93 (1986).
12. J. L. Middlebrook, *J. Toxicol. Toxin Rev.* **5,** 177 (1986).
13. J. O. Dolly, A. C. Ashton, D. M. Evans, P. J. Richardson, J. D. Black, and J.

Melling, *in* "Cellular and Molecular Basis for Cholinergic Function" (M. J. Dowdall and J. N. Hawthborne, eds.), p. 517. Ellis Horwood, Chichester, England, 1987.

14. L. C. Sellin, *Asia Pac. J. Pharmacol.* **2,** 203 (1987).
15. A. De Paiva and J. O. Dolly, *FEBS Lett.* **277,** 171 (1990).
16. F. Dreyer, A. Mallart, and J. L. Brigant, *Brain Res.* **270,** 373 (1983).
17. M. Gansel, R. Penner, and F. Dreyer, *Pfluegers Arch.* **409,** 533 (1987).
18. A. W. Clark, S. Bandyopadyah, and B. R. DasGupta, *J. Neurosci. Methods* **19,** 285 (1987).
19. A. Mallart, J. Molgo, D. Angaut-Petit, and S. Thesleff, *Brain Res.* **479,** 167 (1989).
20. J. Molgo, L. S. Siegel, N. Tabti, and S. Thesleff, *J. Physiol. (London)* **411,** 195 (1989).
21. L. L. Simpson, *J. Pharmacol. Exp. Ther.* **212,** 16 (1980).
22. F. Dreyer and A. Schmitt, *Pfluegers Arch.* **399,** 228 (1983).
23. S. Bandyopadhyay, A. W. Clark, B. R. DasGupta, and V. Sathyamoorthy, *J. Biol. Chem.* **262,** 2660 (1987).
24. E. A. Maisey, J. D. F. Wadsworth, B. Poulain, C. C. Shone, J. Melling, P. Gibbs, L. Tauc, and J. O. Dolly, *Eur. J. Biochem.* **177,** 683 (1988).
25. D. W. Pumplin and T. S. Reese, *J. Physiol. (London)* **273,** 443 (1977).
26. F. Dreyer, F. Rosenberg, C. Becker, H. Bigalke, and R. Penner, *Naunyn-Schmiedeberg's Arch. Pharmacol.* **335,** 1 (1987).
27. J. D. Black and J. O. Dolly, *J. Cell Biol.* **103,** 521 (1986).
28. J. D. Black and J. O. Dolly, *J. Cell Biol.* **103,** 535 (1986).
29. J. Marsal, C. Solsona, X. Rabasseda, J. Blasi, and A. Casanova, *Neurochem. Int.* **10,** 295 (1987).
30. C. Solsona, G. Egea, J. Blasi, C. Casanova, and J. Marsal, *J. Physiol. (Paris)* **84,** 174 (1990).
31. B. Poulain, L. Tauc, E. A. Maisey, J. D. F. Wadsworth, M. Mohan, and J. O. Dolly, *Proc. Natl. Acad. Sci. U.S.A.* **85,** 4090 (1988).
32. B. Poulain, J. D. F. Wadsworth, C. C. Shone, S. Mochida, S. Lande, J. Melling, J. O. Dolly, and L. Tauc, *J. Biol. Chem.* **264,** 21928 (1989).
33. B. Poulain, S. Mochida, J. D. F. Wadsworth, U. Weller, E. Habermann, J. O. Dolly, and L. Tauc, *J. Physiol. (Paris)* **84,** 247 (1990).
34. S. Mochida, B. Poulain, U. Eisel, T. Binz, H. Kurazono, H. Niemann, and L. Tauc, *Proc.Natl. Acad. Sci. U.S.A.* **87,** 7844 (1990).
35. D. E. Knight, *FEBS Lett.* **207,** 222 (1986).
36. R. Penner, E. Neher, and F. Dreyer, *Nature (London)* **324,** 76 (1986).
37. B. Stecher, U. Weller, E. Habermann, M. Gratzl, and G. Ahnert-Hilger, *FEBS Lett.* **255,** 391 (1989).
38. M. A. Bittner, B. R. DasGupta, and R. W. Holz, *J. Biol. Chem.* **264,** 10354 (1989).
39. C. McInnes and J. O. Dolly, *FEBS Lett.* **261,** 323 (1990).
40. G. Dayanithi, G. Ahnert-Hilger, U. Weller, J. J. Nordmann, and M. Gratzl, *Neuroscience* **39,** 711 (1990).
41. I. MacKenzie, G. Burnstock, and J. O. Dolly, *Neuroscience* **7,** 997 (1982).
42. H. Bigalke, I. Heller, B. Bizzini, and E. Habermann, *Naunyn-Schmiedeberg's Arch. Pharmacol.* **316,** 244 (1981).

43. H. Bigalke, G. K. Bergey, and F. Dreyer, *Brain Res.* **360,** 319 (1985).
44. E. Habermann, H. Müller, and M. Hudel, *J. Neurochem.* **51,** 522 (1988).
45. A. C. Ashton and J. O. Dolly, *J. Neurochem.* **50,** 1808 (1988).
46. R. Nakov, E. Habermann, G. Herting, S. Wurster, and C. Allgaier, *Eur. J. Pharmacol.* **164,** 45 (1989).
47. P. Janicki and E. Habermann, *J. Neurochem.* **41,** 395 (1983).
48. R. S. Williams, C. K. Tse, J. O. Dolly, P. Hambleton, and J. Melling, *Eur. J. Biochem.* **131,** 437 (1983).
49. D. M. Evans, R. S. Williams, C. C. Shone, P. Hambleton, J. Melling, and J. O. Dolly, *Eur. J. Biochem.* **154,** 409 (1986).
50. T. Agui, B. Syuto, K. Oguma, H. Iida, and S. Kubo, *J. Biochem. (Tokyo)* **94,** 521 (1983).
51. S. Murayama, B. Syuto, K. Oguma, H. Iida, and S. Kubo, *Eur. J. Biochem.* **142,** 487 (1984).
52. J. D. F. Wadsworth, M. Desai, H. S. Tranter, H. J. King, P. Hambleton, J. Melling, J. O. Dolly, and C. C. Shone, *Biochem. J.* **268,** 123 (1990).
53. S. Kozaki, *Naunyn-Schmiedeberg's Arch. Pharmacol.* **308,** 67 (1979).
54. L. L. Simpson, Y. Kamata, and S. Kozaki, *J. Pharmacol. Exp. Ther.* **255,** 227 (1990).
55. J. O. Dolly, A. C. Ashton, C. McInnes, J. D. F. Wadsworth, B. Poulain, L. Tauc, C. C. Shone, and J. Melling, *J. Physiol. (Paris)* **84,** 237 (1990).
56. C. C. Shone, P. Hambleton, and J. Melling, *Eur. J. Biochem.* **151,** 75 (1985).
57. C. Montecucco, *Trends Biochem. Sci.* **11,** 314 (1986).
58. G. Schiavo, P. Bocquet, B. R. DasGupta, and C. Montecucco, *J. Physiol. (Paris)* **84,** 188 (1990).
59. P. Marxen, U. Fuhrmann, and H. Bigalke, *Toxicon* **27,** 849 (1989).
60. S. Kozaki, G. Sakaguchi, M. Nishimura, M. Iwamori, and Y. Nagai, *FEMS Microbiol. Lett.* **21,** 219 (1984).
61. L. L. Simpson, *J. Pharmacol. Exp. Ther.* **245,** 867 (1988).
62. J. J. Donovan and J. L. Middlebrook, *Biochemistry* **25,** 2872 (1986).
63. R. O. Blaustein, W. J. Germann, A. Finkelstein, and B. R. DasGupta, *FEBS Lett.* **226,** 115 (1987).
64. C. C. Shone, P. Hambleton, and J. Melling, *Eur. J. Biochem.* **167,** 175 (1987).
65. S. G. Cull-Candy, H. Lundh, and S. Thesleff, *J. Physiol. (London)* **260,** 177 (1976).
66. J. Molgo, M. Lemeignan, and S. Thesleff, *Muscle Nerve* **10,** 646 (1987).
67. H. Lundh, *Muscle Nerve* **6,** 56 (1983).
68. J. Molgo and S. Thesleff, *Brain Res.* **297,** 309 (1984).
69. J. Molgo, H. Lundh, and S. Thesleff, *Eur. J. Pharmacol.* **61,** 25 (1980).
70. J. Molgo, B. R. DasGupta, and S. Thesleff, *Acta Physiol. Scand.* **137,** 497 (1989).
71. L. C. Sellin, S. Thesleff, and B. R. DasGupta, *Acta Physiol. Scand.* **119,** 127 (1983).
72. J. A. Kauffman, J. F. Way, L. S. Siegel, and L. C. Sellin, *Toxicol. Appl. Pharmacol.* **79,** 211 (1985).
73. S. Thesleff, *Int. Rev. Neurobiol.* **28,** 59 (1986).

74. J. Molgo, J. X. Comella, D. Angaut-Petit, M. Pécot-Dechavassine, N. Tabti, L. Faille, A. Mallart, and S. Thesleff, *J. Physiol. (Paris)* **84,** 152 (1990).
75. M. T. Lupa, *Synapse* **1,** 281 (1987).
76. J. Molgo, D. Angaut-Petit, and S. Thesleff, *Brain Res.* **410,** 385 (1987).
77. C. B. Gundersen, B. Katz, and R. Miledi, *Proc. R. Soc. London B* **216,** 369 (1982).
78. Y. Ohashi and S. Narumiya, *J. Biol. Chem.* **262,** 1430 (1987).
79. K. Aktories, S. Rösener, U. Blaschke, and G. S. Chhatwal, *Eur. J. Biochem.* **172,** 445 (1988).
80. A. C. Ashton, K. Edwards, and J. O. Dolly, *Toxicon* **28,** 963 (1990).
81. X. Guitart, G. Egea, C. Solsona, and J. Marsal, *FEBS Lett.* **219,** 219 (1987).

[5]   Botulinum Toxin as a Tool in Neurobiology

Lance L. Simpson

Introduction

Botulinum neurotoxin is potentially a valuable tool for studying mechanisms that relate to storage and release of chemical mediators. It possesses characteristics that make it well suited for analyzing transmitter release at the mammalian neuromuscular junction, and it has additional properties that make it a candidate for examining exocytosis in a wide range of secreting cells. In spite of these favorable qualities, the toxin has one substantial drawback that has limited its utility. Botulinum neurotoxin is extremely potent—indeed, it is the most poisonous substance known—and this has diminished enthusiasm for employing it as a research tool.

The perceived hazards in handling the toxin have caused it to be largely overlooked by neurobiologists. This is unfortunate, for a variety of reasons. First, the technical aspects of using the toxin are simple and straightforward, often involving little more than adding it to solutions that bathe excised tissues or cultured cells. Second, the toxin is indeed poisonous, but it is also manageable; there are clear and effective means for storing and using the material in a relatively safe manner. And third, there are many ways in which the toxin can be safely and effectively exploited to help unravel mechanisms that would otherwise be difficult to explore. Thus, there is something of an irony in the concept of using the toxin as a tool. The methodological obstacles to employing the toxin in various research paradigms are minimal; the greater obstacles are the lack of widespread appreciation for its potential value and the lack of familiarity with procedures for safe handling.

This chapter is prepared in a way that takes into account the true obstacles to using botulinum neurotoxin as a tool in neurobiology. The chapter begins with a brief discussion of the toxin, including comments on its origin, structure, and biological activity. This is followed by a survey of the various ways in which the toxin has been, or could be, used as a tool. Finally, there is a presentation of the major guidelines that apply to safe handling of the toxin.

Origin and Structure

Botulinum neurotoxin is one of three substances produced by *Clostridium botulinum* that have profound effects on eukaryotic cell function. The other two are the botulinum binary toxin, which acts somewhat ubiquitously to

Methods in Neurosciences, Volume 8

alter the cytoskeleton of cells (1), and the botulinum exoenzyme, which alters cell growth and development (2). The neurotoxin is synthesized in seven different serotypes designated A, B, C, D, E, F, and G (3). In most cases individual strains of bacteria produce only one serotype of toxin, although in a small number of cases bacteria have been found to produce two serotypes. Organisms that make type C or type D neurotoxin also make the binary toxin and the exoenzyme.

The location of the genetic material that encodes synthesis of the neurotoxin varies with serotype. For example, the genetic material that encodes type A is found in the host genome, the material that encodes type G is found in a plasmid, and that which encodes types C and D is found in a phage that infects the organism. It has been found that organisms cured of their viral infection cease to produce serotypes C and D, but they continue to grow and multiply normally. This suggests that the neurotoxin plays no essential role in the economy of the organism. It should be noted that organisms other than *C. botulinum* are capable of making the toxin. For example, when *Clostridium novyi* is appropriately infected, it produces serotypes C and D. In addition, some wild-type strains of *Clostridium barati* and *Clostridium butyricum* have been found to make the toxin.

All serotypes are synthesized as 150,000-Da proteins that are relatively inactive (4, 5). These molecules undergo posttranslational modification ("nicking") to give a dichain structure in which a heavy chain ($\sim$100,000 Da) is linked by a disulfide bond to a light chain ($\sim$50,000 Da). It is in this state that the toxin is fully active and capable of blocking transmitter release from nerve endings. Neither chain by itself can block exocytosis from intact cells (but see below), and intact toxin that has been subjected to disulfide bond reduction is almost without effect.

The complete primary structures of most of the serotypes have been determined, and there is significant homology among them. Work has begun on the secondary and tertiary structure of the toxins, but as yet this has not helped to clarify the basis for toxin activity.

Mechanism of Action

Botulinum neurotoxin acts at the cholinergic neuromuscular junction to block release of acetylcholine (3, 6). A wealth of data show that the toxin does not interfere with synthesis or storage of transmitter, nor does it block propagation of nerve impulses into the nerve ending. The action of the toxin is to uncouple depolarization from exocytosis. Apparently calcium can enter poisoned nerve endings, but it cannot trigger the process that culminates in vesicle membranes melding with the plasma membrane.

An emerging body of evidence provides some insight into the structure–function relationships in the toxin molecule. The toxin proceeds through a sequence of three steps in blocking transmitter release, including an initial binding step, an internalization step, and an intracellular poisoning step. The heavy chain of the toxin appears to play an important role in tissue targeting the molecule and in promoting internalization (namely, receptor-mediated endocytosis), and the light chain acts inside the cell to block exocytosis. As noted above, the intact toxin is needed to poison cells, but there is an exception to this rule. When techniques are used to introduce the light chain directly into the cell interior, this polypeptide alone is enough to block mediator release.

Research Strategies Involving Toxin

The major action of the toxin is to block acetylcholine release from motor nerve terminals, and thus its potential as a research tool is most obvious when one wishes to study the consequences of having a morphologically intact but functionally disconnected neuromuscular junction. However, there are many additional experimental uses for the toxin that go beyond this obvious paradigm. The selection below provides a representative list of the ways in which the toxin has been, or could be, used as a pharmacological tool.

Ligand

Botulinum neurotoxin binds with high affinity to cholinergic nerves in the voluntary system, with lesser affinity for cholinergic nerves in the autonomic system, and with little or no meaningful affinity for noncholinergic nerves. This suggests that the toxin can be envisioned as an agent that recognizes a membrane determinant that is relatively or absolutely unique to cholinergic nerve endings.

As noted above, current information on structure–function relationships in the toxin molecule suggests that the heavy chain is the tissue-targeting component. This has an important methodological implication. Investigators can utilize the heavy chain as a ligand to isolate and characterize a membrane determinant that may be unique to cholinergic nerves, and this can be done with little risk. The heavy chain by itself cannot poison transmission, and therefore it poses no hazard to investigators.

Chimeric Molecules

During the recent past there has been a surge of interest in the construction of synthetic toxins, mainly in the hope that these novel substances could act as antineoplastic drugs. This area of research has been heavily influenced by the availability of potent, multicomponent toxins.

Botulinum neurotoxin is believed to possess three functional domains: one that tissue targets the molecule, one that promotes internalization, and one that produces intracellular poisoning. In reality, an entire host of protein toxins possess the same or similar domains. These include such substances as the plant lectins abrin and ricin and the bacterial products diphtheria toxin and *Pseudomonas* exotoxin. The fact that there are so many toxins with conceptually similar components has led to the synthesis of chimeric, or unnatural, toxins. The common approach has been to dissociate two toxins into their respective tissue-targeting and poisoning domains. Standard techniques in protein chemistry are then used to link the tissue-targeting domain of one toxin to the poisoning component of another. Interestingly, most of these chimeric toxins are biologically active and quite potent.

The finding that components from different toxins can be linked to generate novel substances prompted investigators to question whether it was necessary to use the constituent parts of toxins in creating new agents. As an alternative, monoclonal antibodies directed against cell-surface antigens have been tested as tissue-targeting domains, and this is the origin of many putative anticancer drugs. When the antibody in question recognizes a determinant on a cancer cell, and when this antibody is linked to a toxin that causes cell death, the resulting drug is conceivably useful for attacking cancer cells.

Chimeric drugs are being considered for their potential role in the treatment of many diseases, not just cancer (namely, an antibody against a component in thrombotic plaques linked to an enzyme that degrades the deposits would be an agent for clearing clogged arteries). Beyond this, chimeric toxins are also being touted as tools in cell biology. One could enhance or disrupt any cellular process merely by linking the appropriate tissue-targeting, internalizing, and cell-modifying components.

Botulinum neurotoxin appears to be well suited for the construction of chimeric molecules. It is one of only a small number of compounds that act selectively on cholinergic nerve endings and that possess the constituent parts for creating a chimeric molecule. The toxin, or certain of its components, could be used to ferry a variety of substances to the interior of nerve endings.

Endocytic Pathways

A substantial literature describes the melding of vesicle membranes with plasma membranes to achieve exocytosis, and an associated literature describes the budding of plasma membranes to regenerate vesicles. However, the relationship between the latter process and receptor-mediated endocytosis is unclear. Indeed, a rather thin literature describes the various endocytic pathways that exist in nerve endings.

Studies on clostridial neurotoxins suggest that there are at least two endocytic paths in cholinergic nerves, one that delivers substances that act locally and one that transports substances in retrograde fashion to the cell body. Botulinum neurotoxin uses the local route to produce blockade of transmitter release, and tetanus toxin uses the retrograde route to reach cell bodies in the central nervous system. It is unclear how the pathways for the various endocytic pathways are marked. One possibility is that the receptor molecule involved in receptor-mediated endocytosis directs the endosome; alternatively, a molecule embedded in the endosome membrane may serve a trafficking function. Whatever the underlying mechanism, the fact remains that clostridial neurotoxins could be useful tools for producing segregation of endosome pools. The isolated pools could then be analyzed to determine their distinguishing features.

As before, a point of methodologic importance pertains to this proposed use of the toxin. It appears that the heavy chains of clostridial toxins are sufficient to bind to cells and be internalized. This means that a relatively nontoxic agent could be exploited to help resolve various aspects of endocytosis.

Denervation Supersensitivity

Perhaps the most well-known use of botulinum neurotoxin is as a tool to produce pharmacologic denervation. Local injection of the toxin in the vicinity of nerve terminals produces sustained (weeks to months) blockade of transmission, and in many respects the phenomenon mimicks surgical denervation. Toxin-induced denervation and surgical denervation are similar in the sense that both cause supersensitivity, both lead to an increase in the number and distribution of nicotinic cholinergic receptors, and both trigger the appearance of tetrodotoxin-resistant sodium channels. The two forms of denervation differ in the sense that the surgical process causes marked loss of cholinesterase, whereas the pharmacologic approach causes only minimal loss of the enzyme.

Botulinum toxin is the agent of choice when one wishes to produce denervation supersensitivity while retaining morphologically intact nerve endings. For example, if an investigator were interested in decoding the signals that a nerve releases at a dysfunctional junction, or wanted to know whether a nerve increases its endocytic activity (namely, to receive messages from nonstimulated muscle), a pharmacologically denervated preparation would be desirable. There is no evidence that nerve terminals become resistant to multiple exposures to the toxin, and the toxin can be administered at doses below those that trigger the immune response, so botulinum neurotoxin can be used to produce functional denervation of an extended duration.

Nerve Sprouting and Disuse Atrophy

There are two ways in which toxin-induced denervation mimics nerve severance, both of which have clinical implications. Sustained blockade of transmission causes terminal portions of the axon to sprout new nerve endings, some of which will make functional contact with underlying muscle. Also, if blockade is sustained and if sprouting produces only minimal neural input, the affected muscle will atrophy.

This use of the toxin to produce these effects can be envisioned as a model for neurological disorders, such as trauma-induced severance of nerves, but recently this area of research has assumed an altogether different meaning. Botulinum neurotoxin has been approved for the treatment of three neurological disorders characterized by involuntary muscle contractions: blepharospasm, stabismus, and hemifacial spasm. In each case, administration of the toxin is intended to diminish or abolish excessive efferent activity in motor nerves. In these disorders, nerve sprouting and muscle atrophy are not research findings but instead therapeutic concerns. The rate at which poisoned nerves generate functional sprouts may govern the duration of therapeutic benefit provided by the toxin, and the rate and extent of muscle atrophy may influence the desirability of long-term administration of the toxin. It would appear that there are now multiple reasons for wanting to gauge the chronic effects of toxin on nerve and muscle.

Types of Transmitter Release

In mammalian motor nerve endings, acetylcholine is stored in synaptic vesicles. When a single vesicle discharges its contents, the response evoked postsynaptically is a miniature end-plate potential (MEPP). Nerve impulses cause synchronous release of acetylcholine from many synaptic vesicles, and the summed response of these quanta is an end-plate potential that triggers an action potential.

The poisoning of neuromuscular junctions with botulinum toxin leads to the emergence of a class of MEPPs that are uncommon at normal junctions. These MEPPs have two distinguishing characteristics: (1) a delayed time to peak and (2) highly variable but occasionally very large amplitudes. These delayed and sometimes giant MEPPs are so large that they can evoke action potentials.

The emergence of the slow class of MEPPs is reversible; when poisoning due to the toxin has waned, slow MEPPs become progressively less common and the natural class of MEPPs reappears. Unlike normal MEPPs, slow MEPPs are not influenced by rate of nerve stimulation or by ambient levels of calcium. The two classes of MEPPs also differ in their responses to various pharmacologic (e.g., 4-aminoquinoline) and physical (e.g., temperature) manipulations.

There is suggestive evidence that slow MEPPs may occur at normal junctions, but at a very low frequency. There are no credible hypotheses about the functional significance of these slow MEPPs, and even their origin is a matter of debate. The ability of botulinum neurotoxin to promote slow MEPPs makes it an ideal pharmacologic tool for studying the origin and significance of these phenomena.

Mechanisms of Transmitter Release

Botulinum neurotoxin is highly potent and selective in blocking transmitter release from mammalian neuromuscular junctions. The fact that it can be utilized as a tool to study exocytosis is therefore somewhat self-evident. If, as is commonly assumed, the toxin is an enzyme that modifies a substrate that governs transmitter release, then identification of the substrate, a determination of its subcellular localization, and a clarification of its mechanism of action all contribute to an understanding of normal neuromuscular transmission. However, the potential value of the toxin for studying mechanisms of release goes beyond the self-evident. Subtleties of toxin action tend to magnify its potential value.

Botulinum neurotoxin is a generic expression that refers to seven serotypes designated A to G. The various serotypes are similar but not identical in their neuromuscular blocking actions. It is their apparent dissimilarities that attract attention to the serotypes as potential tools. More precisely, serotype A possesses properties that are distinct from those of other serotypes, and the distinctions suggest that the underlying bases for neuromuscular blockade are not the same.

Botulinum neurotoxin type A markedly diminishes the frequency of spontaneous MEPPs and nerve stimulus-induced MEPPs. However, if preparations are not totally paralyzed, the blocking actions of the toxin can be slightly overcome. Rapid rates of nerve stimulation, the addition of potassium channel blockers, or treatment with agents that normally promote transmitter release (e.g., black widow spider venom) increase the rate of spontaneous MEPPs. Nerve stimulation in the presence of potassium channel blockers will occasionally lead to muscle action potentials. The latter observation provides the basis for distinguishing serotype A from other serotypes.

The reason why drugs such as 4-aminopyridine increase the likelihood that nerve stimulation will evoke a muscle response in a type A-poisoned preparation is that quanta are released synchronously. The summed actions of the MEPPs lead to an end-plate potential and then to an action potential. This is quite different from the outcome obtained with other serotypes, such as B and D. These neurotoxins have a lesser effect in diminishing the rate of spontaneous MEPPs. However, procedures that would be expected to increase the likelihood that nerve stimulation would evoke a muscle response are largely ineffective. The reason is that these procedures do increase the likelihood of MEPPs, but the MEPPs are uncharacteristically asynchronous. The lack of synchrony precludes the summation of MEPPs to evoke a full-scale muscle response.

Electrophysiologic findings with botulinum neurotoxin suggest that these substances should be seen as a group, all of which block transmitter release, but with individual members having distinct properties. The use of these toxins individually or in combination can be a valuable adjunct to the study of neuromuscular transmission. This is especially true for those serotypes that produce asynchronous transmitter release. The fact that these toxins produce sustained blockade means that they can be used to create stable preparations from which data on synchronous and asynchronous transmitter release can be collected over an extended period of time.

Universal Blockade of Mediator Release

There is a widely held belief that the mechanisms for transmitter release are similar or perhaps even identical in various types of nerve endings, and these similarities may extend to mediator release from nonneuronal cells, such as glands or blood cells. This belief could be tested by examining the effect of an agent that acts intracellularly to block exocytosis in one cell type, then determining whether the effect is observed in other cell types. Botulinum neurotoxin appears ideally suited to this task.

The holotoxin is tissue targeted to cholinergic nerve endings, and it acts there because of the presence of receptors and mechanisms for endocytosis. In the absence of a cellular basis for binding and internalization, the toxin ordinarily would not be able to act. However, this limitation can be overcome by employing techniques that circumvent the need for binding and endocytic uptake. Three such mechanisms are the following.

1. Cell membranes can be rendered leaky by treatment with agents such as digitonin. This detergent creates pores that are large enough to accommodate the passage of proteins such as botulinum neurotoxin. When cells are permeabilized, the toxin no longer relies on customary mechanisms for gaining access to the cell interior; the toxin merely diffuses to its site of action. This approach has been used to show that adrenal cells are susceptible to the blocking action of botulinum and tetanus toxins.

2. Large proteins can be injected directly into the cell interior. When this is done with nerve cells, the injection pipette must be remote from nerve endings because of their small size. With other secreting cells, the toxin can be injected local to the site of exocytosis. This technique has been used to study toxin action on transmitter release from neuronal cells and glandular cells.

3. The nucleic acid that encodes synthesis of the toxin can be injected into cells, with the same provisos that apply to injection of protein. This technique has been used to study toxin action on neuronal cells, but it has not yet been attempted with nonneuronal cells.

In summary, botulinum neurotoxin has an impressive set of credentials as a tool for the study of mediator release from neuronal and other cells. The full potential of the toxin as a research tool has yet to be realized.

Prudent Policies and Procedures

Methodological issues that pertain to use of the toxin as a research tool are rather mundane. They involve little more than adding toxin to the medium bathing a tissue or injecting toxin in the region of neuromuscular junctions. These are technically trivial matters. The greater concern is to establish policies and procedures for safe handling of the toxin. These practices can be implemented in a way that poses relatively little burden on investigators while safeguarding the health and welfare of those who handle the toxin and those who are in the surrounding environment. For the sake of convenience, these practices can be broken down into three categories: preventive medicine, containment, and disposal.

Preventive Medicine

Four major steps should be taken to safeguard the welfare of persons who handle the toxin. These four guidelines should be adopted without exception.

1. An institutional physician knowledgeable about the diagnosis and treatment of botulism should be notified that research with botulinum toxin is in progress. This physician should have the names of all personnel who handle the toxin.

2. All personnel doing research with botulinum toxin, and ideally those personnel who are in close proximity to this research, should be immunized. Pentavalent toxoid, which is available from the Centers for Disease Control (CDC; Atlanta, GA) can be administered under the supervision of an institutional physician.

3. Material safety data sheets, as well as current scholarly publications, should be available in the laboratory and to all interested persons. Investigators who do not feel qualified to prepare a material safety data sheet on botulinum toxin can obtain one from the Division of Safety, National Institutes of Health (NIH; Bethesda, MD).

4. Laboratory personnel and the institutional physician should know the telephone number to contact their state health departments and the Centers for Disease Control (404-639-2888) when there are questions or concerns about the toxin. The latter telephone number is used to report suspected cases of botulism and to obtain antitoxin suitable for human administration.

Containment

There are two dimensions to the concept of containment: (1) within the laboratory, one must use procedures that restrict access to the toxin and minimize its potential for causing immediate harm, and (2) beyond the laboratory, one must adopt procedures that prevent spread of biologically active toxin. The major guidelines for containment within the laboratory are as follow.

1. Doors to the laboratory should be clearly marked to indicate the presence of a biohazard. These doors should remain locked at all times, and only properly authorized personnel should have access.

2. The laboratory itself should conform to the requirements of a BL-2 or BL-3 facility, depending on the exact nature of the intended work. A detailed description of such facilities can be found in the CDC-NIH "Biosafety in Microbiological and Biomedical Laboratories" booklet.

3. Stock solutions of toxin should be stored in a refrigerator/freezer that is marked to indicate the presence of a biohazard. Ideally, stock solutions should be diluted to create working solutions that have the lowest level of toxicity consistent with the scholarly work in progress.

4. Laboratory personnel should wear gloves and appropriate protective garments while handling the toxin. Similarly, laboratory counters should be covered with absorbent material.

5. To the fullest extent practical, toxin should be transported, diluted, and used in disposable pipettes and containers.

6. To the fullest extent practical, toxin should be handled by mechanical means (e.g., automatic pipettes). Care should be taken to avoid creation of aerosols, and the toxin must not be allowed to come into contact with the mouth or broken skin.

The guidelines for ensuring that biologically active toxin does not go beyond the research laboratory are as follow.

1. Toxin should be transported outside the research laboratory only when there is good justification (i.e., transport to another research facility).

2. Steps should be taken to ensure that toxin is contained within the research laboratory. The techniques for preventing escape are inherent in the design of BL-2 and BL-3 facilities (see above). For example, air from the laboratory should not be recirculated into nonlaboratory areas.

3. As indicated above, no unauthorized persons should be allowed access to areas where they might accidentally come into contact with the toxin and inadvertently carry it out of the laboratory.

4. As indicated below, toxin and contaminated materials that are intended for disposal should be handled as a biohazard and, whenever practical, treated to rid them of toxicity.

Disposal

Techniques that have been widely adopted for disposing of the toxin or contaminated materials are as follow.

1. Solutions of toxin are inactivated by heat, strong bases, or formaldehyde. A practical approach is to add solutions of toxin (i.e., spent media

from tissue baths) to a container that has sodium hydroxide (pH > 12). When the container is full, it can be autoclaved. Questions about residual toxicity can be resolved by neutralizing the mixture and performing a bioassay.

2. Potentially infectious waste, such as material from tissue cultures, should be autoclaved and prepared for disposal by incineration.

3. Animal carcasses, bedding, and absorbent material from bench tops should be wrapped in biohazard containers and prepared for disposal by incineration.

4. Disposable labware, such as pipettes, should be autoclaved and placed in biohazard containers. Nondisposable labware should be retained in the facility until it has been decontaminated (i.e., heated, washed with alkaline solution).

5. Iodinated toxin that has been used for research purposes should be stored both to handle radiation and to diminish toxicity. Iodinated material should be retained until radioactivity has fallen to background levels; nonradioactive material (e.g., solution, carcass) can then be prepared for disposal as described (points 1 to 3).

The various guidelines enumerated above should not be seen as all inclusive. They are general guidelines that are likely to apply to most research facilities. Additional precautionary steps may be needed, depending on the amount of toxin and type of work involved. However, all of the guidelines can be implemented in a way that safeguards personnel while still permitting vigorous and scholarly research.

Acknowledgment

This work was supported in part by NIH Grant NS-22153 and by DOA Contracts DAMD17-86-C-6161 and DAMD17-90-C-0048.

References

1. R. V. Considine and L. L. Simpson, *Toxicon* **29,** 913 (1991).
2. K. Aktories and A. Hall, *Trends Pharmacol. Sci.* **10,** 415 (1989).
3. L. L. Simpson (ed.), "Botulinum Neurotoxin and Tetanus Toxin." Academic Press, San Diego, California, 1989.
4. G. Sakaguchi, *Pharmacol. Ther.* **19,** 165 (1983).
5. B. R. DasGupta, *in* "Botulinum Neurotoxin and Tetanus Toxin" (L. L. Simpson, ed.), p. 53. Academic Press, San Diego, California, 1989.
6. L. L. Simpson, *Annu. Rev. Pharmacol. Toxicol.* **26,** 427 (1986).

[6] α-Bungarotoxin Receptor from Chick Optic Lobe: Biochemical, Immunological, and Pharmacological Characterization

C. Gotti, A. Esparis-Ogando, M. Moretti, and F. Clementi

The nicotinic acetylcholine receptor is a cation channel, the aperture of which is modulated by nicotinic agents. The nicotinic receptor family includes a series of molecules, such as muscle and neuronal acetylcholine receptors and neuronal α-bungarotoxin receptors, that share some similarities as far as ionic channel properties are concerned, but which differ in terms of molecular structure and pharmacological and functional characteristics (1, 2). In this chapter, we will give a brief description of the properties of these receptors and of the neurotoxins that are instrumental for their purification and characterization. We will then describe in detail our method for the purification of one member of this family, the α-bungarotoxin receptor from chick optic lobe.

Neurotoxins

Neurotoxins have played a fundamental role in isolating nicotinic receptors and in understanding their key features. It is perhaps worth beginning by summarizing some of those properties that are relevant to the isolation of α-bungarotoxin receptors (BgTXRs).

The venom from the snakes of the Elapidae family is a complex mixture of biologically active polypeptides. This mixture includes a family of homologous proteins, known as postsynaptic neurotoxins, that are partially responsible for the neurotoxic action of the venom. More than 60 highly homologous snake neurotoxins have been sequenced and classified, according to their size, into two distinct groups: short toxins of 60–62 amino acids with 4 disulfide bonds, and long toxins of 71–74 amino acids with 5 disulfide bonds (3, 4).

α-Bungarotoxin (α-BgTX), which is a basic polypeptide belonging to the group of long neurotoxins (74 amino acids, M_r 8000), is the major protein of *Bungarus multicinctus* venom. It binds to muscle nicotinic acetylcholine receptors (AChRs) and blocks nicotinic transmission in skeletal muscle.

α-Bungarotoxin contains two tyrosyl amino acids, one of which (Tyr-54) can be selectively iodinated in such a way as to retain all of its biological activity. Thus, iodinated α-BgTX provides a simple and specific tool for the assay of AChR in both membrane-bound and solubilized form. For these reasons, α-BgTX is routinely used to localize and quantify muscle AChRs and to study their pharmacological response.

Elapidae venom also contains two other groups of neurotoxins that have pharmacological effect on neuronal AchRs. In fact, a number of the effects on neuronal nicotinic synapses reported in the past were, in reality, due to these other toxins that were normally copurified with α-BgTX (for reviews, see Refs. 5 and 6).

One of these toxins, now called neuronal toxin (although it has also been variously referred to as K toxin, F toxin, or toxin 3.1), blocks neuronal AChRs in various tissues (7–9). Neuronal toxin is a minor component of the venom of *B. multicinctus,* where it represents only 0.1% of total venom protein. It has 66 amino acids (internally cross-linked by 5 disulfide bridges), a molecular weight of 6500, an isoelectric point of 9.1, and greater sequence homology with the class of long neurotoxins. This toxin exists in physiological solutions as a dimer of identical subunits and it seems that this dimer is the active state of the toxin.

Three laboratories have identified a second family of related neurotoxins from the venom of *B. multicinctus* that are specific for neuronal AchRs. These toxins, known as BgIIS1, P4-bungarotoxin, or p15, have a molecular weight of 15,000 and a potent phospholipase activity, which, however, is not involved in their pharmacological effect on neuronal AChRs (10–12).

Purified toxins can now be purchased from several suppliers or relatively easily purified from the snake venom itself. Reliable methods of purification have been published by Ravdin and Berg (9) for α-BgTX, by Loring *et al.* (8) for neuronal toxin, and by Quik and Lamarca (10) for BgIIS1.

Muscle Acetylcholine Receptor

Muscle AChR is a pentameric glycoprotein with a molecular weight of 250,000–300,000, consisting of four different subunits present in the stoichiometry of $\alpha_2\beta\gamma\delta$ and belonging to a superfamily of ligand-gated ionic channels defined by DNA sequence homology. The primary amino acid sequence of the individual AChR subunits has been determined for several species by means of DNA cloning. There is a high degree of homology between subunits, both within a species and among different species (for reviews, see Refs. 13–15).

Several studies have localized the α-BgTX binding to the α subunit of the AChR by using ^{125}I-labeled toxin binding to the denatured α subunit, and its proteolytic fragments, or to the synthetic peptides corresponding to the primary sequence of the α subunit itself (16, 17). The more important toxin-binding site has been localized to an α subunit peptide that includes the cysteine amino acids 192–193, which affinity-labeling studies have shown to be very close to the ACh-binding site.

α-Bungarotoxin blocks nicotinic transmission at the vertebrate neuromuscular junction by binding to postsynaptic nicotinic receptors with high specificity and high affinity (K_d 10^{-9}–10^{-12} M), thus preventing the opening of the associated AChR ion channel. α-Bungarotoxin binding to muscle AChR is only slowly reversible and it is also temperature and pH independent. These characteristics make the toxin a useful tool for AChR affinity purification. In fact, Sepharose-bound α-BgTX has allowed muscle AChR to be biochemically purified and has subsequently led to the cloning of the genes of all of the receptor subunits.

Neuronal Acetylcholine Receptors and α-Bungarotoxin Receptors

The high-affinity binding of nicotine to nicotinic receptors in the central nervous system (CNS) has already been described. The distribution of nicotinic receptors, as well as their physiological and pharmacological properties, have been extensively reviewed (18, 19) and, very recently, their molecular structure has been identified by cDNA cloning techniques. At least eight genes ($\alpha2$, $\alpha3$, $\alpha4$, $\alpha5$, $\alpha7$, $\beta2$, $\beta3$, $\beta4$) coding for subunits of rat and chicken neuronal nicotinic receptors are found to encode proteins that are homologous to the related subunits assembled in the muscle receptor.

When messenger RNAs encoding certain combinations of subunits are injected into frog oocytes, functional neuronal nicotinic receptors are expressed on the oocytes surface. Each functional neuronal receptor consists of at least one type of agonist-binding subunit (the α subunit) and one type of structural subunit (the β subunit) arranged according to an unknown stoichiometry (20).

At least seven rat neuronal receptor combinations have been reconstituted into oocytes. Two of them are blocked by neuronal toxin but none by α-BgTX and only one (which is made by injecting $\alpha7$ cDNA alone) is blocked by α-BgTX (21).

Besides these molecules, α-BgTX-binding sites have also been reported in brain and ganglia. α-Bungarotoxin binds with high affinity and in a saturable fashion to a number of vertebrate and invertebrate neuronal tissues, but the relationship between α-BgTX-binding sites and the nicotinic receptor is unclear. In fact, although α-BgTX binds to mammalian neurons, it does not block all neuronal synaptic transmission. In addition its binding sites have a regional distribution that is different from that of nicotine and, in certain brain areas, α-BgTX binding occurs in the apparent absence of cholinergic innervation (for reviews, see Refs. 18 and 19).

By means of α-BgTX affinity chromatography, high-affinity α-bungarotoxin receptors (BgTXRs) have been isolated from the rat pheochromocytoma cell line, the human neuroblastoma cell line, and chick, rat, and mouse brains (18, 22). The N-terminal sequence of the lower molecular weight subunit of the chick brain-purified receptor has revealed a high degree of homology with muscular AChR (23). Using this sequence, two cDNA clones encoding for α subunits of chick BgTXR (α1 and α2) have been cloned. Furthermore, the use of monoclonal antibodies (MAbs) that are specific for these two subunits has revealed the existence of two different BgTXR subtypes, thus indicating a heterogeneity of BgTXRs (24). From all of these studies, recently reviewed by Lindstrom (18), it is possible to conclude that brain BgTXRs are members of the AChR supergene family, although in most cases their functional role is unknown.

It is important to find a function for the BgTXR and also to understand whether the structure of the BgTXRs associated with a cationic channel is similar to that of the BgTXRs that do not have such an association.

Here we give reports of an improved purification protocol for obtaining a very pure BgTXR from chick optic lobe. We have recently demonstrated (25) that this BgTXR behaves as a functional nicotinic channel and here we report the biochemical, immunological, and pharmacological characterization of this receptor.

Experimental Procedures

α-Bungarotoxin Receptor Purification Protocol

Purification of BgTXRs from neuronal membranes is difficult because they are present in only very small quantities and are highly sensitive to protease degradation. It is therefore necessary to carry out the purification of this protein in the presence of several protease inhibitors while maintaining the temperature between 0 and 4°C.

Preparation of Chick Optic Lobe Membranes

Chick optic lobes (COLs) are dissected from 1-day-old chickens, immediately frozen in liquid nitrogen, and stored at -80°C for later use. No differences in the binding properties of fresh and frozen tissues have been observed.

To obtain at least 150–250 pmol of purified BgTXR, 36 g of frozen COLs must be used for every experiment. They are homogenized in 80 ml of 50 mM sodium phosphate, pH 7.4, 1 M NaCl, 2 mM ethylenediaminetetraacetic acid (EDTA), 2mM ethylene glycol bis(β-aminoethyl ether)-N,N,N',N'-tetraacetic acid (EGTA), and 2 mM phenylmethylsulfonyl fluoride (PMSF) (buffer II) for 2 min in an Ultraturrax homogenizer (Janke and Kunkel, Staufen, Germany). The homogenate is then diluted to 1.5 liter of buffer II and centrifuged for 1 hr at 60,000 g and 4°C.

This procedure of homogenization, dilution, and centrifugation is done three times, after which the pellets are collected, rapidly rinsed with 50 mM sodium phosphate, 50 mM NaCl, 2 mM EDTA, 2 mM EGTA, 2 mM PMFS (buffer I) and then resuspended in the same buffer I containing a final concentration of 2% Triton X-100 (v/v) (Sigma, St. Louis, MO) and a mixture of 10 μg/ml of each of the following protease inhibitors: leupeptin, bestatin, pepstatin A, and aprotinin (Sigma).

Step I: Cytochrome c-Sepharose Incubation

The purification of BgTXRs by means of a single passage on a Sepharose α-BgTX column gives a BgTXR that is highly contaminated with α- and β-tubulins. Since tubulins are proteins that have a similar pI to that of BgTXR, it is possible that such contamination is due to an interaction between the basic α-BgTX and acidic tubulins. Consequently, it was thought that prior incubation with a high volume of a resin to which a basic protein, such as cytochrome c (cyt c), is bound would lead to the absorption of some of these tubulins (see Preliminary Experiments, below). For this reason, the extract obtained by incubating the membrane with detergent for 90 min at 4°C is centrifuged for 1 hr at 100,000 g and then incubated at 4°C with cyt c bound to Sepharose.

Cytochrome c (Sigma), at a concentration of 1 mg or 5 mg/ml of resin is bound to activated Sepharose 4B-CNBr (Pharmacial, Piscataway, NJ) according to the instructions of the manufacturer.

Preliminary experiments were undertaken in which no differences in terms of tubulin binding were found if the extract was incubated with either cyt c bound to Sepharose 4B at a concentration of 1 mg of protein/ml of resin, or with cyt c at 5 mg/ml, diluted 1 : 5 with Sepharose 4B. Because of the high cost of activated Sepharose 4B-CNBr, we chose the second method.

The extract (approximately 170 ml) is incubated with 35 ml of cyt c-sepharose 4B (5 mg/ml of resin) and 140 ml of Sepharose 4B for 12 hr with mild agitation, and then recovered.

Step II: α-Bungarotoxin-Sepharose Incubation

After incubation with cyt c-sepharose 4B the extract is passed over the α-BgTX-Sepharose 4B affinity column. α-BgTX (purchased from Sigma), at a concentration of 1 mg/ml, is bound to the activated Sepharose 4B-CNBr resin according to the instructions of the manufacturer.

The extract is passed over the 5-ml affinity column at least three times. After these passages, the beads are rapidly washed in a funnel first with 200 vol of buffer I plus 0.1% Triton X-100, then with 400 vol of buffer II plus 0.1% Triton X-100, and finally with 100 vol of buffer I plus 0.1% Triton.

The flow of the extract on the affinity column should be very fast in order to avoid the absorption of tubulins, because we have observed that the longer the time of passage the greater the tubulin absorption. It is also important to wash the resin-bound receptor with very large volumes of buffers of different ionic strength as quickly as possible in order to block the dissociation of the receptor from the resin.

Step III: Elution of bound α-Bungarotoxin Receptor

In preliminary experiments, we tested which concentration of a cholinergic drug gave the best recovery in terms of BgTXR eluted from the affinity column. Two different drugs (one of which was at two different concentrations) were tested: carbamylcholine chloride (Carb) (Sigma) (0.1 or 1 M) and d-tubocurarine (Sigma) (2.5 mM) dissolved in buffer I plus protease inhibitors and 0.1% Triton X-100.

Given that the best recovery was obtained by using 1 M Carb, after the passage over the α-BgTX affinity column and the washings, the BgTXR bound to beads is routinely eluted by incubation for 5 hr with 1 vol of 1 M Carb. The Carb eluate is then twice dialyzed against 5 liters each of a buffer containing 10 mM sodium phosphate, pH 7.4, 0.5 mM EDTA, 0.5 mM EGTA, 0.5 mM PMFS, and 0.1% Triton X-100 and then against 5 liters of 5 mM sodium phosphate, pH 7.4, 0.25 mM EDTA, 0.25 mM EGTA, 0.5 mM PMFS, and 0.1% Triton X-100.

The purification procedure described above gave consistent and reproducible results for at least 30 purifications. The purified BgTXR is stored in aliquots at −20°C.

^{125}I-Labeled α-Bungarotoxin-Binding Assay

Binding to Membranes

α-Bungarotoxin is iodinated by the chloramine-T method at a specific activity of 20–35 Ci/nmol. Preliminary saturation and kinetic experiments are performed in order to calculate the K_d and B_{max} of the ^{125}I-labeled α-BgTX to COL membrane. For the saturation experiments ^{125}I-labeled αBgTX in concentrations ranging from 5×10^{-10} to 5×10^{-8} mol/liter is used. Nonspecific binding is determined in the presence of 5 μM α-BgTX. The K_d of the binding is 5 nM and the B_{max} 400–500 fmol/mg of protein. This binding is maximal after 1 hr and only slowly dissociable.

In order to detect the ^{125}I-labeled α-BgTX binding to COL membrane at every step of the purification, the binding is performed using 100–200 μg of protein and a saturating concentration of ^{125}I-labeled α-BgTX of 20 nM.

After 2 hr of incubation at room temperature, binding is determined by the addition of 1 ml of ice-cold 10 mM sodium phosphate, pH 7.4, 50 mM NaCl (wash buffer), and 1 mg/ml of bovine serum albumin (BSA). The samples are then centrifuged for 5 min at 4°C in a Beckman (Palo Alto, CA) 2B microcentrifuge at 10,000 g. The pellets are washed twice and bound radioactivity is counted.

Binding to Extracted and Purified Receptor

α-Bungarotoxin binding to solubilized and purified receptor is determined by means of the DE-81 DEAE disk assay (26). This assay makes use of the differences between the isoelectric points of the toxin (9.1) and the toxin–receptor complex (5.3). In fact, at neutral pH the receptor–toxin complex binds to the anion-exchange DEAE-cellulose paper while the basic toxin cannot because, like the paper, it is positively charged.

Aliquots of detergent extract are diluted in wash buffer plus 0.1% Triton X-100 and incubated with increasing concentrations of ^{125}I-labeled α-BgTX (between 5×10^{-10} to 5×10^{-8} M) for 2 hr at room temperature.

Nonspecific binding of both the extract and the disk is determined by incubation in the presence of excess (5 μM) nonradioactive toxin. Normally the nonspecific binding ranged between 5 and 30% of the specific binding.

After incubation, the incubation mixture is absorbed onto a DEAE-cellulose disk (DE-81, diameter 2.3 cm; Whatman, Clifton, NJ) and unbound toxin is removed by rapid washing with wash buffer plus 0.1% Triton X-100. From these experiments the K_d of the binding to the extract and the purified receptor is calculated to be 5 nM. For routine detection of the amount of BgTXR present in the extract, samples of unknown BgTXR content are incubated with a saturating concentration of ^{125}I-labeled α-BgTX of 20 nM for 2 hr at room temperature with or without 5 μM α-BgTX.

Binding to Purified Denatured Bungarotoxin Receptor

Purified BgTXR and *Torpedo* AChR are run on sodium dodecyl sulfate-polyacrylamide gel electrophoresis (SDS-PAGE) [9% (w/v) acrylamide] and then electrotransferred to nitrocellulose (for a detailed description of the procedure see below). Lanes of electroblotted purified BgTXR are incubated with 150 nM ^{125}I-labeled α-BgTX for 3 hr at room temperature in incubation buffer [10 mM Tris-HCl, pH 7.4, 0.9% (w/v) NaCl, 15% (w/v) BSA, 0.2% (w/v) polyvinylpyrroliclone (PVP), and 0.2% (w/v) Ficoll]. Nonspecific binding is measured in parallel, using 20 μM cold α-BgTX. After incubation, the lanes are quickly washed with 10 mM Tris-HCl, pH 7.4, plus 0.9% NaCl and exposed for autoradiography.

Pharmacological Experiments with Purified Receptor

Ligands are dissolved in wash buffer plus 0.1% Triton X-100 just before use. Purified receptor (50 μl) is incubated in a final volume of 75 μl with serial dilutions of the different cholinergic drugs to be tested. After 30 min at room temperature, ^{125}I-labeled α-BgTX is added to the mixture at a final concentration of 20 nM. After the time necessary to reach equilibrium (1.5 hr), the samples are transferred to the DE-81 DEAE disks and processed as described above.

Protein Determination

The protein concentration of the samples is determined either by Lowry's method (27) or by using the BCA protein assay reagent (Pierce, Rockford, IL). Bovine serum albumin is used as standard for both methods, and the standard sample contains the same concentration of Triton X-100 and buffer as the test samples. When the Lowry method is used in the presence of Triton X-100, a precipitate that does not contain proteins is found after the addition of the Folin reagent. This precipitate is removed from both the test samples and the standard samples by means of centrifugation at 5000 g for 5 min prior to reading the absorbance at 750 nm at room temperature.

Blotting of Proteins Separated by SDS-PAGE

SDS-PAGE was performed essentially as described by Laemmli (28) on 1-mm thick 9% polyacrylamide slab gels. Samples are dissolved in a solubilization mixture containing 60 mM DL-dithiothreitol, 4.5% SDS, 0.0015% (w/v) bromphenol blue, 0.2 M Tris-HCl, pH 8.9, 0.35 M sucrose, boiled for 2 min, and then a 10-fold excess of iodoacetamide over DL-dithiothreitol is added. After electrophoresis, gels are either fixed and stained with Coomassie Brilliant Blue or subjected to the blotting procedure described by Towbin *et al.* (29). The transfer onto nitrocellulose paper is carried out at 100 V (initial current, 0.5 A) in a water-cooled apparatus for 90 min.

Detection of α- and β-Tubulins

The samples (either differently washed COL membranes, or purified BgTXRs obtained by different experimental procedures) are separated on SDS-PAGE (9% acrylamide) and then transferred to nitrocellulose paper.

Lanes of electroblotted samples are incubated for 2 hr with anti-α- and anti-β-tubulin antibodies (purchased from Amersham, Arlington Heights, IL), diluted 1 : 250, washed with 10 mM Tris-HCl, pH 7.4, plus 0.9% NaCl and then incubated with anti-mouse IgG diluted 1 : 100 for 2 hr. The lanes are then washed again and bound antibodies are revealed by incubation for 1.5 hr at 4°C with ^{125}I-labeled protein A (200,000 cpm/ml) (Amersham). The antibodies and ^{125}I-labeled protein A are diluted in incubation buffer.

Immunoprecipitation of ^{125}I-Labeled α-Bungarotoxin Receptor from Chick Optic Lobe by Different Antisera

Aliquots of 1% (v/v) extract of COL membrane, or purified COL BgTXR, are incubated with varying amounts (0.1-1–5 μl) of the serum to be tested. Then in order to reach the same immunoglobulin concentration in all samples, normal rabbit serum is added to a final volume of 5 μl. Enough goat anti-rabbit IgG is added to precipitate all of the immunoglobulin present in the samples and left for 2 hr at room temperature. The samples are then centrifuged for 15 min in a microcentrifuge (10,000 g, 4°C). The pellets are washed twice with wash buffer plus 0.1% Triton X-100, and then counted by means of a γ counter. The titer of the serum obtained by using ^{125}I-labeled α-BgTX is expressed as nanomoles of precipitated ^{125}I-αBgTX/liter of serum.

Purification of Torpedo and Fetal Calf Acetylcholine Receptor and Neuroblastoma Bungarotoxin Receptor

Torpedo AChR is routinely purified from 100 g of frozen *Torpedo* electric organs by affinity chromatography on cobra toxin-Sepharose, according to Gotti *et al.* (30), with some minor modifications. The specific activity of the purified receptor is between 6000 and 8000 pmol of α-BgTX binding sites/mg of protein.

Fetal calf AChR is routinely purified from 500 g of frozen fetal calf muscles according to Gotti *et al.* (30). The specific activity of the purified receptor is between 4000 and 5000 pmol αBgTX binding sites/mg of protein. Bungarotoxin receptor from IMR32 neuroblastoma cells is purified as previously described (22). The purified receptor has a specific activity ranging between 1500 and 2500 pmol/of α-BgTX binding sites per milligram of protein.

Production of Antisera against Receptors

Three rabbits are immunized three times at 2-week intervals with intact AChR purified from *Torpedo* electric organs. For every immunization 100 μg (diluted to 500 μl with wash buffer) of *Torpedo* AChR is emulsified in 500 μl of complete Freund's adjuvant and given by intradermal injection. Fifteen days after the third injection, the rabbits are bled and the sera tested for anti-*Torpedo* AChR titer. A similar procedure is followed for the preparation of antisera against purified fetal calf AChR, neuroblastoma, and COL BgTXRs. In this case, only two rabbits are immunized for each receptor and every rabbit receives 70 μg of either fetal calf AChR or COL BgTXR or 20–30 μg of purified neuroblastoma BgTXR for every immunization.

The titers of the pooled sera, tested in an immunoprecipitation assay as described above, are as follows: 200 mM for anti-*Torpedo* AChR antisera, 390 nM for anti-fetal calf AChR antisera, 240 nM for anti-COL antisera, and 100 nM for neuroblastoma BgTXR antisera.

Results

Preliminary Experiments

Since the purified COL BgTXR obtained by means of the routine purification protocol (passing the detergent membrane extract over an α-BgTX-Sepharose column and subsequently washing it with high and low ionic strength buffers and recovering it with Carb) is contaminated with α- and β-tubulins (Fig. 1, lane 1), we have designed a new purification protocol that provides tubulin-free BgTXR. First, we devised a method that led to COL membranes containing the highest quantity of BgTXR with the lowest tubulin content.

The membranes were subjected to three different washing protocols: (1) washing with a pH 11 buffer, (2) repeated washings with a buffer of physiological ionic strength (buffer I), and (3) repeated washings with a buffer of high ionic strength (buffer II).

As can be seen from Table I, the best results were obtained with the pH 11 washings, but only 30% of the BgTXR present in pH 11-treated membranes could be extracted.

Washings with a buffer of high ionic strength gave a membrane fraction with lower specific activity than pH 11, but allowed 70–80% of the BgTXR to be recovered after the detergent extraction. Consequently, membrane washings with a buffer of high ionic strength were adopted.

The second series of experiments was aimed at discovering whether a prior passage of the washed membrane extract over a Sepharose column different

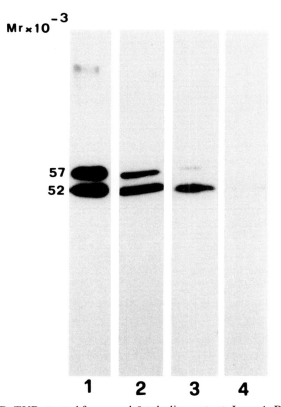

FIG. 1   Purified BgTXRs tested for α- and β-tubulin content. Lane 1, BgTXR purified only by passage of the detergent membrane extract over an α-BgTX-Sepharose column. Lane 2, BgTXR purified by passage over an α-BgTX-Sepharose column of the detergent extract obtained from membrane repeatedly washed with high ionic strength buffer. Lane 3, BgTXR purified by incubation of the detergent extract (prepared as sample in lane 2) with an excess of resin-Sepharose 4B and then passed over an α-BgTX-Sepharose column. Lane 4, BgTXR purified by incubation of the detergent extract (prepared as sample in lane 2) with an excess of cyt c-Sepharose 4B resin, and then passed over an α-BgTX-Sepharose column. The purified BgTXRs (30 pmol/sample) are separated on 9% SDS-PAGE, transferred onto nitrocellulose, incubated with anti-α- and anti-β-tubulin MAbs diluted 1 : 250, anti-mouse IgG diluted 1 : 100, and then with ^{125}I-labeled protein A.

from that of α-BgTX-Sepharose would lead to an even purer BgTXR (see Experimental Procedures).

The extract obtained from high ionic strength membrane washings was divided into three aliquots and treated by (1) not adding resin, (2) incubation

TABLE I   Tubulin Content of Washed Membranes

Sample	Specific activity (pmol/mg protein)	Bound tubulines[a] (%)	Receptor extracted from membranes[b] (%)
Tissue homogenate	0.44	100	80
Membrane washed with pH 11 buffer	1.6	9	30
Membrane washed repeatedly with physiological ionic strength buffer	1.1	25	75
Membrane washed repeatedly with high ionic strength buffer	1.4	16	75

[a] Tubulin content was determined by loading 25 μg of protein for every sample on 9% SDS-PAGE, transferring the protein to nitrocellulose, and incubating with anti-α- and anti-β-tubulin antibodies and ^{125}I-labeled protein A. From each sample bound radioactivity was counted and multiplied by the amount of protein present in membranes. The amount of tubulins present on tissue homogenate was taken as 100% and the other values are expressed as percentages of this.

[b] The differently washed membranes were treated with 2% Triton and the amount of solubilized receptor was assayed by means of DE-81 disks. The values shown represent the percentages of receptor solubilized by the detergent, taking the amount of BgTXR present in tissue homogenate membrane as 100%.

with 60 ml of Sepharose 4B (Pharmacia), and (3) incubation with 60 ml of cyt C-Sepharose 4B. The aliquots were then incubated for 12 hr at 4°C and then separately passed over three identical α-BgTX-Sepharose columns. The three resins were identically processed, the BgTXRs recovered, and the receptors analyzed for their tubulin content. Figure 1 shows the results obtained from the incubation of electroblotted purified BgTXRs (30 pmol for every sample) with anti-α- and β-tubulin MAbs and ^{125}I-labeled protein A.

The BgTXR purified from the extract preincubated with cyt C-Sepharose was found to be completely devoid of α- and β-tubulins and was present in almost undetectable quantities (Fig. 1, lane 4). α- And β-tubulins were still present in the BgTXR not preincubated with Sepharose resins (Fig. 1, lane 2) and, although to a lesser extent, also in the extract preincubated with Sepharose 4B (Fig. 1, lane 3).

Properties of Purified Chick Optic Lobe Bungarotoxin Receptor

Yield and Specificity

A summary of the yield of the BgTXR at the major steps of purification obtained in 10 different experiments is given in Table II. Between 70 and

TABLE II   Purification of Bungarotoxin Receptor from Chick Optic Lobe[a]

Step	Protein (mg)	Receptor (pmol)	Specific activity
Tissue homogenate	3050 ± 200	1350 ± 120	0.44
Membrane washed with buffer II	940 ± 140	1391 ± 94	1.47
Detergent extract	650 ± 35	1066 ± 179	1.64
Detergent extract after incubation with cyt c-Sepharose	534 ± 41	1086 ± 133	2.03
Carb eluate from α-BgTX-Sepharose column	0.03 ± 0.008	263 ± 45	8766

[a] Mean ± SD of the recoveries obtained from 10 different BgTXR purifications. For every purification 36 g of COL is used.

80% of the BgTXR contained in membranes is solubilized by 2% Triton X-100. Neither a longer extraction time nor an increased detergent concentration increased the amount of BgTXR solubilized by the detergent. No absorption of BgTXR to cyt c-Sepharose column was ever determined.

Between 60 and 70% of the BgTXR present in the extract is retained by the α-BgTX affinity column and about 30–40% of the absorbed BgTXR is specifically eluted with 1 M Carb. When 2.5 mM d-tubocurarine is used, only 10 to 15% of the absorbed BgTXR is eluted. The BgTXR eluted with d-tubocurarine has the same peptide composition as that eluted with 1 M Carb (not shown).

The purified BgTXR is a glycoprotein that binds concanavalin A (Con A) and, when run on a 5–20% sucrose gradient, has a sedimentation coefficient of 10S. Isoelectric focusing of the purified BgTXR gave a single peak with a pI of 5.3 (data not shown). This method gives a purified BgTXR with a very high specific activity (7000–9000 pmol of bound ^{125}I-labeled α-BgTX/mg of protein), thus indicating an overall purification of approximately 20,000 times (Table II). Assuming from the sedimentation coefficient value of 10S that the native BgTXR has a molecular weight of 250,000–300,000 and two binding subunits, the pure protein should bind approximately 8000 pmol of α-BgTX/binding sites per milligram protein. Our preparation can thus be considered as more than 90% pure.

Subunit Composition

On SDS gel electrophoresis, different preparations always contained three major components, the molecular weights of which were 67,000, 57,000, and

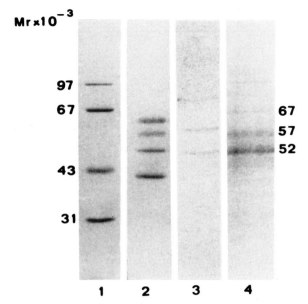

FIG. 2   SDS-PAGE analysis of the subunit composition of purified COL BgTXR. Purified receptors are separated on 9% acrylamide gel and stained with Coomassie Brilliant Blue. Lane 1, standard proteins; lane 2, 20 μg of purified *Torpedo* AChR; lane 3, 5 μg of purified neuroblastoma BgTXR; lane 4, 10 μg of purified COL BgTXR.

52,000 (see Fig. 2, lane 4) and, sometimes, a component with a molecular weight of 60,000 that migrated as a diffuse faint band. Other faint bands with molecular weights of as much as M_r 87,000 are sometimes present, possibly because of a cross-linking of the BgTXR subunits.

In order to determine which subunit(s) of the purified receptor bind(s) ^{125}I-labeled α-BgTX, purified COL BgTXR is run on SDS gel electrophoresis, electroblotted onto nitrocellulose membrane, and then incubated with ^{125}I-labeled α-BgTX. In the same experiment, purified *Torpedo* AChR is run and tested for use as a positive control. The results of the binding are shown in Fig. 3. The COL BgTXR subunit of M_r 57,000 (lane 2) as well as the α subunit of *Torpedo* AChR of M_r 42,000 (lane 4) are labeled by ^{125}I-labeled α-BgTX. In the same experiment, both bindings are inhibited by an excess of cold α-BgTX (lanes 1 and 3).

$M r \times 10^{-3}$

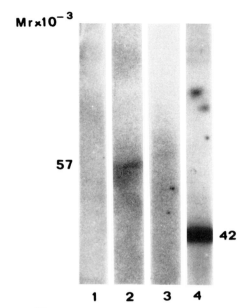

FIG. 3   Localization of ^{125}I-labeled α-BgTX-binding subunits on the Western blots of purified receptors. Chick optic lobe BgTXR (lanes 1 and 2) and *Torpedo* AChR (lanes 3 and 4), 10 μg of purified receptor for each lane, are run on 7.5% SDS-PAGE blotted on a nitrocellulose membrane and then incubated with 20 μM cold α-BgTX and 150 nM ^{125}I-labeled αBgTX (lanes 1 and 3) and 150 nM ^{125}I-labeled α-BgTX (lane 2 and 4). After washing, the nitrocellulose membranes are autoradiographed for 48 hr.

Immunological and Pharmacological Characterization

In order to determine whether COL BgTXR shares any antigenic determinants with other known AchRs, different polyclonal antibodies raised against purified muscle AChRs or neuronal BgTXRs together with two sera of myasthenic patients are tested in an immunoprecipitation assay for their ability to precipitate the labeled ^{125}I-labeled α-BgTX receptor.

In addition, this immunoprecipitation assay is also used to test the ability of MAb 35 to precipitate this BgTXR; MAb 35 is raised against the AChR purified from *Electrophorus electricus* that, in chick brains, recognizes a neuronal nicotinic AChR that does not bind α-BgTX (18). Table III shows the titers obtained from this immunoprecipitation assay. As can be seen, COL BgTXR is specifically recognized by fetal calf AChR antiserum, IMR-32 BgTXR antiserum, COL BgTXR antiserum, but not by *Torpedo* AChR antiserum, MAb 35, or the sera from the myasthenic patients. Although this

TABLE III   Immunoprecipitation by Different Antibodies[a] of
Chick Optic Lobe α-Bungarotoxin Receptor[b]

Antibody	Titer against immunogen	Titer against COL BgTXR
Anti-*Torpedo* AChR antiserum	200	0
Anti-fetal calf AChR antiserum	390	45
Anti-IMR-32 BgTXR antiserum	100	30
Anti-COL BgTXR antiserum	240	230
Serum of myasthenic patient 1	45	0
Serum of myasthenic patient 2	95	0
MAb 35	18,400[c]	0

[a] Titer $\times$ 10^{-9} M.
[b] Labeled with ^{125}I-labeled α-BgTX.
[c] Value from S. J. Tzartos, D. E. Rond, B. L. Einarson, and J. Lindstrom, *J. Biol. Chem.* **256**, 8635 (1981).

molecule has some epitopes in common with muscular AChR and neuronal BgTXR, it is also clearly immunologically different from muscular AChR and from the neuronal AChR with high affinity for nicotine, which is recognized by MAb 35.

The pharmacological profile of the purified BgTXR appears to be similar to that reported for the COL homogenate (31), thus indicating that at least the major component of BgTXR present in COL is purified.

Dose–response curves were generated to test the ability of nicotinic and muscarinic cholinergic drugs to inhibit the high-affinity binding of ^{125}I-labeled α-BgTX to purified BgTXR. The IC$_{50}$ and K_1 values for all of the ligands tested are shown in Table IV. The most powerful inhibitor of ^{125}I-labeled α-BgTX binding is unlabeled α-BgTX (IC$_{50}$ 5 $\times$ 10^{-9} M), followed by agonists such as L-nicotine (IC$_{50}$ 2 $\times$ 10^{-6} M) and antagonists such as d-tubocurarine (IC$_{50}$ 5 $\times$ 10^{-6} M).

At a concentration of IC$_{50}$ 2.5 $\times$ 10^{-6} M, neuronal toxin inhibits ^{125}I-labeled α-BgTX binding to the purified receptor. Other nicotinic antagonists, such as mecamylamine and hexamethonium, inhibit 50% of specific binding only at very high concentrations (IC$_{50}$ more than 1 $\times$ 10^{-3} M), probably because they are at least in part also channel blockers.

The IC$_{50}$ for the muscarinic antagonist atropine is 1 mM, thus confirming the nicotinic pharmacology of the neuronal BgTXR. The pharmacological profile of this COL BgTXR is similar to that of the α-BgTX-binding sites present in rat brain and PC-12 cells, but distinct from that of the AChR present in *Torpedo* and TE761 cells (32), as far as the K_i values for the bisquaternary ammonium compounds such as decamethonium and succinyl-

TABLE IV   Inhibition of ^{125}I-Labeled α-Bungarotoxin Binding to Purified Chick Optic Lobe Bungarotoxin Receptor by Cholinergic Ligands

Ligand	IC$_{50}$ (M)	K_1 (M)
α-Bungarotoxin	5×10^{-9}	9.8×10^{-10}
L-Nicotine	2×10^{-6}	3.9×10^{-7}
Neuronal toxin	2.5×10^{-6}	4.9×10^{-7}
d-Tubocurarine	5×10^{-6}	9.8×10^{-7}
Acetylcholine	4×10^{-5}	7.8×10^{-6}
Carbamylcholine	2×10^{-4}	3.9×10^{-5}
Decamethonium	5×10^{-4}	9.8×10^{-5}
Atropine sulfate	1×10^{-3}	1.9×10^{-4}
Succinylcholine	2×10^{-3}	3.9×10^{-4}
Hexamethonium	2.5×10^{-3}	4.9×10^{-4}
Mecamylamine	2×10^{-2}	3.9×10^{-3}

choline demonstrate. In fact, these drugs inhibit the binding of the ^{125}I-labeled α-BgTX to muscular receptors much more efficiently than the binding to central receptors.

In addition, the pharmacological profile of this BgTXR is different from that of the neuronal AchRs purified from chick and rat brains (33). In fact, agonists and antagonists are equally potent in displacing ^{125}I-labeled α-BgTX binding from our purified receptor, while agonists are at least two orders of magnitude more potent than antagonists in displacing [^{3}H]nicotine binding from neuronal AChRs purified from rat and chick brains and from the [^{3}H] nicotine high-affinity binding sites present in COL.

Conclusions

We have described here a method for the purification of relatively large amounts of COL BgTXR in a very pure form, as demonstrated by its specific activity.

Several factors are critical for obtaining high yields of pure BgTXRs, but we think that at least two are determinant: (1) the blocking of proteolysis by using protease inhibitors of different specificities and (2) the elimination of tubulin and probably other contaminations by repeated washings with large volumes of buffer of high ionic strength and preincubation of the extract with cyt c-Sepharose.

Tubulin contamination is a serious problem in BgTXR purification from nervous tissues and may lead to tubulin peptides being mistaken for BgTXR peptides.

This protocol is also valuable for the purification of BgTXR from other tissues. We have used a slightly modified form of this protocol for the purification of BgTXR from chick cerebellum and the IMR-32 human neuroblastoma cell line. However, when neuronal tissues other than COL are used, the contaminants of the BgTXR may be slightly different and thus the isolation procedure must be tailored to each type of tissue, although the main features of the protocol remain valid.

References

1. R. M. Stroud, M. P. McCarthy, and M. Shuster, *Biochemistry* **29,** 1009 (1990).
2. H. Nybäck, A. Nordberg, B. Langström, C. Halldin, P. Hartvig, A. Ahlin, C.-G. Swahn, and G. Sedvall, *Prog. Brain Res.* **79,** 313 (1988).
3. B. W. Low, *Handb. Exp. Pharmacol.* **52,** 213 (1979).
4. M. J. Dufton and R. C. Hider, *CRC Crit. Rev. Biochem.* **14,** 113 (1983).
5. V. A. Chiappinelli, *Pharmacol. Ther.* **31,** 1 (1985).
6. R. H. Loring and R. E. Zigmond, *Trends NeuroSci.* **11,** 73 (1988).
7. V. A. Chiappinelli, *Brain Res.* **277,** 9 (1983).
8. R. H. Loring, V. A. Chiappinelli, R. E. Zigmond, and I. B. Cohen, *Neuroscience* **11,** 989 (1984).
9. P. M. Ravdin and D. K. Berg, *Proc. Natl. Acad. Sci. U.S.A.* **76,** 2072 (1979).
10. M. Quik and M. V. Lamarca, *Brain Res.* **238,** 385 (1982).
11. L. Saiani, H. Kageyama, B. M. Conti-Tronconi, and A. Guidotti, *Mol. Pharmacol.* **23,** 327 (1984).
12. C. Gotti, C. Omini, F. Berti, and F. Clementi, *Neuroscience* **15,** 563 (1985).
13. M. P. McCarthy, J. P. Earnest, E. F. Young, S. Choe, and R. M. Stroud, *Annu. Rev. Neurosci.* **9,** 383 (1986).
14. R. M. Stroud and J. Finer-Moore, *Annu. Rev. Cell. Biol.* **1,** 317 (1985).
15. J.-L. Popot and J. P. Changeux, *Physiol. Rev.* **64,** 1162 (1984).
16. P. Wilson, T. L. Lentz, and E. Hawrot, *Proc. Natl. Acad. Sci. U.S.A.* **82,** 8790 (1985).
17. C. Gotti, G. Mazzola, R. Longhi, D. Fornasari, and F. Clementi, *Neurosci. Lett.* **82,** 113 (1987).
18. J. Lindstrom, R. Schoepfer, and P. Whiting, *Mol. Neurobiol.* **1,** 281 (1987).
19. C. W. Luetje, J. Patrick, and P. Séguéla, *FASEB J.* **4,** 2755 (1990).
20. J. H. Steinbach and C. Ifune, *Trends NeuroSci.* **12,** 3 (1989).
21. S. Couturier, D. Bertrand, J. M. Matter, M. C. Hernandez, S. Bertrand, N. Millar, S. Valera, T. Barkas, and M. Ballivet, *Neuron* **5,** 847 (1990).
22. C. Gotti, A. Esparis-Ogando, and F. Clementi, *Neuroscience* **32,** 759 (1989).
23. B. M. Conti-Tronconi, S. M. J. Dunn, E. A. Barnard, J. O. Dolly, D. A. Lai, N. Ray, and M. A. Raftery, *Proc. Natl. Acad. Sci. U.S.A.* **82,** 5208 (1985).

24. R. Shoepfer, W. G. Conroy, P. Whiting, M. Gora, and J. Lindstrom, *Neuron* **5,** 35 (1990).
25. C. Gotti, A. Esparis-Ogando, W. Hanke, R. Schlue, M. Moretti, and F. Clementi, *Proc. Natl. Acad. Sci. U.S.A.* **88,** 3259 (1991).
26. J. Schmidt and M. A. Raftery, *Anal. Biochem.* **52,** 343 (1973).
27. O. H. Lowry, N. J. Rosebrough, A. L. Farr, and R. J. Randall, *J. Biol. Chem.* **193,** 265 (1951).
28. U. K. Laemmli, *Nature (London)* **227,** 680 (1970).
29. H. Towbin, T. Staehelin, and J. Gordon, *Proc. Natl. Acad. Sci. U.S.A.* **76,** 4350 (1979).
30. C. Gotti, B. M. Conti-Tronconi, and M. A. Raftery, *Biochemistry* **21,** 3148 (1982).
31. G. K. Wang, S. Molinaro, and J. Schmidt, *J. Biol. Chem.* **253,** 8507 (1978).
32. R. Lukas, *Proc. Natl. Acad. Sci. U.S.A.* **83,** 5741 (1986).
33. M. Schneider, C. Adee, H. Betz, and J. Schmidt, *J. Biol. Chem.* **260,** 14505 (1985).

[7] Use of Channel Ligands to Probe Role of Voltage-Sensitive Calcium Ion Channels in Neuropeptide Release

Marek Treiman, Karsten Lollike, Johanna Baldvinsdottir, Annette Jørgensen, Bjarne Fjalland, and Jens Dencker Christensen

Introduction

Single-channel recording methods have allowed a detailed description of the properties and the classification into broad categories of the voltage-sensitive Ca^{2+} channels (VSCCs). This current classification has been discussed in authoritative reviews (1, 2). Briefly, the major categories of the VSCCs in neurons include the forms designated as low voltage-activated (LVA) and high voltage-activated (HVA) channels. The LVA channels are also designated T type, while HVA channels are further subdivided into N and L categories (1). Although Ca^{2+} channels not covered by this classification exist, the identification of T, N, and L types of channels has provided a very useful basis for further studies.

Because the release of neurotransmitters and peptides from neurons is critically dependent on the depolarization-activated entry of Ca^{2+} through the plasma membrane (3, 4), interest has focused on defining the involvement of the VSCCs in this process. Such studies have been facilitated by the availability of a steadily growing group of ligands modifying the currents through the VSCCs. We shall be concerned here with the use of two types of such ligands: ω-conotoxin (ω-CgTX), a representative of the naturally occurring peptide toxins, and organic ligands. For specific examples, we shall concentrate on the use of ligands to investigate the properties of the VSCCs involved in the release of peptides from the neurohypophysis. However, we shall include methodological considerations and comments that should be useful for a broader range of experimental systems. In particular, we wish to stress the strong dependence of the Ca^{2+} channel ligand effects, in the context of neuronal release, on the precise conditions of tissue preparation and stimulation.

The neurohypophysis has long served as a useful model system for studies of the molecular and cellular mechanisms in neuronal release (for reviews, see Refs. 5 and 6), including the role of Ca^{2+}. The dominant neuronal constit-

Methods in Neurosciences, Volume 8

uents of the neurohypophysis are the secretory terminals of the peptide-producing magnocellular neurons, the cell bodies of which are located in the hypothalamus (5). High concentrations of vasopressin and oxytocin (the two main secretory products of the hypothalamo-neurohypophyseal system), about 1 μg/mg tissue, and the absence of cell bodies, are the major advantages in the use of the isolated neurohypophysis for studies of the release mechanisms operating at the level of the secretory terminals, including the involvement of the VSCCs in the Ca^{2+} influx necessary for the triggering of peptide exocytosis (7–9).

To ascertain the role of the individual types of VSCCs in the activation of release from neurons, studies of ligand binding as well as of ligand-mediated modulation of the depolarization-evoked release are useful. The organic ligands bind to sites associated with L-type Ca^{2+} channels, whereas ω-CgTX binding sites are present on N- and L-type channels in some neurons, and only on N-type channels in others (10, 11). No selective ligands for the T-type Ca^{2+} channels are presently available. It is useful to establish binding affinities of the ligands in question in a particular system, in order to obtain a basis for comparison with the potencies of these substances in modulation of the release.

Binding Studies: Use of ω-Conotoxin GVIA as a Representative of Peptide Toxins with Blocking Action on Voltage-Sensitive Calcium Ion Channels

The VSCCs are among the molecular targets of peptide neurotoxins isolated from venoms of certain species of marine fish-hunting snails. The origin, structure, and classification according to the predominant actions of these toxins have been reviewed (12, 13). We shall concentrate here on the use of the ω-conotoxin GVIA (ω-CgTX), to date the best characterized of these peptides. Originally isolated from the venom of the species *Conus geographus* L., this 27-amino acid peptide has been synthesized and shown to possess the full activity of the native molecule (12). We have used ω-CgTX from Peninsula Laboratories (Belmont, CA). ^{125}I-Labeled ω-CgTX of high specific activity (about 2000 Ci/mmol) is necessary for binding experiments. This may be prepared by in-house iodination of the cold peptide if appropriate facilities are available, including a high-performance liquid chromatography (HPLC) system for the purification of the radioactive product (14). Commercial ^{125}I-labeled ω-CgTX may be obtained from New England Nuclear Research Products (Boston, MA) or from Amersham (Arlington Heights, IL). This is supplied as a lyophilized solid and is reconstituted in acetic acid [1%

(v/v), approximately 0.17 N] to the original volume, as specified by the manufacturer. A concentrated (e.g., 100 μM) solution of the nonradioactive ω-CgTX is made in 0.1 N acetic acid. These cold and radioactive stock solutions are divided into aliquots sufficient for 1 day of use and stored at $-20°C$ under nitrogen. Under these conditions, the ^{125}I-labeled ω-CgTX may be used for about 6 weeks, and the nonradioactive toxin for about 12 weeks. Dilutions are prepared from these stock solutions directly to the incubation medium (see below).

^{125}I-labeled ω-CgTX binds nonspecifically to storage and assay tubes, pipette tips, filters, and tissue. Binding to the nonbiological materials is minimized by using low-adhesive plastics [Minisorp tubes; Teknunc, Copenhagen, Denmark, of the type employed for radioimmunoassays (RIAs) are appropriate], including bovine serum albumin (BSA) at 1 mg/ml in all solutions, and keeping the number of transfers to a minimum.

The filters (GF/F; Whatman, Clifton, NJ) are soaked before use in a solution of BSA (2 mg/ml) in water for 1 hr. [Alternatively, polyethyleneimine (1%, v/v) in water may be used.] If a new type of filter is used, this should be tested for nonspecific binding of ^{125}I-labeled ω-CgTX. Filter-bound radioactivity may account for most of the total background activity, including the nonspecific binding to the tissue.

Nonspecific binding to the tissue is determined by adding an amount of a nonlabeled ω-CgTX to the assay sufficient to saturate all the high-affinity sites, and measuring the ^{125}I-labeled ω-CgTX bound under these conditions. Note that this method of estimating the nonspecific binding is valid only if a negligible fraction of total ligand is bound under all conditions. Otherwise, an overestimation of the nonspecifically bound counts may occur, particularly at low ligand concentrations. (For a detailed discussion of this aspect of the binding assay, see, for example, Refs. 15 and 16.) As one precaution against this error, a linear dependence of the specific binding on the amount of tissue in the assay should be demonstrated. A time course of binding should be examined to establish a sufficient incubation time for the attainment of the equilibrium or, if the binding is irreversible, to demonstrate that maximal binding capacity has been reached. A difficulty in reaching a plateau with respect to time suggests a problem with the stability of the ligand or the preparation. Instability may be due to the action of proteases on the binding sites or on the toxin itself, particularly if incubations lasting several hours are involved. Inclusion of protease inhibitors is recommended.

As an example, the following protocol shows the procedure for the measurement of the time dependence of the ^{125}I-labeled ω-CgTX binding to plasma membranes from the peptidergic nerve endings of the bovine neurohypophysis. The plasma membranes were prepared as described by Conigrave et al. (17).

1. Fifty microliters of the incubation medium is added to each tube containing 1–2 μg of plasma membrane protein. The incubation medium contains 20 mM Tris(hydroxymethyl)methyl-2-aminoethanesulfonic acid (TES), pH 7.4, 125 mM NaCl, 5 mM KCl, 1.3 mM $CaCl_2$, 1.5 mM Na_2HPO_4, and 0.6 mM $MgSO_4$ in addition to BSA (1 mg/ml) and the protease inhibitors phenylmethylsulfonyl fluoride (0.5 mM), aprotinin (50 units/ml), and leupeptin (5 μg/ml).

2. Twenty-five microliters of incubation medium containing nonradioactive ω-CgTX in a 1000-fold excess of the radioactive ligand (e.g., final assay concentration 0.1 μM) is added to the tubes designated for the measurement of nonspecific binding. The same volume of the medium without the toxin is added to the remaining tubes. (If the experiment involves using different concentrations of the radioactive toxin, the ratio of ω-CgTX to ^{125}I-labeled ω-CgTX should be kept constant for all determinations of the nonspecific binding.)

3. The reaction is started by adding 25 μl of incubation medium containing ^{125}I-labeled ω-CgTX to obtain an appropriate final concentration (e.g., 0.1 nM). The incubation is carried out in a shaking bath at 18°C.

4. The incubation is stopped at the desired times (indicated in Fig. 1) by adding 1 ml of ice-cold wash medium. This contains 20 mM TES (pH 7.4), 160 mM NaCl, 1.5 mM $CaCl_2$, and 0.1 mg/ml BSA. The mixture is filtered through Whatman GF/F filters on a suction manifold. The filters are then washed twice with 5 ml of the wash medium, and the retained radioactivity is counted. Figure 1 shows the results obtained by applying the protocol quoted above.

Comments

Minimizing the nonspecific binding to the tissue is critical for the accuracy and reproducibility of the results. Therefore for any system under investigation it is desirable to choose a preparation as enriched in the specific ^{125}I-labeled ω-CgTX-binding sites as may be obtained. For instance, our attempts to measure the binding of the ^{125}I-labeled ω-CgTX to the nerve endings of the neurohypophysis were frustrated by a very high proportion of nonspecific counts (60%). When the preparation was purified to the stage of plasma membranes, this background was reduced to about 15% of total counts bound.

Specific, high-affinity binding of ^{125}I-labeled ω-CgTX has been found in brain membrane preparations (18, 19), brain synaptosomes (14, 20, 21), and cultured neurons (14). These studies have reported binding affinities ranging from 0.6 pM (21) to about 60 pM (19), with one report of a biphasic binding showing K_d values of 10 and 500 pM (18). The higher values of this range

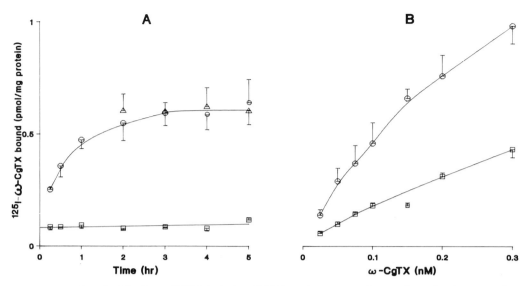

Fig. 1   Binding of ^{125}I-labeled ω-CgTX to plasma membranes from bovine neurohy-pophyseal secretory terminals. (A) Time course of binding with 0.1 nM ^{125}I-labeled ω-CgTX. (○) Total and (□) nonspecific binding; (△) total binding obtained when 0.1 μM ω-CgTX was added after 2 hr of incubation with ^{125}I-labeled ω-CgTX, and the incubation was continued for another 3 hr (means and SEM from three or four experiments). (B) Concentration dependence of ^{125}I-labeled ω-CgTX binding (2-hr incubation). Total and nonspecific binding as in (A) (means and ranges from two experiments). In (A) and (B), 1–2 μg of total membrane protein/tube was used. (Data from Ref. 9, with permission.)

may in part reflect the suboptimal binding conditions. including use of the ^{125}I-labeled ω-CgTX of low specific activity and high tissue/ligand ratios. However, a possibility of a true heterogeneity of the ^{125}I-labeled ω-CgTX-binding sites in the nervous tissue should be kept in mind, as suggested by some of the earlier (18) as well as the recent studies (22). Given the absence of specific antagonist compounds, it is at present not possible to determine definitely the nature of the ω-CgTX-binding sites (and even less so, the particular type of the VSCC responsible for the binding) in a given preparation based on the pharmacological binding data alone.

The binding of the toxin has in most studies been reported to be essentially irreversible, with other reports showing dissociation kinetics with a half-time of 2 (21) to 12 (19) hr. Meaningful K_d estimates can be given only if reversible equilibrium conditions obtain. For the irreversible binding conditions, the concentration dependence can be defined only for specified incubation times, and is more appropriately used (along with the time course experiments) to estimate the kinetic association constant (14).

Studies of Neuropeptide Release: Use of ω-Conotoxin and Organic Ca^{2+} Channel Ligands

The effects of the Ca^{2+} channel ligands on the release of neurotransmitters and neuropeptides are strongly dependent on the conditions of the tissue stimulation determining the functional state of the channels. The experimental protocols presented below may serve to demonstrate this stimulation parameter dependency in the case of peptide release from the neurohypophysis.

Protocol A

Male Wistar rats (200–220 g) are used. Following decapitation, the skull is opened over the dorsal aspect of the brain while taking care to minimize pressing the brain tissue with one branch of the scissors. The brain and the cerebellum are removed. A steel spatula is inserted from behind about 10 mm deep between the base of the skull and the brain stem, and the brain is lifted enough to permit the insertion of a narrow scalpel blade in the rostral direction parallel to the lower surface of the brain. This enables the neurohypophyseal stalk to be cut close to the point of its emergence from the infundibulum, facilitating the subsequent attachment to the electrode. The brain is now carefully removed. Using pointed forceps, the soft meningeal cover over the pituitary gland is now removed. The entire gland is dislodged from its position in the bone recess and transferred to a Petri dish containing the incubation medium (see below). Under the stereomicroscope, the adenohypophysis is separated from the neurointermediate lobe (21-gauge syringe needles are helpful as manipulating tools), and any excess of tissue at the cut end of the stalk is trimmed. The end of the stalk is guided to the opening of the PP10 polyethylene tubing at the tip of the suction electrode (Fig. 2A) and gently drawn into the tip by means of the connected syringe. The electrode with the neurohypophysis attached is now fitted into the opening of the incubation chamber (Fig. 2A, left) to give a tight seal. The reference electrode is positioned permanently at the bottom of the incubation chamber. The chamber is perfused at a rate of 200 μl/min with a medium containing 125 mM NaCl, 5 mM KCl, 19 mM NaHCO$_3$, 1.5 mM Na$_2$HPO$_4$, 0.6 mM MgSO$_4$, 1.3 mM CaCl$_2$, 10 mM D-glucose, 0.1 mg/ml BSA. The medium is saturated

A

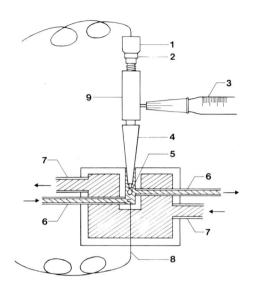
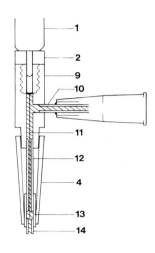

B

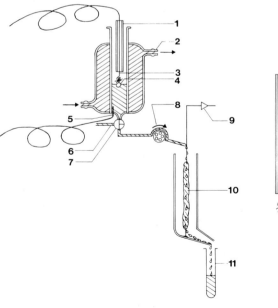
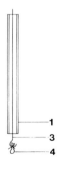

by 95% O_2/5% CO_2 at 37°C, pH 7.4. Fractions of the perfusate are collected every 10 min and the vasopressin or oxytocin content is measured by RIA. Stimuli are delivered at a constant current strength, as specified in Table I (protocol A). Alternatively, stimulation by high K^+ may be employed by suitable changes in the perfusion medium. The release evoked during each stimulation period is defined as the cumulative overflow above the basal release rate during 30 min (three fractions) following the onset of stimulation. For each neurohypophysis, the release is quantified as a ratio (S_2/S_1) between the evoked release values in the second and the first stimulation periods, for the control (no drug added) and the test (drug added before the second stimulation period) conditions, respectively. Figure 3 illustrates the dependence of the ω-CgTX-mediated inhibition of vasopressin release on the stimulation method (electrical versus high K^+ depolarization), using protocol A.

Comments on Protocol A

It is important to establish sufficient time in which the tissue will be exposed to the toxin. A comparison of Figs. 1 and 3 illustrates the importance of testing for a sufficient exposure time. In the binding experiment (Fig. 1), prolonging the incubation time from 1 to 2 hr increases the ^{125}I-labeled ω-CgTX binding by 20% (close to the full binding capacity). In contrast (Fig.

FIG. 2   Diagram of the incubation and stimulation systems for the isolated rat neurointermediate lobes, as used in protocols A and B (parts A and B of the figure, respectively). (A) Closed perfusion system: *left,* suction electrode with the neurointermediate lobe attached at the tip is inserted into the top opening of the incubation chamber. A cross section of the cylindrical chamber is drawn, to show the thermostatting and perfusion compartments (hatched): *right,* the design principle of the suction electrode, cross section. 1, Plug and wire for stimulator connection; 2, plug socket; 3, 1-ml disposable syringe; 4, protective cover and fitting for insertion to the perfusion chamber opening; 5, neurointermediate lobe; 6, 18-gauge stainless steel inlet and outlet for the perfusion medium; 7, inlet and outlet for the thermostatting water jacket; 8, permanent electrode (0.2-mm platinum wire) and stimulator connection; 9, electrode body machined in Perspex; 10, shaft and fitting of an 18-gauge injection needle for syringe connection; 11, 0.15-mm platinum wire; 12, shaft of a 25-gauge injection needle; 13, PP50 polyethylene tubing; 14, PP10 polyethylene tubing for neurohypophysis attachment. The hatched space from the tip to the syringe is filled by the incubation medium. (B) Open immersion system: 1, electrode insulation and holder; 2, water jacket; 3, cathode (0.5-mm platinum wire); 4, neurointermediate lobe tied to the electrode by means of a cotton thread; 5, anode; 6, uterus superfusion medium; 7, three-way stopcock; 8, peristaltic pump; 9, force-displacement transducer; 10, isolated rat uterus; 11, incubation medium collected for RIA.

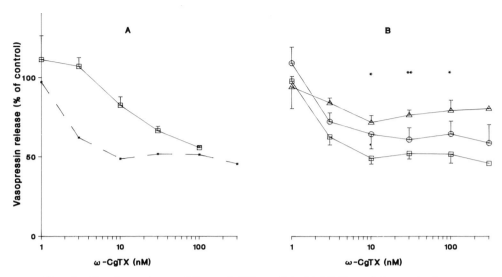

FIG. 3   The dependence of the ω-CgTX-mediated inhibition of the evoked vasopressin release from the isolated rat neurointermediate lobes on the stimulation conditions. (A) The dependence of inhibition on the length of preincubation with the toxin. Preincubation was for 60 (□) or 120 (■) min. (B) Inhibition of evoked vasopressin release by ω-CgTX using electrical stimulation according to protocol A (□), or stimulation by 50 (○) or 100 (△) mM K^+. Preincubation with the toxin was for 120 min. Statistical significance (*, $P < 0.05$; **, $P < 0.01$) was determined for comparisons between the release values obtained with electrical and 100 mM K^+ stimulation in (B). (For details, see Ref. 9, from which the data are quoted with permission.)

3A), with 10 nM ω-CgTX in the perfusion medium, prolonging the presence of the toxin from 1 to 2 hr results in about a 200% increase in the inhibition of vasopressin release (from 16% to the maximal inhibition level of 50%). Similar findings were reported in using ω-CgTX to investigate neurotransmitter release from brain slices (23).

The time for sufficient exposure to the toxin will be dictated both by the necessity to allow for the toxin penetration to its binding sites, and by the binding kinetics itself. A significant inhibition of neurotransmitter or neuropeptide release may require an almost complete saturation of the binding sites if redundant (''spare'') channels exist in the system, further stressing the importance of allowing for sufficient exposure time to the inhibitor.

The toxin concentrations necessary for maximal inhibition of release in an incubated whole tissue (e.g., a brain slice, neurohypophysis) may exceed considerably the toxin concentrations needed for saturation in binding assays

TABLE I   Comparison of Electrical Stimulation Parameters according to Protocols A and B

Parameter	Protocol A	Protocol B
Stimulation period	5 min	2.5 min
Monophasic square pulses	Yes	Yes
Alternating polarity	Yes	No
Pulse width	0.2 msec	0.2 or 2 msec
Pulse strength		
Constant current	0.3 mA	
Constant voltage		0.8 V
Frequency	16 Hz	6.5, 13, or 30 Hz
Pulse train duration	20 sec	10 sec
Intertrain interval	10 sec	10 sec

using the membranes prepared from the corresponding tissue (e.g., an approximately 30-fold increase seen in the data of Fig. 3B vs Fig. 1B). To a large extent, this is likely to reflect different receptor concentrations under the conditions of the two types of experiments. For instance, although only a rough estimate can be given for the concentration of the ω-CgTX-binding sites in an incubated whole-tissue preparation, for the neurohypophysis in Fig. 3 such an estimate would suggest 250 pM, as compared to 6–12 pM in the binding assay.

The selectivity of the ω-CgTX action in any given system must be particularly carefully considered when its use in the micromolar concentrations is contemplated. It has been demonstrated that voltage-dependent K^+ currents in chick dorsal root ganglion neurons were not affected by the toxin at 50 μM, while with 5 μM ω-CgTX there was a 20% reduction of Na^+ current in most of the cells tested (24). On the other hand, the toxin was recently reported to label the subunits of the nicotinic acetylcholine receptor, with a half-maximal displacement in the range of 0.1 to 1.0 μM (22). Therefore it should not be assumed that all of the toxin effects observed would derive from its binding to the VSCCs, in particular at higher toxin concentrations.

Protocol B

We have found this protocol useful in studies of the action of the organic Ca^{2+} channel ligands on vasopressin and oxytocin release from isolated rat neurohypophyses. The three most widely investigated classes of these drugs are 1,4-dihydropyridines (DHPs), e.g., nifedipine, nitrendipine, Bay K 8644,

202-791; phenylalkylamines, e.g., verapamil, D-600; and benzothiazepines, e.g., diltiazem. The organic ligands are included here mainly for the following reasons: (1) they constitute so far the only ligands that, under appropriate conditions, may be considered selective for the L-type channels [however, a new generation of the organic Ca^{2+} channel ligands appears to be underway (25)]; (2) since effects of ω-CgTX may be exerted either through its action on the channels of the L or N type, use of the organic ligands may help to identify the type of channels involved in a given system; and (3) these ligands provide some striking examples of the dependence of the results on the precise method of tissue stimulation. Detailed reviews are available covering the chemistry, and the biochemical, physiological, and behavioral aspects of the pharmacology of the organic Ca^{2+} channel ligands (26–29).

Female Sprague-Dawley rats (250–300 g) in spontaneous estrus are used. The animals are decapitated and the skin and skull overlying the brain removed. After carefully teasing the pituitary free of the surrounding membranes, the whole brain with the intact hypophysis is transferred to a Petri dish containing the medium bubbled with 95% O_2/5% CO_2, pH 7.4, of the following composition: 115 mM NaCl, 6.0 mM KCl, 0.8 mM Na_2HPO_4, 1.5 mM $CaCl_2$, 0.9 mM $MgCl_2$, 22 mM $NaHCO_3$, 10 mM D-glucose. Under stereomicroscope the neurointermediate lobe is separated from the anterior lobe and the neurohypophyseal stalk is cut at the level of the infundibulum. By means of a fine cotton thread the pituitary stalk is tied to a 0.5-mm platinum wire electrode (Fig. 2B) and immersed in 2 ml of the medium at 37°C. The preparation is preincubated for 1 hr, during which time the solution is changed every 15 min. Each neurointermediate lobe is electrically stimulated three times, with 75-min rest periods interposed. The incubation medium is changed every 15 min during these rest periods. Drugs are present 30 min before, and during, the second stimulation period. They are diluted to the incubation medium from freshly prepared stock solutions (1 mg/ml) in ethanol. (Dihydropyridines are highly sensitive to light below 450 nm, particularly when dissolved. The solutions should be protected from light. If incubation chambers or other parts of equipment cannot easily be protected, light may be dimmed in the room during the experiments.) Electrical stimuli are applied between the platinum wire carrying the neurohypophysis and a platinum wire dipped to the incubation medium. The stimulation conditions are summarized in Table I (protocol B). During the stimulation period the gland is raised to the surface of the incubation medium (Fig. 2B, left) and the gas supply is interrupted. The preparation is again immersed into the medium immediately after stimulation and the gas supply is restored. The medium is collected for the RIA (30) after the 10-min period following the stimulation. The response is quantified as a ratio (S_2/S_1) between the amounts of hormone released on the second and the first stimulations, respectively.

To obtain an immediate preliminary measure of the response to the stimulation, we use a semiquantitative bioassay. This is set up as follows. The uteri are dissected out from the above-mentioned rats and freed from fat. A thread is attached at each end and the organ is superfused with the medium at a rate of 1.35 ml/min. This superfusion medium (with a composition identical to that of the neurohypophysis incubation medium) is thermostated at 25–30°C (at 37°C, there is a high spontaneous contractile activity of the uterus). Contractions are recorded isotonically (Grass FT03 transducers, Quency, MA) after the muscle is given a 1-g load. The incubation medium containing the neurohypophyseal hormones is led over the organ at a rate of 1.35 ml/min (90 sec), before the collection for the RIA (Fig. 2B). Standard dose–response curves are obtained by superfusion of the muscle with arginine–vasopressin (0.1–8 mU/ml) or oxytocin (0.05–1.6 mU/ml) for 90 sec. The detectable minimum is about 0.2 mU arginine–vasopressin/ml and 50 μU oxytocin/ml.

Comments on Protocol B

In contrast to the evidence for the presence of the binding sites with nanomolar affinities for DHPs, phenylalkylamines, and benzothiazepines on L channel subunits in neurons (31, 32), it has been rather difficult to demonstrate correspondingly high potencies in the action of these drugs on release from neurons (29, 33–36). At least in part, this appears to be due to the interaction of the organic Ca^{2+} channel ligands with the channels being sensitive to the channel state, which in turn depends both on the membrane potential and on the immediate history of the preceding channel activity. For instance, the DHP antagonists appear to bind with the highest affinity to the inactivated state of the L channel (37, 38). The dependence on membrane potential has also been proposed to explain other complex features of the DHP action, including agonist–antagonist properties (27) and use dependence (33). Figure 4 shows the differences between the results obtained with the same drugs and the same tissue, but using two different stimulation protocols. From the present, methodological point of view, the important point is that the interpretation of such results should take into the àccount not only the relevant physiological mechanisms (e.g., the significance of pulse width and the stimulation frequency for the magnitude of Ca^{2+} influx), but any membrane potential-dependent behavior of the ligands as well. For instance, in protocol B, the shift from the enhancement to the inhibition by BAY K8644 and $S(+)$202-791 of the vasopressin release between 6.5 and 30 Hz (Fig. 4, protocol B) is consistent with the ability of these drugs to shift from the agonist to the antagonist action on increasing depolarization.

Caution should be exercised when using the organic Ca^{2+} channel ligands at concentrations exceeding 1 μM. Around 10 μM, these drugs are known to exert a number of nonspecific effects, including blockade of voltage-

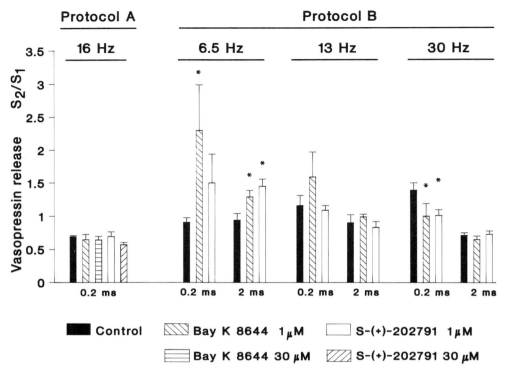

FIG. 4 The dependence of the effects of dihydropyridines Bay K 8644 and S(+)202-791 on the evoked vasopressin release from isolated rat neurointermediate lobes on the stimulation conditions. The results (means ± SEM) are expressed as the ratios (S_2/S_1) of the amount released by the second stimulation (S_2) in the presence or absence of a test substance, to that released by the first stimulation (S_1) in control medium. See Table I and the text for details of stimulation conditions for protocols A and B. Statistical significance (denoted by *): $P < 0.05$, when compared to the corresponding value in the absence of a ligand.

sensitive Na^+ channels (39, 40), blockade of Na^+–Ca^{2+} exchange in the mitochondria, as well as of Ca^{2+}–calmodulin-dependent enzymes (41). To confirm the specific nature of the observed effects, stereoselectivity of their action should be demonstrated whenever possible. This criterion was met using the stimulation according to protocol B, but not according to protocol A (not shown): for instance, the increase in the release of vasopressin due to $S(+)202$-791 (1 μM) was abolished in the presence of the opposite enantiomer $R(-)202$-791 (1 μM), whose antagonistic action on Ca^{2+} channels has been demonstrated (see, e.g., Ref. 42).

Conclusions

ω-Conotoxin and organic Ca^{2+} channel ligands offer a potential for relatively selective probing for the presence of N- and L-type Ca^{2+} channels and determining their involvement in neurotransmitter and neuropeptide release. Design of binding and release studies using ω-CgTX requires attention to the toxin stability, nonspecific binding, sufficient incubation times, irreversible action, and the relationship between the exposure time and effective concentrations. When using ω-CgTX and the organic ligands, any design of release experiments should encompass a range of stimulation conditions before the magnitude and the direction ("agonism" or "antagonism") of ligand action is evaluated. With all the ligands, pharmacological selectivity requirements (concentration limits and stereoselectivity) need to be borne in mind.

Acknowledgments

This work was supported by the Danish Government Biotechnology Program and Nordisk Insulin Foundation. Our thanks are due to Ms. Elin Engberg for excellent technical assistance in many of the quoted experiments.

References

1. R. W. Tsien, D. Lipscombe, D. V. Madison, K. R. Bley, and A. P. Fox, *Trends NeuroSci.* **11,** 431 (1988).
2. R. J. Miller, *Science* **235,** 46 (1987).
3. G. J. Augustine, M. P. Charlton, and S. J. Smith, *Annu. Rev. Neurosci.* **10,** 633 (1987).
4. M. P. Blaustein, *Handb. Exp. Pharmacol.* **83,** 275 (1988).
5. J. F. Morris, J. J. Nordmann, and R. E. J. Dyball, *Int. Rev. Exp. Pathol.* **18,** 2 (1978).
6. M. Treiman, S. Zolnierowicz, K. Allesøe, and P. H. Andersen, *in* "Molecular Mechanisms in Secretion" (N. A. Thorn, M. Treiman, and O. H. Petersen, eds.), p. 230. Munksgaard, Copenhagen, 1988.
7. J. R. Lemos and M. C. Nowycky, *Neuron* **2,** 1419 (1989).
8. G. Dayanithi, N. Martin-Moutot, S. Barlier, D. A. Colin, M. Kretz-Zaepfel, F. Couraud, and J. J. Nordmann, *Biochem. Biophys. Res. Commun.* **156,** 255 (1988).
9. S. Von Spreckelsen, K. Lollike, and M. Treiman, *Brain Res.* **514,** 68 (1990).
10. E. W. McCleskey, A. P. Fox, D. H. Feldman, L. J. Cruz, B. M. Olivera, R. W. Tsien, and D. Yoshikami, *Proc. Natl. Acad. Sci. U.S.A.* **84,** 4327 (1987).
11. M. R. Plummer, D. E. Logothetis, and P. Hess, *Neuron* **2,** 1453 (1989).

12. W. R. Gray, B. M. Olivera, and L. J. Cruz, *Annu. Rev. Biochem.* **57,** 665 (1988).
13. B. M. Olivera, W. R. Gray, R. Zeikus, J. M. McIntosh, J. Varga, J. Rivier, V. de Santos, and L. J. Cruz, *Science* **230,** 1338 (1985).
14. B. Marqueze, N. Martin-Moutot, C. Levêque, and F. Couraud, *Mol. Pharmacol.* **34,** 87 (1988).
15. P. Cuatrecasas and M. D. Hollenberg, *Adv. Protein Chem.* **30,** 251 (1976).
16. P. Seeman, C. Ulpian, K. A. Wreggett, and J. W. Wells, *J. Neurochem.* **43,** 221 (1984).
17. A. D. Conigrave, M. Treiman, T. Saermark, and N. A. Thorn, *Cell Calcium* **2,** 125 (1981).
18. T. Abe, K. Koyano, H. Saisu, Y. Nishiuchi, and S. Sakakibara, *Neurosci. Lett.* **71,** 203 (1986).
19. J. A. Wagner, A. M. Snowman, A. Biswas, B. M. Olivera, and S. H. Snyder, *J. Neurosci.* **8,** 3354 (1988).
20. L. J. Cruz, D. S. Johnson, and B. M. Olivera, *Biochemistry* **26,** 820 (1987).
21. J. Barhanin, A. Schmid, and M. Lazdunski, *Biochem. Biophys. Res. Commun.* **150,** 1051 (1988).
22. W. A. Horne, R. R. Delay, and R. W. Tsien, *Soc. Neurosci. Abstr.* **16,** 957 (1990).
23. D. J. Dooley, A. Lupp, and G. Hertting, *Naunyn-Schmiedeberg's Arch. Pharmacol.* **336,** 467 (1987).
24. D. H. Feldman, B. M. Olivera, and D. Yoshikami, *FEBS Lett.* **214,** 295 (1987).
25. D. Rampe and D. J. Triggle, *Trends Pharmacol. Sci.* **11,** 112 (1990).
26. M. M. Hosey and M. Lazdunski, *J. Membr. Biol.* **104,** 81 (1988).
27. D. J. Triggle and D. Rampe, *Trends Pharmacol. Sci.* **10,** 507 (1989).
28. R. A. Janis, P. J. Silver, and D. J. Triggle, *Adv. Drug Res.* **16,** 311 (1987).
29. R. J. Miller, *in* "Structure and Physiology of the Slow Inward Calcium Channel" (D. J. Triggle and C. J. Venter, eds.), p. 161. Liss, New York, 1987.
30. J. D. Christensen and B. Fjalland, *Acta Pharmacol. Toxicol.* **50,** 113 (1982).
31. R. Cortes, P. Supavilai, M. Karobath, and J. M. Palacios, *J. Neural Transm.* **60,** 169 (1984).
32. A. Skattebøl and D. J. Triggle, *Biochem. Pharmacol.* **36,** 4163 (1987).
33. T. J. Turner and S. M. Goldin, *Ann. N.Y. Acad. Sci.* **522,** 278 (1988).
34. J. J. Woodward, M. E. Cook, and S. W. Leslie, *Proc. Natl. Acad. Sci. U.S.A.* **85,** 7389 (1988).
35. D. N. Middlemiss and M. Spedding, *Nature (London)* **314,** 94 (1985).
36. S. Kongsamut and R. J. Miller, *Proc. Natl. Acad. Sci. U.S.A.* **83,** 2243 (1986).
37. P. B. Bean, *Proc. Natl. Acad. Sci. U.S.A.* **81,** 6388 (1984).
38. G. G. Holz IV, K. Dunlap, and R. M. Kream, *J. Neurosci.* **8,** 463 (1988).
39. J. J. Corcoran and N. Kirshner, *J. Neurochem.* **40,** 1106 (1983).
40. D. A. Nachshen and M. P. Blaustein, *Mol. Pharmacol.* **16,** 579 (1979).
41. G. Zernig, *Trends Pharmacol. Sci.* **11,** 38 (1990).
42. S. Kongsamut, T. J. Kamp, R. J. Miller, and M. C. Sanguinetti, *Biochem. Biophys. Res. Commun.* **130,** 141 (1985).

[8] Modulation of Acetylcholine Release by Calcium Channel Antagonists*

I. Wessler

Introduction

Calcium, which transmits electrical signals into biological events, plays a pivotal role in the regulation of multiple cellular functions, such as the release and liberation of transmitters, hormones, local-operating modulators and cytokines, activation of enzymes, gene expression, differentiation, growth, metabolic activity, and pacemaker activity. One way in which the intracellular calcium concentration can be increased rapidly is by the opening of voltage-operated or receptor-sensitive calcium channels, whereas the second way mobilizes calcium from intracellular stores via the phosphoinositide pathway (1). By using electrophysiological and pharmacological methods distinct voltage-operated calcium channels (T, L, N, and P channels) have been determined (2–4), and it becomes clear now that neurons are endowed with multiple calcium channels allowing a discriminative neuronal activity, when a distinct pattern of calcium channels is activated at a communicating neuron. In the past, the use of toxins has been most fruitful in the characterization of ion channels. When the electrophysiological profile of calcium channels is similar (high threshold-activated channels, similar inactivation kinetics, and gating properties) a pharmacological characterization of those calcium channels becomes particularly important (5). Venoms from snakes, fish-hunting snails, and spiders have largely contributed to the biochemical, electrophysiological, and pharmacological characterization of different calcium channels. ω-Conotoxin isolated from fish-hunting cone snails (6, 7) has forwarded the characterization of neuronal calcium channels. By blocking N-type calcium channels ω-conotoxins have provided the opportunity to investigate the relative significance of N-type calcium channels in the release of various transmitters and hormones. Two different forms of conotoxins have been found, ω-conotoxin GVIA from *Conus geographus* and ω-conotoxin MVIIA from *Conus magus*. Meanwhile, both peptide have been chemically synthesized (6–9), and ω-conotoxin GVIA is the toxin currently used. Most importantly, ω-conotoxin has been shown to target only neuronal voltage-operated calcium channels, whereas calcium channels in cardiac mus-

---

* Dedicated to Professor P. Schölmerich, Mainz, on the occasion of his 75th birthday.

Methods in Neurosciences, Volume 8

TABLE I   Neurotoxins Blocking Calcium Channels

Toxin	Tissue	Species
ω-Conotoxin MVIIA or GVIA	Motor nerve terminals	Fish, frog, avian
	Brain, peripheral autonomic nervous system (N-type channel)	Mammals
	Dorsal root ganglia (N- and L-type channel)	Chick, mammals
Funnel-web spider venom[a,b]	Cerebellum, brain (P-type channel)	Mammals
	Giant synapse	Squid
Type I ω-agatoxin[c]	Neuromuscular junction	Insect, frog
	Sensory neurons	Mammals
TaiCatoxin[d]	Heart	Mammals
Mojave toxin[e]	Brain	Mammals

[a] R. Llinás, M. Sugimori, J.-W. Lin, and B. Cherksey, *Proc. Natl. Acad. Sci. U.S.A.* **86,** 1689 (1989).
[b] J.-W. Lin, B. Rudy, and R. Llinás, *Proc. Natl. Acad. Sci. U.S.A.* **87,** 4538 (1990).
[c] M. E. Adams, V. P. Bindokas, L. Hasegawa, and V. J. Venema, *J. Biol. Chem.* **265,** 861 (1990).
[d] A. M. Brown, A. Yatani, A. E. Lacerda, G. B. Gurrola, and L. D. Possani, *Circ. Res., Suppl.* **61,** I-6 (1987).
[e] J. J. Valdes, R. G. Thompson, V. L. Wolff, D. E. Menking, E. D. Rael, and J. P. Chambers, *Neurotoxicol. Teratol.* **11,** 129 (1989).

cles, smooth muscles, and skeletal muscles are insensitive (10, 11). However, one should realize that ω-conotoxin can also block neuronal L-type channels in sensory neurons (2, 3). Additional neurotoxins are available that block calcium channels in different tissues with high specificity, and which therefore may be helpful in producing a more detailed characterization of distinct calcium channels in different tissues (see Table I).

The present chapter will focus on the effects of ω-conotoxin on the release of the classical transmitters, particularly the effects of ω-conotoxin GVIA on the release of acetylcholine. Release of acetylcholine from neuroeffector junctions (smooth or skeletal muscles) can be monitored indirectly by recording of the electrical (excitatory synaptic potentials; end-plate potentials) or mechanical (contraction) end-organ responses. A more direct approach is the measurement of the release of newly synthesized radiolabeled acetylcholine, which excludes the possibility that any changes in the sensitivity of the postsynaptic detection machinery (nicotine or muscarine receptor) or nonspecific effects of calcium channel antagonists at the postsynaptic cell membranes (see Ref. 12) would complicate the interpretation of the results. Before describing the results observed in release experiments, some results obtained with ω-conotoxin in binding and functional experiments are discussed to compare these data with those obtained in release experiments.

Binding Experiments

Specific binding of ω-conotoxin has been shown to occur in the peripheral and central nervous system. In mammalian brain ω-conotoxin binds to a single site (the α subunit of the channel protein) with high affinity (K_D value within 0.5–60 pM). Specific binding differs markedly from that observed with the L-type calcium channel antagonists and is concentrated at the synaptic zones, where excitation–secretion coupling occurs (10, 13–16). Similar binding characteristics have been found in sympathetic ganglia, cultured neurons, and human neuroblastoma cell lines (15, 17, 18). Binding of ω-conotoxin GVIA to adrenomedullary membranes and brain synaptosomal preparations shows two binding sites [pico- and nanomolar range (13, 19)]. In amphibian neuronal preparations binding differs between ω-conotoxins GVIA and MVIIA, indicating the existence of subtypes of N-type calcium channels; at least three subtypes have been suggested (20). Finally, binding of ω-conotoxin is inhibited by divalent cations (13, 15).

Electrophysiological Experiments

Using patch-clamp recording ω-conotoxin GVIA has been shown to block neuronal L- and T-type calcium channels in sensory, sympathetic, and hippocampal neurons (vertebrates) in a more or less irreversible manner (2, 3, 11, 21). Miniature excitatory synaptic currents evoked in cultured hippocampal neurons by an excitatory amino acid transmitter are also reduced by nanomolar concentrations of ω-conotoxin GVIA. Moreover, amplitudes of evoked end-plate potentials were inhibited in amphibian neuromuscular junctions, and in the electric organ of the ray; likewise, synaptic transmission at the bullfrog sympathetic ganglion is blocked by nanomolar concentrations of ω-conotoxin GVIA (21–23). Evoked end-plate potentials recorded in mammalian skeletal muscles, however, are not affected, even by high concentrations (micromolar) of ω-conotoxin GVIA (22, 24). Likewise, a more recent study recording excitatory postsynaptic potentials in the submandibular parasympathetic ganglia of rats did not find any inhibitory effect of ω-conotoxin GVIA (1 μM), thus showing that the release of acetylcholine from these preganglionic neurons is insensitive to the blockade of N-type calcium channels (12). Nevertheless, whole-cell calcium currents recorded in cultured rat parasympathetic neurons have turned out to be highly sensitive to ω-conotoxin GVIA. This apparent discrepancy should be considered, and it is emphasized that investigations should be made of single biological events coupled to definite neuronal or cellular functions, because one cannot draw conclusions from ''overall effects.'' The calcium channels controlling the depolarization-induced acetylcholine release from these preganglionic neurons appear to contribute only to a small extent to the total calcium influx.

Functional Experiments

ω-Conotoxin is a potent inhibitor of neurally evoked smooth muscle contractions in various mammalian tissues. Stimulated responses in the vas deferens, urinary bladder, stomach fundus, small intestine, uterus, and small mesenteric arteries were blocked by ω-conotoxin, whereas end-organ responses evoked by applied agonists were not affected by the toxin (25–28). In most of these functional experiments ω-conotoxin GVIA has turned out to be a very effective tool: concentrations of 1–10 nM ω-conotoxin GVIA prevented neurally evoked end-organ responses. These results indicate the release of noradrenaline and acetylcholine from postganglionic autonomic neurons to be predominantly controlled by N-type calcium channels.

Release Experiments

Two approaches are currently used to measure the release of acetylcholine, in addition to those methods that monitor the release of acetylcholine by recording the electrical or mechanical end-organ responses. First, unlabeled endogenous acetylcholine can be detected by various methods [bioassay, radioenzymatic assays, gas chromatography combined with mass spectrometry, high-performance liquid chromatography (HPLC) with electrochemical detection]; all these methods require the inactivation of the enzyme acetylcholinesterase. Second, release of acetylcholine, newly synthesized during incubation of the tissue with radioactive choline, can be estimated from the increase in stimulated efflux of radioactivity without blocking the enzyme acetylcholinesterase. An important observation is that multiple unwanted effects are caused by the blockade of the enzyme, such as tipped-up concentrations of acetylcholine in the biophase, increased diffusion radius of acetylcholine, nicotine receptor desensitization, attenuation of the effects of applied agonists at nicotine and muscarine receptors, artificial amplification of the effects of muscarine receptor antagonists, formation of surplus acetylcholine and, possibly, modifications of ions fluxes. Therefore, whenever possible, one should avoid inactivating the enzyme acetylcholinesterase, particularly when presynaptic mechanisms are investigated.

Evaluation of [^{3}H]Acetylcholine Release

So far, the release of newly synthesized acetylcholine has been measured in various tissues from the stimulated increase in radioactive efflux after a preceding incubation with the radioactive precursor choline (airways, brain, heart, intestine, urinary bladder, ganglion cells, motor nerve). Using this method of evaluation, the stimulated tritium efflux reflects exclusively the release of radioactive acetylcholine from cholinergic neurons. This is exemplified for the motor nerve [rat phrenic nerve (29–31)].

End-plate preparations (small muscle strips of 1- to 2-mm width containing the end-plate region of the left rat hemidiaphragm together with the innervating phrenic nerve) are superfused/incubated in 2-ml organ baths with a physiological salt solution (choline, 1 μM) that is gassed with 5% CO_2 in O_2 and warmed to a constant temperature of 36°C. After a 30-min equilibration the tissue is incubated (30–40 min) with [^{3}H]choline (10 μCi/2 ml), and the phrenic nerve is stimulated electrically (biphasic pulses with a pulse width of 0.2 msec; current, 8 mA; potential drop between the electrodes, 0.5 V/mm). Nerve stimulation during labeling accelerates the exchange of newly synthesized [^{3}H]acetylcholine against endogenous acetylcholine and the incorporation of [^{3}H]acetylcholine into the releasable vesicular pool (30, 32, 33). After the labeling period the end-plate preparations are superfused at a high rate (12 ml/min) to wash out the excess radioactivity. Hemicholinium-3 (10 μM) is added to the medium from the washout period onward to block the uptake of choline and to allow the subsequent assay of [^{3}H]choline originating from the hydrolysis of released [^{3}H]acetylcholine. After a 60-min washout period tritium efflux from the organ bath is measured at 2-, 3-, or 5-min intervals. Release of [^{3}H]acetylcholine is elicited during 2 periods (S_1 and S_2, 39–45 min apart) of electrical nerve stimulation (100–300 pulses at 1, 3, or 10 Hz); the stimulation parameters are identical for S_1 and S_2. Substances (calcium channel antagonists) are added 15–21 min before S_2, and their effects can be analyzed by the comparison of the amounts of [^{3}H]acetylcholine released by S_2 and S_1, respectively (S_2/S_1 ratio). Comparable experimental protocols have been set up for experiments with myenteric plexus and brain cortical slices (29, 31, 34, 35).

Significant amounts of [^{3}H]acetylcholine have been shown to be synthesized in innervated end-plate preparations, whereas [^{3}H]acetylcholine synthesis in preparations in which the phrenic nerve was surgically removed 6 days prior to the release experiments (chronically denervated end-plate preparations) declined 4% compared to innervated preparations (30). Electrical stimulation of the phrenic nerve (100 pulses, 1–100 Hz) causes an increased tritium efflux that is abolished by the removal of extracellular calcium or by the application of 0.3 μM tetrodotoxin (see Fig. 1). Electrical field stimulation of a chronically denervated end-plate preparation, however, did not produce any release of tritium (30), indicating that neither choline nor choline metabolites [i.e., phosphorylcholine (36)] are liberated in response to the electrical nerve stimulation.

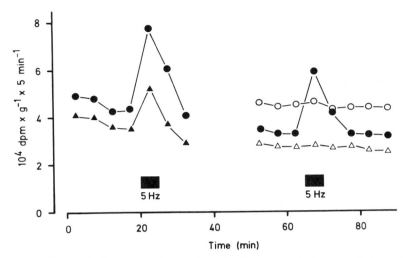

FIG. 1   Abolition of stimulated tritium efflux by the removal of extracellular calcium or by the application of tetrodotoxin. After incubation with 10 μCi [³H]choline and a subsequent 60-min washout, tritium efflux was measured at 5-min intervals. (●, ▲: extracellular calcium 1.8 ml.) The phrenic nerve was stimulated (5 Hz, 5 min) twice at the indicated times. In some experiments extracellular calcium (○) was removed or 300 nM tetrodotoxin (△) added 30 min before the second stimulation. Both modifications abolished the stimulated increase in tritium efflux. [From I. Wessler and H. Kilbinger, *Naunyn-Schmiedeberg's Arch. Pharmacol.* **334,** 357 (1986).]

In some control experiments cholinesterase is inactivated by 10 μM neo-stigmine to identify [³H]acetylcholine biochemically and to investigate whether the stimulated efflux of total tritium is balanced by the stimulated release of [³H]acetylcholine. Acetylcholine can be separated from different radioactive compounds (see above) and detected either by ion-pair extraction followed by thin-layer chromatography (37) or, with a high recovery rate, by reversed-phase HPLC followed by liquid scintillation spectrometry (31). Figure 2 shows the spontaneous tritium efflux from the phrenic nerve end-plate preparation to be composed mainly of phosphorylcholine and choline; at rest, [³H]acetylcholine is only a minor fraction. Importantly, the efflux of choline and phosphorylcholine is not affected by electrical nerve stimulation [sum of both compounds, 260 disintegrations per minute (dpm)/200 μl at rest vs 270 dpm/200 μl during stimulation], whereas the release of [³H]acetylcho-line increased considerably in response to electrical nerve stimulation (15 dpm/200 μl vs 120 dpm/200 μl; Fig. 2). A detailed analysis of the samples collected immediately before, during, and after nerve stimulation demon-

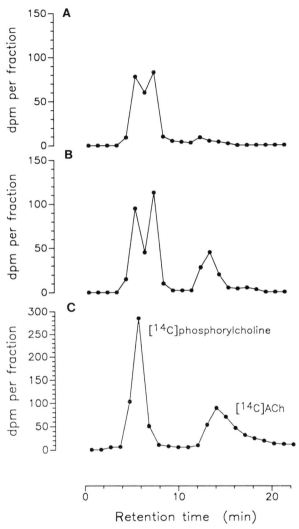

FIG. 2   Separation of radioactive compounds liberated spontaneously or in response to electrical stimulation of the phrenic nerve. After the labeling and washout period the enzyme acetylcholinesterase was inactivated by 10 μM neostigmine. Tritium efflux was obtained (A) at rest (spontaneous) or (B) after electrical nerve stimulation (10 Hz, 200 pulses) was assayed, and 200 μl of each sample was injected onto a reversed-phase HPLC column (31). (C) ¹⁴C-Labeled phosphorylcholine and acetylcholine (ACh) were used as internal standards for the identification of the retention times. Stimulation of the phrenic nerve does not affect the outflow of phosphorylcholine or choline, but causes the release of acetylcholine.

strates the stimulated tritium efflux to be balanced by the enhanced release of [³H]acetylcholine (30); a similar conclusion has been drawn from experiments with the small intestine [plexus myentericus (29, 31)]. All the "control experiments" described so far have provided fairly convincing evidence that, after a preceding labeling with the precursor choline, the stimulated tritium efflux indicates the calcium-dependent release (exocytosis) of radiolabeled acetylcholine from cholinergic nerve terminals; this release can be detected in the presence of active acetylcholinesterase: [³H]acetylcholine, after escaping the neuronal membrane (exocytosis), is hydrolyzed to [³H]choline and acetate; [³H]choline diffuses into the incubation medium and can be assayed, because uptake of choline into the tissue is blocked by hemicholinium-3.

Some limitations of the present radiotracer method, however, should be considered. The use of hemicholinium-3 and subsequent blockade of choline uptake prevents synthesis of acetylcholine. Thus, all the mechanisms controlling the synthesis of acetylcholine cannot be investigated by this method. To avoid any limitation of the stimulated release of [³H]acetylcholine that might occur due to the pool of [³H]acetylcholine being fixed and blockage of synthesis after the labeling period, one should use very moderate stimulation parameters. The stimulation conditions currently used in experiments with the motor nerve, the small intestine, or the brain cortex cause the release of less than 5% of the tissue store of radioactive acetylcholine, which excludes exhaustion of the releasable [³H]acetylcholine pool. Finally, one must consider the possibility of a different regulation between endogenous, preformed acetylcholine and radiolabeled, newly synthesized acetylcholine. Concerning the modulatory effects of presynaptic receptors there is, however, excellent agreement in the regulation of the release of both endogenous and radiolabeled acetylcholine; only in one report, describing the release of acetylcholine from *Torpedo* synaptosomes, have differences between endogenous and radiolabeled acetylcholine been found (38).

Modulation of [³H]Acetylcholine Release

Effects of Calcium Channel Antagonists on Stimulated Acetylcholine Release from Rat Brain Cortex, Small Intestine, and Motor Nerve

Nerve terminals, particularly motor nerve endings, are so far not directly accessible to electrophysiological methods such as patch-clamp techniques. However, the investigation of the effects of calcium channel antagonists on stimulated transmitter release can help to evaluate the role of different calcium channels regulating transmitter release from the nerve terminals.

ω-Conotoxin GVIA inhibited in a concentration-dependent manner the release of [³H]acetylcholine evoked electrically (3 Hz, 2 min) from the rat small intestine (myenteric plexus–longitudinal muscle preparation) or rat cortical slices (see Fig. 3). ω-Conotoxin GVIA appeared very effective; already a concentration of 1 nM caused a significant inhibition in the myenteric plexus. In contrast, neither verapamil nor nifedipine, even at high concentrations (micromolar), affected the release of acetylcholine from the myenteric plexus or from brain cortical neurons (35, 39). These results fairly convincingly show N-type calcium channels to be dominantly involved in the regulation of stimulated acetylcholine release from cortical and postganglionic autonomic neurons. Interestingly, a homology between the cortex and the myenteric plexus has been already proposed on the basis of ultrastructural and electrophysiological studies (40) and led Brooks to suggest that the enteric nervous system resembles "scattered little brains" (41).

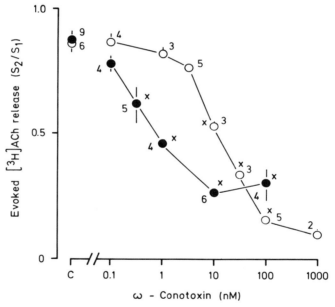

FIG. 3   Inhibition of [³H]acetylcholine release from the rat myenteric plexus and brain cortical slices by ω-conotoxin GVIA. After the labeling and washout period, release of [³H]acetylcholine was elicited by two stimulation periods (S_1, S_2; 3 Hz, 2 min); ω-conotoxin GVIA was added to the organ bath 15–21 min before S_2. The effect of ω-conotoxin GVIA is indicated by the ratio S_2/S_1. (●) Experiments with myenteric plexus. (○) Experiments with cortical slices. Values given are the means ± SEM of the number of experiments indicated. Significance of differences: $x < 0.01$ [From I. Wessler, D. J. Dooley, J. Werhand, and F. Schlemmer, *Naunyn-Schmiedeberg's Arch. Pharmacol.* **341,** 288 (1990).]

ω-Conotoxin GVIA inhibited [^{3}H]acetylcholine released from the myenteric plexus (IC$_{50}$ value, 0.7 nM) more potently than that released from cortical slices (IC$_{50}$ value, 13 nM), although the experiments with both tissues were performed under quite similar experimental conditions (35) (see Fig. 3). This difference can, of course, reflect tissue-specific differences such as the diffusion of the toxin to the binding sites or its enzymatic degradation. One should, however, also consider the possibility of subtypes of N-type calcium channels that have already been proposed (3). Cruz and colleagues (20), performing animal studies as well as binding and calcium-uptake experiments in different species with both forms of ω-conotoxin (GVIA, MVIIA), found evidence for the existence of three different subtypes of N-type calcium channels. Likewise, the present results suggest the N-type calcium channels regulating acetylcholine release from cortical and myenteric neurons to represent two subtypes of N-type calcium channels.

In contrast to the experiments with the myenteric plexus and cortical neurons, ω-conotoxin GVIA, even at high concentrations (0.1 μM), did not inhibit the stimulated release of [^{3}H]acetylcholine from the motor nerve. Inhibition was also not observed when different stimulation frequencies were applied (1, 3, and 10 Hz). Likewise, neither verapamil (0.1, 1, and 10 μM) nor nifedipine (0.1 and 1 μM) produced any significant inhibitory effect on transmitter release from the rat phrenic nerve (35). Thus the calcium channel(s) regulating the stimulated release of acetylcholine from motor nerves differ from the corresponding channels operating at the endings of myenteric and cortical neurons. The calcium channel(s) triggering the depolarization-induced transmitter release from the mammalian motoneuron have not yet been classified. It is important, however, to evaluate whether the release of acetylcholine from the motor nerve is inhibited by neurotoxins that block the P-type calcium channel [funnel-web spider venom; type I ω-agatoxin (4, 42)]. Nevertheless, motor nerve terminals are also endowed with N-type calcium channels; evidence for the existence of N-type calcium channels is obtained under two distinct experimental conditions: first, after stimulation of presynaptic adrenoreceptors (see below), and second, after reduction of the extracellular calcium concentration and a prolonged exposure to the toxin. Under this latter condition (extracellular calcium concentration, 0.9 mM; 42-min exposure to the toxin) ω-conotoxin GVIA significantly inhibited [^{3}H]acetylcholine release by about 47%, whereas under the same experimental conditions nifedipine was ineffective (35). This observation indicates the existence of N-type calcium channels, which are, however, only marginally involved in the regulation of transmitter release from motor neurons. The increased potency of ω-conotoxin GVIA occurring with a reduced extracellular calcium concentration can be explained by two mechanisms. First, toxin binding is inversely related to the concentration of divalent cations (15, 17), thus allowing increased toxin binding at decreasing calcium concentrations. Second, reduction of extracellular calcium reduces the driving force for calcium influx through voltage-operated calcium channels and thereby the calcium availability for stimulus-secretion coupling. Under this condition, blockade of N-type calcium channels contributing less to the total calcium influx may become critical and consequently may mediate a reduced transmitter release.

The present experiments have demonstrated a clear difference in the regulation of the stimulated release of acetylcholine from autonomic neurons and from motor neurons: N-type calcium channels are critically involved in the former but not in the latter nervous system. This difference is even more remarkable as the motor nerve terminals are endowed with N-type calcium channels. In contrast to autonomic neurons, these channels do not transmit the depolarization-induced calcium influx at those spots critically involved in triggering the evoked release of acetylcholine.

Effects of Calcium Channel Antagonists on Receptor-Sensitive Calcium Channels at Rat Motor Nerve Terminal (Phrenic Nerve)

Facilitation of transmitter release is caused by an increase in the intraneuronal calcium availability that can be mediated by the opening of calcium channels, either directly via regulatory G proteins or indirectly via second messengers. For example, β_1-receptor stimulation and, consequently, the enhanced formation of cyclic AMP in cardiac cells is thought to mediate phosphorylation of a protein close to or in calcium channels and thereby to increase or prolong the events of channel opening. At motor nerve terminals presynaptic α_1- and β_1-receptors have been shown to enhance the stimulated transmitter release either under in vivo (43) or in vitro conditions (44, 45). The facilitatory effects of phenylephrine, stimulating α_1-receptors at phrenic nerve terminals, and of noradrenaline, stimulating β_1-receptors, were investigated in the presence of ω-conotoxin GVIA and nifedipine. In this context it should be kept in mind that both calcium channel antagonists alone did not affect the electrically evoked [³H]acetylcholine release (see above). Thus any effect of nifedipine or ω-conotoxin GVIA observed in the presence of sympathomimetic amines indicates the calcium channel antagonists interact with the signal transduction activated by the stimulation of facilitatory α_1 or β_1 receptors. In these experiments sympathomimetic amines and ω-conotoxin GVIA were added to the organ bath 21 min before S_2, and, in the respective experiments, nifedipine was already present 30 min before S_1 and onward.

ω-Conotoxin GVIA (1–100 nM) prevented the facilitatory effect of noradrenaline, and nifedipine (0.1 and 1 μM) abolished the effect of phenylephrine (see Figs. 4 and 5). In contrast, nifedipine did not inhibit the enhancing effect of noradrenaline, and ω-conotoxin GVIA did not inhibit the enhancing effect of phenylephrine (46) (see Fig. 5). These results indicate the α_1 recep-

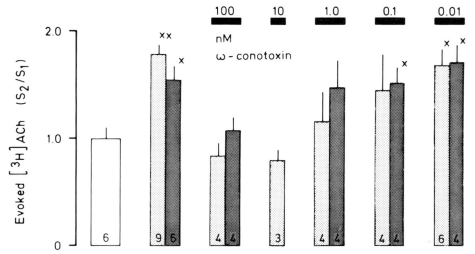

Fig. 4 Facilitatory effect of noradrenaline (stimulation of β_1 receptors) at phrenic nerve terminals in the absence and presence of ω-conotoxin GVIA. After the labeling and washout period, release of [^{3}H]acetylcholine was elicited by two stimulation periods (S_1, S_2; 10 Hz, 200 pulses). ω-Conotoxin GVIA and noradrenaline (black bars, 10 μM; patterned bars, 1 μM) were added to the organ bath 21 min before S_2. Noradrenaline considerably enhanced transmitter release in the absence of the toxin, whereas already low concentrations of ω-conotoxin GVIA prevented the facilitatory effect. Values given are the means $\pm$SEM of the number of experiments indicated. Significance of differences: $x < 0.05$; $xx < 0.01$. [From I. Wessler, D. J. Dooley, H. Osswald, and F. Schlemmer, *Neurosci. Lett.* **108**, 173 (1990).]

tors are linked to dihydropyridine-sensitive calcium channels (L-like calcium channels), whereas the β_1 receptors are associated with N-type calcium channels. Whether the presynaptic α_1 and β_1 receptors are linked directly or indirectly to the calcium channels remains to be elucidated. The dihydropyridine-sensitive calcium channel, activated by α_1-receptor stimulation, appears not to be a typical neuronal L-type calcium channel, because ω-conotoxin GVIA was ineffective; these calcium channels resemble more the L-type calcium channels present in skeletal or heart muscle fibers, in which the inefficiency of ω-conotoxin GVIA has already been shown.

The results obtained in the release experiments are in excellent agreement with the results obtained in electrophysiological and contraction experiments. ω-Conotoxin GVIA does not inhibit evoked end-plate potentials at mammalian neuromuscular junctions, but reduces neurally evoked contrac-

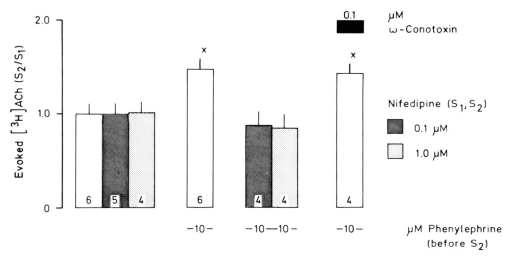

FIG. 5   Facilitatory effect of phenylephrine (stimulation of α_1 receptors) at phrenic nerve terminals in the absence and presence of nifedipine. After the labeling and washout period, release of [³H]acetylcholine was elicited by two stimulation periods (S_1, S_2; 10 Hz, 200 pulses). Nifedipine was added 30 min before S_1 and phenylephrine (concentrations indicated) 21 min before S_2. Phenylephrine enhanced transmitter release; this effect was abolished by nifidepine but not by ω-conotoxin GVIA. Values given are the means ±SEM of the number of experiments indicated. Significance of differences: $x < 0.05$. [From I. Wessler, D. J. Dooley, H. Osswald, and F. Schlemmer, *Neurosci. Lett.* **108,** 173 (1990).]

tions in various smooth muscle preparations (intestine and urinary bladder). Likewise, acetylcholine released from the electric organ of fishes or from the amphibian neuromuscular junction has been shown in electrophysiological studies to be inhibited by ω-conotoxin GVIA (22, 23, 47). Obviously, release experiments have contributed to our present knowledge about the role of different presynaptic calcium channels; particularly, at the endings of the phrenic nerve at least four different calcium channels have been described (46). It is understood that the different calcium channels must be characterized on the basis of both their electrical and pharmacological properties; neurotoxins have contributed considerably to the characterization of calcium channels critically involved in the regulation of acetylcholine release at different parts of the nervous system. The calcium influx through different channels appears to serve as a basic mechanism by which neuronal communication, adaptation, and regulation can be differentially controlled by one cation.

Comparison to Other Transmitters

A dominant role of N-type calcium channels in regulating the stimulated noradrenaline release from the central and peripheral nervous system has been repeatedly shown (28, 48–50), whereas adrenomedullary secretion is dominantly regulated by L-type calcium channels (51). Release of dopamine from striatal slices is also inhibited by ω-conotoxin GVIA, i.e., controlled by N-type calcium channels (52); similar results have been obtained with vasopressin released from the isolated hypophysis (53) and with excitatory amino acid transmitters released from hippocampal neurons (54); particularly, single-channel recordings in isolated hypophyseal neurosecretosomes (nerve endings) have revealed evidence for the existence of N- and L-type calcium channels (55). However, the release of other peptides, such as substance P and vasoactive intestinal polypeptide, appears insensitive to ω-conotoxin (25, 56), whereas the release of serotonin from the enterochromaffin cells was inhibited by both ω-conotoxin GVIA and nifedipine (57). Thus, a large degree of heterogeneity appears to exist among different neurons and secreting cells, and the distinction between different calcium channels or channel subtypes is regarded as an important aim for further research. In the future, the possibility of modulating neuronal and nonneuronal cell activity by subtype-specific calcium channel antagonists or agonists will enlarge the area for therapeutic intervention.

Conclusion

Release of radioactive acetylcholine from the brain, postganglionic autonomic neurons, and the motor nerve can be measured by a radiolabeling technique in the presence of active acetylcholinesterase. This method allows the pharmacological characterization of calcium channels critically involved in the regulation of transmitter release, while at the same time possible postsynaptic effects of calcium channel antagonists do not interfere with the detection method. ω-Conotoxin GVIA inhibited acetylcholine release evoked from the brain and postganglionic autonomic neurons but not that evoked from the motor nerve. N-Type calcium channels control the stimulated release of acetylcholine in the brain and the autonomic nervous system (postganglionic), whereas the corresponding calcium channel(s) at motor nerve terminals have not yet been characterized. Motor nerve terminals are, however, endowed with N-type calcium channels, and facilitatory β_1 receptors are coupled directly or indirectly to these channels. The release studies show, in excellent agreement with functional studies, the stimulated release of both classical transmitters acetylcholine and noradrenaline from the mammalian peripheral autonomic nervous system to be controlled by N-type calcium channels. The opening of different calcium channels having a very particular sphere of influence at the soma and at the terminal is regarded as a discriminative property of communicating neurons.

References

1. M. J. Berridge, *Annu. Rev. Biochem.* **56,** 159 (1987).
2. R. J. Miller, *Science* **235,** 46 (1987).
3. R. W. Tsien, D. Lipscombe, D. V. Madison, K. R. Bley, and A. P. Fox, *Trends NeuroSci.* **11,** 431 (1988).
4. R. Llinás, M. Sugimori, J.-W. Lin, and B. Cherksey, *Proc. Natl. Acad. Sci. U.S.A.* **86,** 1689 (1989).
5. E. Carbone and H. D. Lux, *Pfluegers Arch.* **413,** 14 (1988).
6. B. M. Olivera, J. M. McIntosh, L. J. Cruz, F. A. Luque, and W. R. Gray, *Biochemistry* **23,** 5087 (1984).
7. B. M. Olivera, W. R. Gray, R. Zeikus, J. M. McIntosh, J. Varga, J. Rivier, V. de Santos, and L. J. Cruz, *Science* **230,** 1338 (1985).
8. B. M. Olivera, L. J. Cruz, V. de Santos, G. W. LeCheminant, D. Griffin, R. Zeikus, J. M. McIntosh, R. Galyean, J. Varga, W. R. Gray, and J. Rivier, *Biochemistry* **26,** 2086 (1987).
9. J. Rivier, R. Galyean, W. R. Gray, A. Azimi-Zonooz, J. M. McIntosh, L. J. Cruz, and B. M. Olivera, *J. Biol. Chem.* **262,** 1194 (1987).
10. L. J. Cruz and B. M. Olivera, *J. Biol. Chem.* **261,** 6230 (1986).
11. E. W. McCleskey, A. P. Fox, D. H. Feldman, L. J. Cruz, B. M. Olivera, R. W. Tsien, and D. Yoshikami, *Proc. Natl. Acad. Sci. U.S.A.* **84,** 4327 (1987).
12. G. R. Seabrook and D. J. Adams, *Br. J. Pharmacol.* **97,** 1125 (1989).
13. T. Abe, K. Koyano, H. Saisu, Y. Nishiuchi, and S. Sakakibara, *Neurosci. Lett.* **71,** 203 (1986).
14. L. J. Cruz, D. S. Johnson, and B. M. Olivera, *Biochemistry* **26,** 820 (1987).
15. J. A. Wagner, A. M. Snowman, A. Biswas, B. M. Olivera, and S. H. Snyder, *J. Neurosci.* **8,** 3354 (1988).
16. M. Takemura, H. Kiyama, H. Fukui, M. Tohyama, and H. Wada, *Neuroscience* **32,** 405 (1989).
17. E. Sher, A. Pandiella, and F. Clementi, *FEBS Lett.* **235,** 178 (1988).
18. B. Marqueze, N. Martin-Moutot, C. Levêque, and F. Couraud, *Mol. Pharmacol.* **34,** 87 (1988).
19. J. J. Ballesta, M. Palmero, M. J. Hidalgo, L. M. Gutierrez, J. A. Reig, S. Viniegra, and A. G. Garcia, *J. Neurochem.* **53,** 1050 (1989).
20. L. J. Cruz, D. S. Johnson, J. S. Imperial, D. Griffin, G. W. LeCheminant, G. P. Miljanich, and B. M. Olivera, *Curr. Top. Membr. Transp.* **33,** 417 (1988).
21. L. M. Kerr and D. Yoshikami, *Nature* (*London*) **308,** 282 (1984).
22. K. Sano, K. Enomoto, and T. Maeno, *Eur. J. Pharmacol.* **141,** 235 (1987).
23. K. Koyano, T. Abe, Y. Nishiuchi, and S. Sakakibara, *Eur. J. Pharmacol.* **135,** 337 (1987).

24. A. J. Anderson and A. L. Harvey, *Neurosci. Lett.* **82,** 177 (1987).
25. C. A. Maggi, R. Patacchini, P. Santicioli, I. T. Lippe, S. Giuliani, P. Geppetti, E. Del Bianco, S. Selleri, and A. Meli, *Naunyn-Schmiedeberg's Arch. Pharmacol.* **338,** 107 (1988).
26. P. M. Lundy and R. Frew, *Eur. J. Pharmacol.* **156,** 325 (1988).
27. S. Ichida, H. Oka, A. Masada, T. Fujisue, T. Hata, and N. Matsuda, *Jpn. J. Pharmacol.* **48,** 395 (1988).
28. D. Pruneau and J. A. Angus, *Br. J. Pharmacol.* **100,** 180 (1990).
29. H. Kilbinger and I. Wessler, *Neuroscience* **5,** 1331 (1980).
30. I. Wessler and H. Kilbinger, *Naunyn-Schmiedeberg's Arch. Pharmacol.* **334,** 357 (1986).
31. I. Wessler and J. Werhand, *Naunyn-Schmiedeberg's Arch. Pharmacol.* **341,** 510 (1990).
32. I. Wessler and O. Steinlein, *Neuroscience* **22,** 289 (1987).
33. I. Wessler, *Trends Pharmacol. Sci.* **10,** 110 (1989).
34. I. W. Richardson and J. C. Szerb, *Br. J. Pharmacol.* **52,** 499 (1974).
35. I. Wessler, D. J. Dooley, J. Werhand, and F. Schlemmer, *Naunyn-Schmiedeberg's Arch. Pharmacol.* **341,** 288 (1990).
36. I. Wessler and J. Sandmann, *Naunyn-Schmiedeberg's Arch. Pharmacol.* **335,** 231 (1987).
37. I. von Schwarzenfeld, *Neuroscience* **4,** 477 (1979).
38. S. Luz, I. Pinchasi, and D. M. Michaelson, *J. Neurochem.* **45,** 43 (1985).
39. K. Starke, L. Späth, and T. Wichmann, *Naunyn-Schmiedeberg's Arch. Pharmacol.* **325,** 124 (1984).
40. J. D. Wood, *in* "Integrative Functions of the Autonomic Nervous System" (C. Brooks, K. Koizumi, and A. Sato, eds.), p. 177. Univ. of Tokyo Press, Tokyo, 1979.
41. J. D. Wood, *Annu. Rev. Physiol.* **43,** 33 (1981).
42. M. E. Adams, V. P. Bindokas, L. Hasegawa, and V. J. Venema, *J. Biol. Chem.* **265,** 861 (1990).
43. W. C. Bowman, *Handb. Exp. Pharmacol.* **54,** 47 (1981).
44. I. Wessler and A. Anschütz, *Br. J. Pharmacol.* **94,** 669 (1988).
45. I. Wessler, E. Ladwein, and E. Szrama, *Eur. J. Pharmacol.* **174,** 77 (1989).
46. I. Wessler, D. J. Dooley, H. Osswald, and F. Schlemmer, *Neurosci. Lett.* **108,** 173 (1990).
47. S. N. Ahmad and G. P. Miljanich, *Brain Res.* **453,** 247 (1988).
48. D. J. Dooley, A. Lupp, and G. Hertting, *Naunyn-Schmiedeberg's Arch. Pharmacol.* **336,** 467 (1987).
49. L. D. Hirning, A. P. Fox, E. W. McCleskey, B. M. Olivera, S. A. Thayer, R. J. Miller, and R. W. Tsien, *Science* **239,** 57 (1988).
50. B. Clasbrummel, H. Osswald, and P. Illes, *Br. J. Pharmacol.* **96,** 101 (1989).
51. C. R. Artalejo, M. G. López, C. F. Castillo, M. A. Moro, and A. G. Garcia, *in* "The Calcium Channel: Structure, Function and Implications" (M. Morad, W. G. Nayler, S. Kazda, and M. Schramm, eds.), p. 347. Springer-Verlag, Berlin, 1988.

52. H. Herdon and S. R. Nahorski, *Naunyn-Schmiedeberg's Arch. Pharmacol.* **340,** 36 (1989).
53. G. Dayanithi, N. Martin-Moutot, S. Barlier, D. A. Colin, M. Kretz-Zaepfel, F. Couraud, and J. J. Nordmann, *Biochem. Biophys. Res. Commun.* **156,** 255 (1988).
54. D. M. Finch, R. S. Fisher, and M. B. Jackson, *Brain Res.* **518,** 257 (1990).
55. J. R. Lemos and M. C. Nowycky, *Neuron* **2,** 1419 (1989).
56. J. L. Martin and P. J. Magistretti, *Neuroscience* **30,** 423 (1989).
57. H. H. Schwörer, A. Reimann, and K. Racké, *J. Physiol. (London),* Cambridge Meeting (1991), in press (abstr.).

[9]   Capsaicin: A Probe for Studying Specific Neuronal Populations in Brain and Retina

Sue Ritter and Thu T. Dinh

Introduction

Peripheral Actions

Capsaicin (8-methyl-*N*-vanillyl-6-nonenamide), the pungent principle in hot peppers, is a valuable tool in neurobiology because it selectively stimulates and damages primary somato- and viscerosensory neurons possessing fine caliber, unmyelinated afferent processes (C fibers). An extensive recent literature testifies to the emerging role of capsaicin in defining the anatomy and function of specific sensory subsystems that could not otherwise be independently investigated due to their anatomical intermingling with other elements of the peripheral nervous system. The directions and results of this work have been summarized in a number of excellent and comprehensive review articles (1–6).

Neurotoxicity of Capsaicin in Brain and Retina

Until recently the neurotoxicity of capsaicin was thought to be limited to primary sensory neurons. Nevertheless, results from several studies suggested that capsaicin also has central effects (7–14). Recently, we examined this possibility using a cupric–silver stain (15) for labeling degenerating neurons. We discovered that, contrary to the general belief, systemic administration of capsaicin does cause degeneration of nerve terminals at specific sites along the entire neuraxis. Some of these sites are not known to be innervated by primary sensory neurons. In addition, some cell bodies intrinsic to the brain are destroyed by capsaicin. Capsaicin-induced degeneration in the brain is not diffuse. Rather, it is consistently and reproducibly localized in specific nuclei or subnuclei. Capsaicin causes degeneration in adult rats (16) and in rat pups (17), although age-related differences are observed. The loss of cell bodies and terminals appears to be permanent since no degeneration is present in capsaicin-treated rats given a second capsaicin dose 9 months after the initial treatment.

Methods in Neurosciences, Volume 8

In addition to the degeneration in the brain itself, capsaicin also causes degeneration of subpopulations of retinal bipolar and ganglion cell bodies. Ganglion cells destroyed by capsaicin appear to be a subset of those projecting to the suprachiasmatic nucleus, the magnocellular portion of the ventrolateral geniculate nucleus, the intergeniculate leaflet, and the medial pretectal and olivary pretectal nuclei. Prior unilateral ocular enucleation reduces or eliminates capsaicin-induced degeneration in these sites. Other retinofugal projections, notably the remaining pretectal and tectal and the dorsolateral geniculate projections, are not affected by capsaicin (18).

Our results indicate that capsaicin may be a valuable tool for chemical dissection of highly specific neural subsystems within the brain and retina. This chapter will emphasize procedures we have found useful in our investigation of the central effects of capsaicin in rats, the only species in which the central effects of capsaicin have been investigated.

Capsaicin Administration

Hazards to Investigators

Avoid inhaling capsaicin powder or getting it into the eyes, as this will cause extreme discomfort or choking. Wear gloves when handling capsaicin or solutions containing it and use Luer-lock syringes for capsaicin injections. Accidental contamination is easier to avoid if the capsaicin is in liquid form. A stock solution can be made in the vendor bottle by addition of a known volume of the desired solvent [ethanol or dimethyl sulfoxide (DMSO)] to the capsaicin powder.

Forms of Capsaicin

Capsaicin and dihydrocapsaicin together constitute 90% or more of the total pungent principle of hot peppers (19, 20). Commercial preparations containing various ratios and purities of capsaicin and dihydrocapsaicin are available. In addition, a number of capsaicin analogs have been synthesized and screened for their neural toxicity (21), their ability to release substance P or other peptides from spinal cord (22, 23), their pain-producing properties (24), and desensitizing actions (25). Our work has been done with preparations containing 80–98% capsaicin or 90% dihydrocapsaicin.

Systemic Treatment

Capsaicin Dose and Route of Administration

Intraperitoneal injection is usually the preferred route for administration for high systemic doses of capsaicin to adult rats. However, subcutaneous administration is also effective and may be more convenient for treatment of rat pups. To produce neurotoxic effects by these routes, capsaicin is usually administered in the milligram per kilogram range (10–100 mg/kg). Lethality is much greater with intravenous rather than with subcutaneous or intraperitoneal capsaicin injections; intravenous injection is generally reserved for studies examining acute stimulatory effects of capsaicin, which require much lower doses (in the microgram per kilogram range).

When the experimental protocol permits, the total capsaicin dose can be divided and administered in a series of increasing doses spaced over a 24–48 hr (or longer) period. A typical series would be 10, 25, 50, and 50 mg/kg capsaicin [intraperitoneal (ip)]. The desensitization (see Acute Reactions, below) that occurs with the initial lower doses improves survival following the injection of the higher doses and allows a higher total dose to be administered. It is not known whether the total dose or the highest dose administered in a series is most important in determining the amount of capsaicin-induced neurotoxicity.

Injection Vehicle

Capsaicin is nearly insoluble in water. For subcutaneous or intraperitoneal administration a typical injection vehicle is 10% (v/v) ethanol and 10% (v/v) Tween 80 in 0.9% (w/v) saline. Capsaicin can also be mixed with DMSO to which an equal volume of saline is added immediately before injection. Typically, we calculate the injection volumes so that the desired dose can be injected in a volume of 0.1–0.2 ml/100 mg of body weight. Toxic reactions to capsaicin, as assessed behaviorally or with the cupric–silver stain, appear to be similar with both injection vehicles. However, we prefer ethanol/Tween 80 as a vehicle because it produces a more homogeneous and physically stable suspension than DMSO.

Anesthesia

Capsaicin injections are potentially painful and produce physiological reactions necessitating respiratory assistance during the immediate postinjection period. Therefore, animals must be anesthetized during the injection and for the duration of the acute postinjection effects. Anesthesia must be used for both systemic and local capsaicin treatments. When treating adult rats, it may be helpful to atropinize animals prior to treatment to reduce respiratory tract secretions (2 mg, 30–60 min before capsaicin injection). Atropine is not required for rat pups, and may interfere with suckling. We prefer the inhalation anesthetic, methoxyflurane (Metofane; Pitman Moore, Mundelein, IL), because it provides excellent analgesia and better control of anesthetic depth than do injectable anesthetic agents. Anesthesia is induced initially by placing the rat in a covered jar containing gauze pads moistened with anesthetic liquid. To maintain the desired anesthetic level during and after capsaicin treatment, anesthetic is administered through a nose cone containing a gauze pad moistened with Metofane and positioned so that the rat breathes a combination of room air and anesthetic vapor. Utilization of a fume hood is recommended with inhalation anesthetics such as methoxyflurane.

Acute Reactions

Immediately after systemic capsaicin injection rats will display a characteristic series of reactions, including laryngeal spasms, apnea, and cutaneous vasodilation, resulting in intense reddening of the ears, nose, tongue, and feet. Deaths following capsaicin treatment appear to be largely due to respiratory arrest. However, deaths from this cause can usually be avoided by careful attention to the animal. Unless an endotracheal tube has been positioned prior to capsaicin injection, laryngospasm may prevent artificial ventilation during the initial apneic phase. Rats must be carefully watched while apneic for the first sign of cyanosis. At this point, the larynx relaxes and rats can be given positive pressure ventilation with an external breathing tube positioned over the nose and mouth. Following the initial respiratory crisis, rats must be carefully watched for about an hour in case apneic episodes recur.

Activation of vagal circuits plays an important role in the acute apneic and cardiac responses to capsaicin (26, 27). These responses also occur after fourth ventricular injections of systemically ineffectual capsaicin doses, presumably due to direct activation of vagal sensory nerve endings in the nucleus of the solitary tract (see Local Administration of Capsaicin in Central Nervous System) (28).

Systemic reactions are diminished and often disappear with repeated dosings, suggesting that they are initiated by capsaicin-induced activation of sensory neurons that subsequently degenerate or are "desensitized" by other mechanisms. The relative contributions of neuronal degeneration, peptide depletion, and other transient mechanisms of desensitization to loss of capsaicin responsivity are not known. However, there is some evidence to suggest that desensitization may involve mechanisms additional to those producing capsaicin-induced degeneration (25, 29). Desensitization is the basis for the common practice of administering capsaicin in a graded series of injections, as described in Capsaicin Dose and Route of Administration (above).

Delayed Side Effects

Capsaicin-treated rats maintain normal body weights under standard laboratory conditions and are remarkably healthy. However, two delayed side effects may occur. These are corneal ulceration and scarring (30) and patchy hair loss, especially behind the ears (31). Animals may irritate these areas during grooming due to loss of corneal and cutaneous pain sensation. However, loss of C-fiber innervation also contributes in other ways to the development of these lesions. Skin and corneal lesions occur most frequently, but in our experience not exclusively, in rats treated with capsaicin as neonates. Corneal ulcers should be treated with an antibiotic ophthalmic ointment, whereas the skin lesions are usually self-limiting and heal spontaneously.

Age of Treatment

The greater sensitivity of somatosensory C fibers to capsaicin in rat pups compared to adult rats has been repeatedly noted (2). Our studies clearly indicate that the central effects of capsaicin are also age related. Using silver stains we compared the degeneration observed in the brains of rats injected systemically with capsaicin at 10, 15, 20, 25, 30, or 75 days, or 11 months of age (32). We found that capsaicin-induced degeneration does not differ between the two adult age groups (75 days and 11 months). However, there are major differences in both the amount and distribution of capsaicin-induced degeneration seen in rat pups 30 days old or less compared to the adults. At sites where capsaicin caused degeneration in both rat pups and adults, the amount of degeneration is typically greater in pups. In addition, there are a number of brain sites in which degeneration is present until 30 days, but is totally absent in adults (Fig. 1). Finally, in some brain regions capsaicin sensitivity is lost between 10 and 30 days of age. Thus, loss of capsaicin sensitivity is not progressive throughout the life of the animal but reflects the influence of developmental factors. Loss of sensitivity occurs with a discrete time course that may be different for different brain sites. Whatever the mechanism for these changes, our experience to date is that even very high capsaicin doses in adults do not cause degeneration in brain areas where sensitivity is lost during development.

Clearly, age at time of treatment is an important factor in studies of central capsaicin effects. Age at time of capsaicin administration must be carefully controlled for uniformity of effect, especially when treating rat pups. In addition, the strategic placing of capsaicin treatments at different ages may be a useful approach for functional dissection of various capsaicin-sensitive systems. Finally, the changing sensitivity to capsaicin of certain projections within the brain suggests that capsaicin may be useful in the study of normal developmental events in these systems.

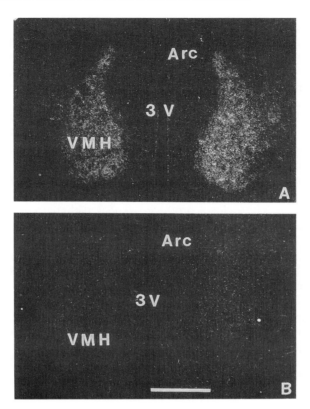

Fig. 1 Dark-field photomicrographs of cupric–silver stained brain sections (horizontal plane) showing ventromedial hypothalamic nucleus (VMH) of a 20-day-old rat (A) and an 80-day-old rat (B). Rats were treated systemically with capsaicin (100 mg/kg) and sacrificed 6 and 18 hr (respectively) later. The postcapsaicin survival times were chosen for rats of each age to coincide with the time of maximal argyrophilia. Significant capsaicin-induced degeneration is present in the VMH at 20 days of age, but none is present in the VMH of the adult rat. Bar: 400 μm. Arc, Arcuate nucleus; 3V, third ventricle.

Local Administration of Capsaicin in Central Nervous System

In the peripheral nervous system, neurons damaged by systemic capsaicin are also susceptible to damage by local capsaicin administration (1–6). This also appears to be the case with central capsaicin administration. Although the number of studies using local capsaicin injections within the brain or spinal cord is still small, results indicate that administration of capsaicin by intraventricular (28, 33), intracisternal (34), intraparenchymal (7, 11, 28), and intrathecal routes (22, 28) damages known capsaicin-sensitive terminals in the vicinity of the treatment. However, many questions regarding selectivity, duration, and localization of effect and influence of treatment age are still unanswered for local injections and must be assessed by the investigator.

For local injections capsaicin can be administered in either ethanol/Tween 80 or DMSO, as described for systemic treatment. South and Ritter (28) gave a total dose of 300 μg of capsaicin in the 50% (v/v) DMSO vehicle into the fourth ventricle using four separate doses (50 μg/5 μl, 100 μg/7.5 μl, 75 μg/5 μl, and 75 μg/5 μl) over a 50-hr period. For intrathecal injections a total dose of 300 μg was administered in four doses of 75 μg/7.5 μl over a 50-hr period. These doses produced expected changes in substance P-like immuno-reactivity and capsaicin-sensitive behaviors mediated by neurons in the vicinity of the treatments. For intraparenchymal injections in the region of the nucleus of the solitary tract and area postrema, 25 μg of capsaicin in 5 μl of vehicle (50% DMSO in 0.9% saline) was injected bilaterally at a rate of 1 μl/min or slower (9).

Our silver stain results indicate that when capsaicin is administered by intraventricular or intrathecal injection, the damage produced is selective for areas where capsaicin-induced damage is observed after systemic injections (Fig. 2A, A', B, and B'). However, the penetrance of capsaicin from a ventricular injection site into brain tissue may be very limited. After a single fourth ventricular injection of 40 μg of capsaicin damage was limited to the nucleus of the solitary tract and the spinal trigeminal nucleus. No degeneration was present in the inferior olivary nucleus, a capsaicin-sensitive site located more ventrally in the same rostrocaudal plane as the injection cannula. Lateral ventricular injection of 80 μg of capsaicin damaged only a small proportion of the capsaicin-sensitive terminals in the forebrain. Damaged terminals were restricted to the lateral septal nucleus and accumbens shell ipsilateral to the injection. In addition, the lateral ventricular capsaicin caused terminal degeneration in the nucleus of the solitary tract and spinal trigeminal nucleus, but the damage was very slight. In the nucleus of the solitary tract, damage was limited to an area on the ventricular floor just rostral to the area postrema (Fig. 2C). No degeneration was found in portions of the nucleus of the solitary tract ventral to the area postrema (Fig. 2C'). Intraparenchymal injections into the interpeduncular nucleus produced less damage in that structure than systemic capsaicin injections and vehicle effects appeared to account for a significant amount of the degeneration. Nevertheless, argyrophilia was relatively well localized to the known capsaicin-sensitive terminals in that area and to tissue damaged by cannula penetration.

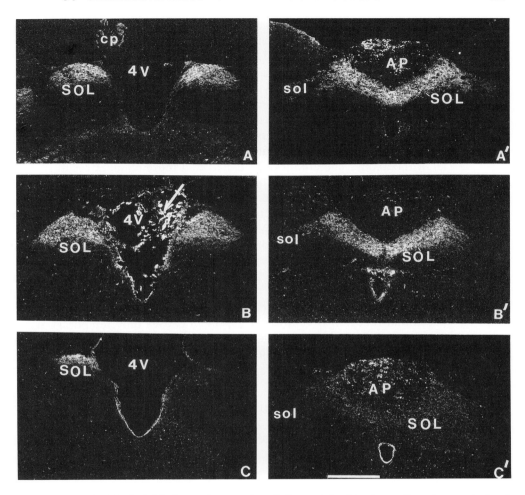

FIG. 2 Dark-field photomicrographs of silver-stained brain sections (coronal plane) showing two regions of the nucleus of the solitary tract (SOL, sol) from each of three capsaicin-treated rats. Rats were sacrificed 18 hr after capsaicin treatment. Degeneration induced by fourth ventricular (4V) capsaicin injection (40 μg) (B and B') was selective for areas also damaged by systemic capsaicin (75 mg/kg, ip) (A and A'). Injection of capsaicin (120 μg) into the lateral ventricle produced much less damage than 4V injection in this same area, despite the larger dose (C, C'). The arrow in (B) indicates disruption of the choroid plexus (cp) from cannula penetration. *Note:* silver precipitate is frequently trapped in the area postrema (A' and C') and choroid plexus (B), presumably due to the heavy vascularization or to poor adherence of these tissue areas to the slide. This artifact also occurs in controls. Bar: 400 μm. AP, Area postrema; sol, solitary tract; SOL, nucleus of the solitary tract.

Special attention must be given to vehicle effects when DMSO or ethanol vehicle is used for intraparenchymal, intrathecal, or intraventricular injections. Petsche *et al.* (35) found that the standard 10% ethanol, 10% Tween 80, and 80% saline blocked action potentials from both A and C fibers when applied directly to the rat coccygeal nerve. Caution should also be used with DMSO, which is frequently used as a 50% solution for capsaicin administration. Donoso *et al.* (36) reported that a 5% concentration of DMSO applied directly to the cat cervical vagus nerve blocked fast axoplasmic transport in many axons and a 10% concentration blocked fast axoplasmic transport in all of the axons. The authors speculated that these changes result from the effect of DMSO on polymerization of microtubules. Dimethyl sulfoxide also caused complex changes in the size of unmyelinated vagal axons. Because of the potential for vehicle effects, we advocate the use of the lowest possible vehicle concentration for central administration.

Whether central capsaicin administration is capable of producing permanent deficits is not known. The potential for recovery would depend in part on the severity of damage, if any, to the cell bodies of affected nerve terminals and there is no direct evidence on this point. In one of the few experiments to examine the time course of centrally produced deficits, South and Ritter (28) found that fourth ventricular capsaicin causes only temporary deficits (persisting 2–3 months) in cholecystokinin-induced suppression of feeding. In contrast, intraperitoneal injections produce permanent deficits in this vagally mediated behavioral response.

Assessment of Effects of Capsaicin

With all methods of capsaicin administration it is important to include in the experimental protocol physiological or histological tests of treatment efficacy that are independent of the response being measured. Verification of the effects of capsaicin is important for several reasons. In the first place, commercial preparations may vary in potency. In our work we have observed considerable variability between capsaicin preparations, especially with regard to behavioral indices of toxicity. In some cases the variability was traced to poor quality control by the supplier. In other cases, the causes were obscure. Differences in animal sensitivity to capsaicin (e.g., due to age or strain differences) and the potential for recovery are also important reasons to verify the effect of capsaicin within any experimental protocol. Several methods for assessing the toxicity of capsaicin will be discussed. In assessing capsaicin toxicity, it is important to keep in mind that the sensitivity of particular populations of neurons to capsaicin may differ. Thus, the degree of damage assessed in one capsaicin-sensitive system may not ensure that damage to another system has occurred.

Behavioral and Physiological Screening Tests

The occurrence of acute effects after capsaicin injection provides some assurance of drug efficacy. However, it is quite clear that these immediate responses are due in large part to the stimulatory effects of capsaicin and are not necessarily correlated with the extensiveness of C-fiber damage or central nerve terminal degeneration from a particular capsaicin dose. When capsaicin-treated rats are scheduled for long-term studies, we therefore advocate the use of screening tests to assess the effect of the capsaicin treatment on different C-fiber populations. Use of one such test before and after the main experiments can provide an estimate of the initial deficit and an assessment of possible recovery during the testing period.

Suppression of feeding by cholecystokinin (CCK) is dependent on capsaicin-sensitive sensory neurons (37) with fibers traveling primarily in the gastric branches of the vagus nerve (38). Therefore, CCK-induced suppression of feeding is a convenient screening test for capsaicin-induced damage to visceral C-fiber afferents. In controls, CCK (1–2 μg/kg, ip) suppresses food intake 50–90%, depending on dose. In rats with capsaicin-induced damage to vagal sensory fibers, CCK suppresses intake less or not at all (37).

A benign and very sensitive test for capsaicin-induced damage to trigeminal C-fiber afferents is the corneal chemosensory response (24, 39). Deficits can be assessed by instilling a drop of 1% (v/v) ammonium hydroxide (1 ml 30% concentrated ammonium hydroxide solution in 99 ml doubly distilled water) or another mild irritant onto the corneal surface of the eye of capsaicin-treated and vehicle-treated rats (28). The normal response to this stimulus is a brief (less than 15 sec) wiping of the eye with the forepaw. Rats with capsaicin-induced damage of the afferent limb of this reflex will exhibit a deficient wiping response or no response. Both eyes should be tested. The hot plate test for thermal nociception has also been used by some investigators to assess somatosensory C-fiber damage (40), but is less reliable as a screening test than the corneal chemosensory response. Finally, in acute anesthetized preparations, the selective diminution of the C-fiber component of the compound action potential in a peripheral nerve can be used as an index of the damage of capsaicin to somatosensory C fibers (35, 41).

Histological Approaches

Silver Impregnation Techniques

Silver stains are still the major light microscopic procedure for direct demonstration of neuronal degeneration. They are based on the fact that degenerating neurons become argyrophilic. In order for these stains to be useful, however, it is critical to sacrifice animals when neuronal degeneration is occurring and before phagocytosis of degenerating neural elements occurs. Although silver stains may be difficult to use for a number of reasons, they seem to be ideally suited for the study of capsaicin-induced degeneration in the brain. Systemically administered capsaicin appears to damage neurons along their entire extent, resulting in simultaneous degeneration of all portions of the neuron. Therefore, soma, axon, and terminal degeneration can be observed over the same time course and potentially in the same tissue sections. In addition, capsaicin-sensitive neurons found in various brain regions appear to undergo degeneration at similar rates. Finally, capsaicin-induced argyrophilia is clearly visible in nerve terminals, despite their small caliber, because these terminals are concentrated within specific brain loci.

A number of specific staining protocols can be used to study capsaicin-induced degeneration in the central nervous system. Jancso and Kiraly (42) used the Fink–Heimer (43) silver stain to demonstrate degeneration of primary sensory nerve terminals in the central nervous system. Our preference is for the Carlsen–de Olmos (15) cupric–silver stain. An advantage of the cupric–silver technique is that it produces excellent staining of all portions of the degenerating neuron: nerve terminals, soma, and processes. In addition, silver impregnation of normal tissue is minimal. Thus, degenerating neurons appear black against a nearly clear background of normal tissue. We modified the technique slightly by staining slide-mounted, as opposed to floating, sections. This improves the quality of the tissue and reduces staining artifact. The absence of background staining and artifact enhances the visibility of small-caliber terminals and permits high-quality dark-field photomicrographs. In our experience, once sources of artifact were identified and eliminated, the cupric–silver stain has yielded highly reproducible results. For aid in anatomical localization, selected sections can be counterstained with thionin without loss of silver grains or suitability of the section for dark-field photomicrography. The cupric–silver technique has been an invaluable tool for investigating the central effects of capsaicin. For this reason, a protocol for this stain is included at the end of this section.

A second silver stain we have found useful is the Gallyas (44) procedure. With this stain, the normal neural tissue is light brown and the degenerating neurons are darker brown or black. Because of the darker background staining, the Gallyas procedure at times produces ambiguous results and there is a risk that the very fine capsaicin-sensitive terminals might be missed. For the same reason, the degenerating neural elements are not as easily distinguishable in black-and-white photomicrographs as with the cupric–silver stain. Nevertheless, the background staining in the Gallyas procedure facilitates recognition of anatomical landmarks and cytomorphology. In addition, the Gallyas stain is simpler, less time consuming, and less expensive (since it uses less silver nitrate) than the cupric–silver stain.

We have examined the brain with silver stains at intervals between 2 hr and 1 month and the retina between 2 and 48 hr after systemic capsaicin. Capsaicin-induced degeneration and subsequent phagocytosis of neurons in brain, retina, and peripheral nervous system are remarkably rapid. For rat pups, argyrophilia can be observed by about 2 hr after systemic capsaicin injection and is maximal 6–8 hr postinjection. By 18–24 hr after capsaicin, very little evidence of degeneration can be observed. In adult rats, the maximum argyrophilic response occurs between 12 and 18 hr after capsaicin but diminishes rapidly thereafter. Very little staining is present at survival times longer than 24 hr. Therefore, when using silver stains to evaluate capsaicin-induced degeneration, the timing of posttreatment survival must be very precise due to the very rapid progression of the degeneration and phagocytosis. Unless this is done, effects cannot be compared across animals or doses and might even be missed altogether. For the same reasons, the entire dose of capsaicin must be administered in a single injection to see the fullest effect of the treatment with silver stains.

Electron Microscopy

Capsaicin-induced degeneration has been studied using electron microscopic techniques in the spinal cord dorsal horn, the dorsal root ganglion, the nucleus of the solitary tract, and various peripheral nerves and terminal organs (45–47). Recently we examined several areas of the central nervous system in which capsaicin-induced degeneration has been observed with the silver stain, including the nucleus of the solitary tract (NTS) and retina. For brain, the desired areas were dissected from vibratome sections under the microscope. It is clear that in these areas capsaicin leads to rapid condensation of intracellular organelles and ultimately necrosis of the entire terminal, axonal or dendritic processes, or perikarya. Capsaicin treatment also results in rapid infiltration of microglia and appearance of numerous phagocytic profiles. In 20-day-old rat pups, these events are already apparent at 3 hr and quite advanced by 6 hr after systemic capsaicin treatment. A similar time course for appearance of capsaicin-induced degenerative changes was observed in electron microscope studies of the dorsal root ganglia (48).

Challenge Dose

Silver stain and electron microscopy are not useful for assessing capsaicin-induced damage in chronic experiments requiring survival periods exceeding the period of active neuronal degeneration immediately following drug administration. In such cases, we have used a "challenge dose" procedure. Rats are initially injected systemically with capsaicin or the injection vehicle (16). After a specified interval during which various physiological or behavioral tests might be conducted, half of the capsaicin-treated and half of the vehicle-treated rats are injected with the same capsaicin dose used in the initial treatment and the other half of each group are injected with the vehicle. If no degeneration is observed in the rats receiving their second (i.e., challenge) dose of capsaicin, this is interpreted as indicating that the neurons sensitive to that particular capsaicin dose were destroyed by the initial dose and did not recover. Conversely, degeneration in response to the challenge dose could indicate either that recovery had occurred or that the initial lesion was incomplete. The capsaicin–vehicle group is included to demonstrate that evidence of the first treatment is no longer visible at the time of the challenge dose. The vehicle–capsaicin group confirms the effectiveness of the capsaicin in capsaicin-naive rats of the same age and laboratory history as the challenged rats. The vehicle–vehicle group is simply a control for the stain. An additional group of capsaicin-treated rats is sacrificed after the initial treatment to verify its neurotoxicity.

Other Histological Tests of Efficacy

Transport of horseradish peroxidase (HRP) or retrograde tracers such as fluorogold (49) are also techniques that may be useful for assessing capsaicin-induced neuronal damage at long intervals after treatment. Horseradish peroxidase conjugated to cholera toxin (CT–HRP) or to lectins such as wheat germ agglutinin (WGA–HRP) is transported both retrogradely and anterogradely. When applied to the terminal areas of a mixed peripheral nerve, these conjugates can simultaneously demonstrate the effects of capsaicin on sensory neurons and the absence of its effect on motor neurons (50). We have found this procedure particularly useful in confirming capsaicin-induced damage to the vagus nerve after systemic injections or after local application to the vagal trunks. This nerve contains both sensory and motor fibers and the majority of sensory neurons contributing to the subdiaphragmatic vagus nerve in the rat are capsaicin sensitive. In vehicle-treated rats, injection of HRP into the stomach wall results in labeling of cell bodies in the dorsal motor nucleus of the vagus and sensory terminals in the nucleus of the solitary tract (Fig. 3A). In capsaicin-treated rats, vagal motor neurons are heavily labeled but very little labeling is evident in the nucleus of the solitary tract (Fig. 3B).

Although this general approach could be applied to systems other than the vagus, it is not useful for assessing degeneration in all systems. In the visual system, for example, loss of capsaicin-sensitive neurons cannot be easily

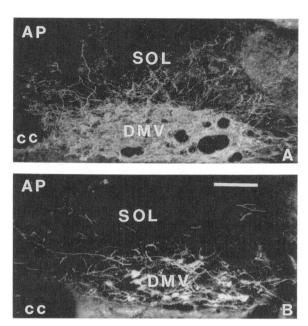

FIG. 3   Dark-field photomicrograph of coronal brain section showing cholera toxin conjugated to horseradish peroxidase (CT–HRP) in the dorsal motor nucleus of the vagus (DMV) and the nucleus of the solitary tract (SOL) 3 days after injection of a total dose of 100 μl CT–HRP [0.1% (w/v) solution] into eight loci in the stomach wall. The rat in (A) was treated intraperitoneally with the 10% ethanol/10% Tween 80 injection vehicle. The rat in (B) was treated with 75 mg/kg capsaicin. Capsaicin treatment greatly reduced labeling of terminals in SOL and DMV. In contrast, cell bodies of vagal motor neurons in the DMV contained significant amounts of CT-HRP, even after capsaicin treatment. Bar: 100 μm. cc, Central canal; AP, area postrema.

detected in retinofugal projections by this technique due to the profuse CT–HRP labeling of capsaicin-insensitive neurons (18). In the latter case, the results with CT–HRP were nevertheless useful in demonstrating that capsaicin damages only a subset of the total population of ganglion cells projecting to the particular subcortical nuclei under investigation.

Finally, receptor autoradiography or peptide immunohistochemistry could be used to assess capsaicin-induced degeneration in specific neuronal populations in the brain and spinal cord, or to assess penetrance of capsaicin into specific areas from a distant injection site as a means of defining localization of effect (28).

Protocol for Carlsen–de Olmos (15) Cupric–Silver Stain

Perfusion

After exsanguination of a deeply anesthetized rat, the rat is perfused by gravity flow through a 20-gauge needle inserted into the left cardiac ventricle. Reservoirs containing perfusion solutions are elevated 1.3 m to achieve a hydrostatic head approximating the arterial pressure. Perfusion of 100–200 ml of sodium phosphate-buffered saline (0.01 M) is followed by perfusion of approximately 200 ml of 4% (v/v) paraformaldehyde solution (see Solutions). The brain is removed and soaked in the paraformaldehyde solution for 3 or 4 days. The brain is then cryoprotected in a 30% sucrose solution made with 0.01 M sodium phosphate buffer diluted from stock with doubly distilled H_2O. The brain is refrigerated in the sucrose solution just until the brain sinks. Mounted cryostat sections are then prepared as described below.

Tissue Sections

Cryostat sections (10–40 μm thick) are cut at $-16°C$ and mounted directly on subbed slides. The mounting solution is applied to the subbed slide with a camel hair brush immediately before lifting the section from the knife blade. The sections are dried on the slide 3 hr to overnight before staining. Mounted sections are not postfixed. To do so causes a significant decrease in staining. Mounted sections can be stored for up to 1 week prior to staining, if care is taken to prevent dehydration of the tissue. Longer storage decreases the quality of the tissue and amount of staining.

Subbing Slides

Slides are loaded into slide carrier, soaked in chromic sulfuric acid for 5 min, and rinsed in tap water five times. They are then soaked in hot soapy water, rinsed with tap water to remove all soap, and, finally, rinsed twice in doubly distilled water. Slides are then dipped in freshly made subbing solution (see Solutions) and dried in a 37°C oven or overnight. Subbed slides may be stored about 1 month.

Acid Wash for Glassware and Plastics

We use white Tissue-Tek R II staining dishes (VWR Scientific, Philadelphia, PA). These require a volume of 170 ml of solution to stain 25 slides. Before staining, the glassware, staining dishes, and racks are cleaned with 1 M HNO_3 made in doubly distilled H_2O (1 min) and rinsed with doubly distilled H_2O (five times). Staining dishes and rack are then soaked in 1% (v/v) H_2O_2 for 1 min to prevent reduction of silver on the vessel walls. This is followed by three additional rinses in doubly distilled H_2O. Dishes and rack are left in the last rinse until ready to use. Nitric acid can be saved and reused about five times.

Solutions

Solutions are calculated for a 250-ml staining dish, where applicable.

> Paraformaldehyde: To 1 liter doubly distilled H_2O, add 40 g paraformaldehyde and 12.5 g Na_2HPO_4
>
> Chromic sulfuric acid: Combine 1800 ml sulfuric acid and 5 ml Chromerge (chromic sulfuric acid cleaning solution, J. T. Baker Chemical Co., Phillipsburg, NJ). Reuse until solution turns green
>
> Subbing solution [1% (w/v) gelatin, 0.1% (w/v) chrome alum]: To 1 liter doubly distilled H_2O, add 10 g gelatin (heated to dissolve). Then add 1 g chromium potassium sulfate (chrome alum)
>
> Mounting solution: Combine 1 ml subbing solution with 9 ml doubly distilled H_2O
>
> Concentrated (0.25 *M*) sodium phosphate buffer stock solution: Combine 30 g Na_2HPO_4 and 5.35 g $NaH_2PO_4 \cdot H_2O$ and bring to 1000 ml with doubly distilled H_2O. Store refrigerated up to 3 months
>
> Sodium phosphate-buffered saline (0.01 *M*, working solution): Combine 40 ml concentrated sodium phosphate buffer stock, 8.5 g NaCl, and 960 ml doubly distilled H_2O. Bring to pH 7.4 with HNO_3 or NaOH
>
> Boric acid/sodium tetraborate buffer (0.2 *M*): Bring 0.2 *M* boric acid (0.62 g in 50 ml doubly distilled H_2O) to pH 8.5 with 0.05 *M* sodium tetraborate (0.95 g sodium tetraborate in 50 ml doubly distilled H_2O). Store at room temperature 1–3 months
>
> Cupric–silver–allantoin: Combine, in the following sequence:
>
> > 166.5 ml doubly distilled H_2O
> > 11.4 mg allantoin
> > 3 ml boric acid/sodium tetraborate buffer, pH 7.5
> > 20.2 mg cupric nitrate
> > 1.2 g silver nitrate
> > 6.4 ml pure pyridine
>
> > Pour into washed container, wrap in aluminum foil, and place in 40°C water bath for 20–30 min before adding slides
>
> Ammoniacal silver: Dissolve 18 g silver nitrate completely in 97.65 ml doubly distilled H_2O; add
>
> > 47.7 ml 0.4% (w/v) sodium hydroxide (NaOH)
> > 19–21 ml concentrated ammonia hydroxide (30% w/v)
> > 4.5 ml acetone

Note: Add just enough ammonia to clear the solution. Ammonia may lose its potency over time, so the precise amount required may vary. This is a critical step since it determines the degree of silver impregnation. Too much ammonia prevents silver impregnation and too little can cause impregnation of normal tissue

Reducing Bath: Combine the following:

12 ml 10% (v/v) formalin
7 ml 1% (w/v) citric acid
100 ml 100% (v/v) ethanol
881 ml neutralized doubly distilled H_2O

Sodium thiosulfate: 250 ml of a 1.0% (w/v) solution
Potassium ferricyanide: 250 ml of a 0.5% (w/v) solution
Sodium hydroxide: 250 ml of a 0.4% (w/v) solution
Citric acid: 250 ml of a 1.0% (w/v) solution
Formalin (10%, v/v): Add 2 ml 37% commercial formaldehyde solution
to 18 ml doubly distilled H_2O

Preparation for Staining

Acid wash glassware and plastics. Turn on water bath to 40°C. Prepare 4 liters of neutralized doubly distilled H_2O, titrated to pH 7.0 with 1 M NaOH or 1 N HNO_3. Prepare fresh staining solutions. Except as noted, all solutions must be made just prior to use.

Staining Procedure

Transfer slide rack through the following solutions: doubly distilled H_2O (five changes, 1 min each); Cu–Ag–allantoin, 40°C (30 min, agitating); Cu–Ag–allantoin, 25°C (30 min, agitating); acetone (30 sec); ammoniacal silver (30 min); reducing bath 1 (one dip); reducing bath 2 (five dips); reducing bath 3 (10 min); reducing bath 4 (15 min); doubly distilled H_2O (five changes, 1 min each); 0.5% (w/v) potassium ferricyanide (3–20 min); doubly distilled H_2O (five changes, 1 min each); 1% (w/v) thiosulfate (1 min); doubly distilled H_2O (five changes, 1 min each); 80% (v/v) ethanol (1 min); 95% ethanol (1 min); isopropyl alcohol (2-propanol) (1 min); isopropyl (1 min); Histo-Clear (1 min); Histo-Clear (1 min–1 hr); coverslip.

Note: Bleaching occurs in the 0.5% potassium ferricyanide bath. The time required to produce the desired amount of bleaching must be determined empirically by visual inspection during the bleaching process. To decrease the rate of bleaching, decrease the concentration of potassium ferricyanide.

Prospectus

Capsaicin has provided a new window through which to discover the organization and basic biological functions of specific classes of somato- and viscerosensory neurons. The discovery of capsaicin-induced degeneration within the brain and retina should greatly extend the usefulness of this toxin for studies of neural function. Although much additional work is necessary to fully describe the effects of capsaicin on the brain and retina, work already begun predicts that the central effects of capsaicin will be especially useful in the characterization of subcortical visual pathways and functions (18), in parceling out the central and peripheral mechanisms and pathways for thermoregulatory responses to heat (10, 12, 13, 51), in the isolation of neural substrates monitoring nutrient availability in the interest of food intake (52, 53), and in examining integration of sensory signals in higher order neurons of brain and spinal cord (54). Finally, the molecular basis for the selective toxicity of capsaicin for specific central and peripheral neural subpopulations and the developmental events that alter sensitivity of certain neurons to capsaicin should be particularly fruitful areas of investigation.

References

1. N. Jancso, in "Pharmacology of Pain—Proceedings of the Third International Congress on Pharmacology" (R. K. S. Lim, ed.), p. 33. Pergamon, Oxford, England, 1968.
2. S. H. Buck and B. T. Burks, *Pharmacol. Rev.* **38,** 179 (1986).
3. Y. Monsereenusorn, K. Sathapana, and P. D. Pezalla, *CRC Crit. Rev. Toxicol.* **10,** 321 (1982).
4. P. Holzer, *Neuroscience* **24,** 739 (1988).
5. C. A. Maggi and A. Meli, *Gen. Pharmacol.* **19,** 1 (1988).
6. L. C. Russell and K. J. Burchiel, *Brain Res. Rev.* **8,** 165 (1984).
7. Y. Ishikawa, T. Nakayama, K. Kanosue, and K. Matsumura, *J. Therm. Biol.* **9,** 47 (1984).
8. A. E. Panerai, A. Martini, V. Locatelli, and P. Mantegazza, *Pharmacol. Res. Commun.* **15,** 825 (1983).
9. E. H. South and R. C. Ritter, *Brain Res.* **288,** 243 (1983).
10. M. Cormareche-Leydier, S. G. Shimada, and J. T. Stitt, *J. Physiol (London)* **363,** 227 (1985).
11. D. Dawbarn, A. J. Harmar, and C. J. Pycock, *Neuropharmacology* **20,** 341 (1981).
12. M. Hajos, F. Obal, Jr., G. Jancso, and F. Obal, *Neurosci. Lett.* **54,** 97 (1985).
13. M. Hajos, G. Engberg, H. Nissbrandt, T. Magnusson, and A. Carlsson, *J. Neural Transm.* **74,** 129 (1988).
14. J. Szolcsanyi, F. Joo, and A. Jancso-Gabor, *Nature (London)* **229,** 116 (1971).
15. J. Carlsen and J. S. de Olmos, *Brain Res.* **208,** 426 (1981).
16. S. Ritter and T. T. Dinh, *J. Comp. Neurol.* **271,** 79 (1988).
17. S. Ritter and T. T. Dinh, *J. Comp. Neurol.* **296,** 447 (1990).
18. S. Ritter and T. T. Dinh, *J. Comp. Neurol.* **308,** 79 (1991).
19. K. Iwai, T. Suzuki, and H. Fujiwake, *Agric. Biol. Chem.* **43,** 2493 (1979).
20. T. Suzuki, T. Kawada, and K. Iwai, *J. Chromatogr.* **198,** 217 (1980).

21. G. Jancso and E. Kiraly, *Brain Res.* **210,** 83 (1981).
22. K. Jhamandas, T. Yaksh, G. Hartz, J. Szolcsanyi, and V. Go, *Brain Res.* **306,** 215 (1984).
23. P. Micevych, T. Yaksh, and J. Szolcsanyi, *Neuroscience* **8,** 123 (1983).
24. J. Szolcsanyi, A. Jancso-Gabor, and F. Joo, *Naunyn-Schmiedeberg's Arch. Pharmacol.* **287,** 157 (1975).
25. J. Szolcsanyi and A. Jancso-Gabor, *Arzneim.-Forsch.* **26,** 33 (1976).
26. C. C. Toh, T. S. Lee, and A. K. Kiang, *J. Pharmacol.* **10,** 175 (1955).
27. J. Porszasz, G. Such, and K. Porszasz-Giviszer, *Acta Physiol. Acad. Sci. Hung., Suppl.* **12,** 189 (1957).
28. E. H. South and R. C. Ritter, *Peptides* **9,** 601 (1988).
29. J. Szolcsanyi and A. Jancso-Gabor, *Arzneim.-Forsch.* **25,** 1877 (1975).
30. T. Shimizu, K. Fujita, K. Izumi, T. Koja, N. Ohba, and T. Fukuda, *Naunyn-Schmiedeberg's Arch. Pharmacol.* **326,** 347 (1984).
31. R. Gamse, D. Lackner, G. Gamse, and S. Leeman, *Naunyn-Schmiedeberg's Arch. Pharmacol.* **316,** 38 (1982).
32. S. Ritter and T. Dinh, *J. Comp. Neurol.* (in press) (1991).
33. R. Gamse, S. E. Leeman, P. Holzer, and F. Lembeck, *Naunyn-Schmiedeberg's Arch. Pharmacol.* **317,** 140 (1981).
34. G. Jancso, *Neurosci. Lett.* **27,** 41 (1981).
35. U. Petsche, E. Fleischer, F. Lembeck, and H. O. Handwerker, *Brain Res.* **265,** 233 (1983).
36. J. A. Donoso, J.-P. Illanes, and F. Samson, *Brain Res.* **120,** 287 (1977).
37. R. C. Ritter and E. E. Ladenheim, *Am. J. Physiol.* **248,** R501 (1985).
38. G. P. Smith, C. Jerome, and R. Norgren, *Am. J. Physiol.* **249,** R638 (1985).
39. N. A. Jancso, A. Jancso-Gabor, and J. Szolcsanyi, *Br. J. Pharmacol. Chemother.* **31,** 138 (1967).
40. J. I. Nagy, S. R. Vincent, W. A. Staines, A. C. Fibiger, T. D. Reisine, and H. I. Yamamura, *Brain Res.* **186,** 435 (1980).
41. P. D. Wall, *J. Physiol. (London)* **329,** 21 (1982).
42. G. Jancso and E. Kiraly, *J. Comp. Neurol.* **190,** 781 (1980).
43. R. P. Fink and L. Heimer, *Brain Res.* **4,** 369 (1967).
44. F. Gallyas, J. R. Wolff, H. Bottcher, and L. Zaborszky, *Stain Technol.* **55,** 299 (1980).
45. G. Jancso, E. Kiraly, and A. Jancso-Gabor, *Nature (London)* **270,** 741 (1977).
46. J. W. Scadding, *J. Anat.* **131,** 473 (1980).
47. K. Chung, R. J. Schwen, and R. E. Coggeshall, *Neurosci. Lett.* **53,** 221 (1985).
48. G. Jancso, E. Kiraly, F. Joo, G. Such, and A. Nagy, *Neurosci. Lett.* **59,** 209 (1985).
49. T. L. Powley, E. A. Fox, and H.-R. Berthoud, *Am. J. Physiol.* **253,** R361 (1987).
50. R. E. Shapiro and R. R. Miselis, *J. Comp. Neurol.* **238,** 473 (1985).
51. J. Szolcsanyi, *Handb. Exp. Pharmacol.* **60,** 437 (1982).
52. S. Ritter and J. Taylor, *Am. J. Physiol.* **256,** R1232 (1991).
53. D. P. Yox and R. C. Ritter, *Am. J. Physiol.* **255,** R569 (1988).
54. R. C. Ritter, S. Ritter, W. R. Ewart, and D. L. Wingate, *Am. J. Physiol.* **257,** R1162 (1989).

[10]   Charybdotoxin in Study of Voltage-Dependent Potassium Channels

Maria L. Garcia, Margarita Garcia-Calvo, Jesus Vazquez, and Gregory J. Kaczorowski

Introduction

Ion channels are specialized integral membrane proteins that undergo conformational changes to allow transmembrane movement of ions through aqueous filled pores. Several different techniques have helped us to obtain a better understanding of how these proteins function. Biophysical methodologies, such as the patch-clamp technique, have allowed classification of channels into different types based on ion selectivity. Moreover, each group of ion-selective channels has been subdivided into different categories according to single-channel conductance, kinetics of activation and inactivation, and dependence of gating on membrane potential and/or ligand binding. Molecular biology techniques have given information on the amino acid sequence of various channel proteins, their localization in different tissues, and the role that specific residues play in channel function. Biochemical techniques have been used to identify specific receptor sites associated with channels through the use of high-affinity ligands. To be useful, such agents must not only display high affinity for the channel of interest, but also exhibit selectivity. They can then be employed in *in vitro* studies to assess the contribution of a particular channel protein in the physiology of a given tissue. For those channels where molecular biology techniques have failed to identify the species of interest, high-affinity ligands can also be used to aid in the purification of the channel to homogeneity, in order to obtain partial amino acid sequences from which to clone the target protein.

Charybdotoxin (ChTX) is a 37-amino acid basic peptide derived from the venom of the scorpion *Leiurus quinquestriatus* var. *hebraeus* (1). Charybdotoxin was originally described as a potent blocker of the high-conductance Ca^{2+}-activated K^+ channel [$P_{K,Ca}$ (2)]. Subsequently, it was shown that ChTX will also block other types of K^+ channels; namely, an inactivating voltage-dependent K^+ channel ($P_{K,V}$) that is present in rat brain and human T lymphocytes (3, 4). However, ChTX does not block other types of ion channels, including Na^+, Ca^{2+}, and many other members of the K^+ channel family (1, 3, 5).

The mechanism by which ChTX inhibits $P_{K,Ca}$ has been extensively studied using skeletal muscle t-tubule membranes incorporated into artificial lipid bilayers (6, 7). Charybdotoxin binds to the outer face of the channel to block the ion conduction pathway through an electrostatic mechanism that involves positive charges on the toxin molecule and negatively charged residues within the mouth of the channel. This electrostatic attraction mechanism also appears to be involved in the interaction of ChTX with $P_{K,V}$ in human T lymphocytes (4).

In the present article we will focus on methods developed in our laboratory for purification of ChTX to homogeneity and radiolabeling of toxin in order to produce a high specific activity derivative of toxin that retains biological activity. This agent has been used to characterize high-affinity receptor sites associated with two different types of K^+ channels.

Purification of Charybdotoxin

In order to employ ChTX in subsequent radiolabeling protocols, it is essential to obtain a homogeneous peptide preparation. This can be achieved by either of two different means: purification of toxin from a crude venom sample, or synthesis of the peptide using solid-phase methodologies, followed by oxidation of the hexasulfhydryl form to obtain biologically active material.

Several different laboratories have independently reported methods for the purification of ChTX from crude venom of the scorpion *L. quinquestriatus* var. *hebraeus* (1, 8–11). Because of its simplicity, reproducibility, and ability to achieve a homogeneous preparation of peptide, we will discuss the procedure developed in our laboratory (1). This procedure has been repeated many times, with different batches of venom, and has always produced identical results in terms of purity and total yield of toxin. In 1 day, starting with 100 mg of crude venom, it is possible to obtain 250 μg of purified ChTX.

Lyophilized venom from *L. quinquestriatus* var. *hebraeus* can be purchased from several different commercial sources. The first step in purification involves the use of a cation-exchange chromatographic step that takes advantage of the basic nature of ChTX. Venom, ca. 100 mg, is resuspended by vortexing in 20 mM sodium borate, pH 9.0, at a final protein concentration of 5 mg/ml. Due to the presence of much insoluble material, a nonhomogeneous suspension is obtained. This suspension is then subjected to centrifugation for 15 min at 27,000 g, and the soluble material is removed. Because the column employed in the first step is a Pharmacia (Piscataway, NJ) Mono S HR 5/5 fitted to a high-performance liquid chromatography (HPLC) system, the sample to be injected must be filtered through a Millex-GV 0.2-μm pore size filter (Millipore, Bedford, MA) in order to remove particulate material that could obstruct the system and increase the pressure of the column. In initial experiments, the pellet obtained after centrifugation was subjected to a second extraction with the sodium borate buffer. After centrifugation, the soluble material was treated as above, but after injection it was consistently noted that the pressure of the system would increase to the limit of the column. Since a second extraction did not significantly increase the final yield of ChTX, it is no longer performed, nor recommended.

Before injection of sample, the ion-exchange column is equilibrated with 20 mM sodium borate, pH 9.0, at a flow rate of 0.5 ml/min. After sample injection, there is a large amount of material absorbing at 280 nm that is not retained by the column. This material has no biological activity against the channels of interest and can be discarded. Once the absorbance returns to baseline values, the retained material is eluted with a linear gradient of NaCl (0.75 M/hr). The fraction containing the bulk of ChTX-like activity can be easily recognized as a major peak eluting at 320 mM NaCl. This fraction corresponds to the last major absorbance peak eluted during the gradient. This fraction can be stored at $-80°C$, or used immediately in the second and final purification step.

The final step of purification is accomplished with a C_{18} reversed-phase HPLC column (25×0.46 cm, 5-μm particle size; the Separations Group, Hesperia, CA). The column is equilibrated with 10 mM trifluoroacetic acid, and elution is achieved with a linear gradient (0–20%) of 2-propanol/acetonitrile (2 : 1), in 4 mM trifluoroacetic acid, at a flow rate of 0.5 ml/min applied over a 30-min period. Charybdotoxin can be distinguished as the first major absorbance peak, eluting at 9–10% organic solvent, and is easily separated from all other components of the Mono S fraction. It has been found that equilibration of the column in starting buffer, before sample injection, is critical. Failure to do this leads to lack of retention of ChTX by the column. If no retention of material on the column is observed, the column should be reequilibrated before sample reinjection.

Starting with 100 mg of crude venom, it is possible to obtain ca. 250 μg of purified ChTX. Because only minor amounts of toxin are needed for most experiments, ChTX can be lyophilized in small aliquots of ca. 20 μg, and stored at $-80°C$. Toxin stored in this way is stable for many months. When an aliquot of ChTX is needed, toxin is resuspended in any buffer of high ionic strength (i.e., 100 mM salt). Once resuspended, it can be stored at 4°C for several months without loss of biological activity. It is important to note that ChTX is a highly positively charged molecule that will stick to glass surfaces unless a high ionic strength buffer is used to prevent such an interaction. Therefore, if toxin is dried in a glass tube and water is used as the resuspension agent, it is likely that most of the toxin will be lost by absorption onto the surface of the tube. We do not subject the toxin solution to repetitive freeze–thaw cycles, and we have not checked such a procedure with regard to toxin stability.

In addition to the method described above for purification of ChTX, it has recently been possible to synthesize the peptide by solid-phase techniques and oxidize it to yield material that is indistinguishable from that purified from crude scorpion venom (12, 13). In this way, if access to a peptide synthesizer is convenient, large quantities of toxin can be prepared. In addition, a synthetic approach can be useful for obtaining different variants of ChTX, in which one or more amino acids are substituted, in order to determine those residues in the toxin molecule that are responsible for high-affinity binding to various target channels. The chemical synthesis of ChTX was also useful for confirming this peptide as the active component involved in channel-blocking activity, thus discarding the possibility that some minor contaminant in the ChTX preparation was responsible for that activity.

Iodination of Charybdotoxin

Charybdotoxin contains several amino acids that can be subjected to chemical modification in order to obtain radiolabeled derivatives of high specific activity. There are four lysine residues that are potential sites for reaction with a Bolton–Hunter reagent, as well as single tyrosine and histidine residues that could be iodinated. Since the goal of our investigation was to achieve a radiolabeled molecule that displays biological activity, modification at the lysine residues was not pursued because in initial studies all adducts obtained after HPLC purification were devoid of channel-blocking activity. This finding is not unexpected because it is well known that the positively charged residues of ChTX play an important role in the mechanism by which K^+ channels are inhibited (6, 7). Therefore, conditions were found under which the tyrosine residue can be iodinated and the monoiodotyrosine ChTX was purified and shown to retain its biological activity (14).

Iodination of ChTX at its tyrosine residue can be achieved by two methods. Using the Iodogen methodology, 0.5 μg of Iodogen (Pierce Chemical Co., Rockford, IL) prepared in acetone is dried under argon or nitrogen at the bottom of a Reacti-vial. Once dried, the vial is rinsed with buffer to remove any aqueous contaminants. Immediately, 10 μl of a solution containing ca. 5 μg of ChTX in 100 mM sodium phosphate, pH 7.3, is added, followed by the addition of 1 mCi of Na^{125}I (10 μl, 2000 Ci/mmol). After brief mixing, the capped vial is kept at room temperature for 15 min. One minute before injection onto a C_{18} reversed-phase HPLC column, the vial is open to the air, and then the iodination mixture is injected onto a column that has been equilibrated with 10 mM trifluoroacetic acid, at a flow rate of 0.5 ml/min. After washing for 20 min to remove any traces of unreacted iodine, elution of retained material can be achieved with a linear gradient (5–14%) of 2-propanol/acetonitrile (2 : 1), in 4 mM trifluoroacetic acid, applied over a 40-min period at a flow rate of 0.5 ml/ min. By following changes in absorbance at 210 nm, different peaks can be easily discerned and separated.

The results of a typical iodination are shown in the HPLC profile of Fig. 1. The major absorbance peak (A in Fig. 1) corresponds to unreacted toxin, while peak B represents monoiodotyrosine ChTX based on the specific activity of the radiolabeled peptide and on sequence analysis of the modified toxin. Other minor peaks are also present, although these are well separated from the one of interest. Even though they have not been analyzed in detail, because they do not display biological activity, peak C in Fig. 1 most likely represents the diiodotyrosine derivative of ChTX based on the specific activity of this peptide, while peak D in Fig. 1 contains a single iodine per molecule, and may represent a monoiodohistidine derivative of ChTX. The yield of peak B in Fig. 1 is not high, as is evident from the chromatogram; typical yields range from 10 to 20%. However, attempts to increase the yield of the

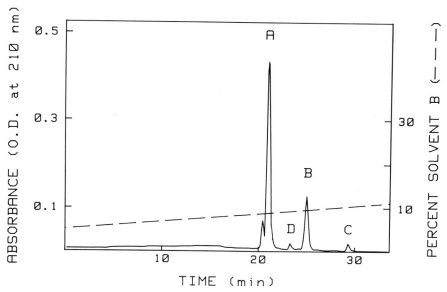

FIG. 1   HPLC purification of ^{125}I-labeled ChTX. Charybdotoxin was subjected to iodination and the reaction mixture injected onto a C_{18} reversed-phase HPLC column equilibrated with 10 mM trifluoroacetic acid. Elution was achieved by applying a linear gradient (5–14%) of 2-propanol/acetonitrile (2 : 1) in 4 mM trifluoroacetic acid at a flow rate of 0.5 ml/min over a 40-min period. Peaks A and B correspond to unmodified ChTX and monoiodotyrosine ChTX, respectively. Peaks C and D are likely to represent diiodotyrosine ChTX and monoiodohistidine ChTX, respectively. [Reprinted with permission from Vazquez *et al.*, *J. Biol. Chem.* (1989) **264**, 20,902–20,909 (14).]

iodination reaction by altering the ratio of NaI to peptide, or by increasing the amount of Iodogen used, were not successful. These modifications did not improve the production of monoiodotyrosine ChTX, but lead to the appearance of other species on reversed-phase chromatography, which makes the isolation of the derivative of interest more difficult. Therefore, when greater amounts of ^{125}I-labeled ChTX are required, the procedure is scaled up proportionally. For storage purposes, the ^{125}I-labeled ChTX fraction is made 0.5% (w/v) in bovine serum albumin, lyophilized, and reconstituted with 100 mM NaCl, 20 mM Tris-HCl, pH 7.4. Aliquots of this material are stored at $-80°C$, and are stable for at least 2 months. When an aliquot is needed, it is thawed at room temperature, and then stored at 4°C. No loss of activity is found by handling the samples in this fashion, and the results obtained from many different iodination reactions have always been highly reproducible. As found with the purification of ChTX, it is important that the HPLC column be equilibrated with 10 mM trifluoroacetic acid before injection. Otherwise, the peptide mixture will not adsorb onto the column.

In addition to the Iodogen methodology, ^{125}I-labeled ChTX can also be produced via a glucose oxidase/lactoperoxidase technique. This reaction has been carried out with beads purchased from Bio-Rad (Richmond, CA) to which the two enzymes are covalently attached. For this purpose, one vial of dried beads is hydrated with 50 μl of 100 mM sodium phosphate, pH 7.3, by incubation with buffer on ice for 30 min. Beads are then transfered to a 0.5-ml Eppendorf tube to which ChTX and Na[125]I are added. The reaction is started by addition of 5 μl of 5% (w/v) β-D-glucose, and incubation is carried out at room temperature for 30 min. At the end of the incubation period, beads are removed by centrifugation and the supernatant is injected onto a C$_{18}$ HPLC column, equilibrated as described above. Elution of retained material is achieved using the same protocol as that described for the Iodogen method, and an identical pattern is obtained. Other methods of iodination have not been attempted since the two procedures described above are simple and reproducible. We prefer the Iodogen method because the entire reaction mixture can be injected directly onto an HPLC column, thus avoiding the centrifugation step. Because the various products of the iodination reaction, although well separated, elute very close to one another, it is crucial that the starting material be homogeneous in order to prevent contaminant peaks from overlapping with the material of interest.

Characterization of Binding Sites for ^{125}I-Labeled Charybdotoxin

When considering a binding reaction involving a peptide with the characteristics of ChTX, several considerations must be taken into account. First, ChTX is a highly basic peptide which blocks K^+ channels in the low-nanomolar range. Although this property defines the toxin as a high-affinity probe, this is not sufficient for characterization of a ChTX receptor, given the relatively low abundance expected of such sites, and the high nonspecific binding component likely at these nanomolar toxin concentrations. Therefore, conditions must be established for enhancing the interaction of toxin with the channel (i.e., increasing toxin affinity). This can easily be accomplished by selecting a reaction medium in which the ionic strength is low, for it is well known that ChTX blocks channel activity through an electrostatic interaction between positively charged residues on the toxin and negatively charged residues within the mouth of the channel. Accordingly, increased ionic strength will screen this electrostatic interaction and weaken toxin affinity. For example, ChTX inhibition of $P_{K,Ca}$ in skeletal muscle t-tubular membranes can be enhanced two orders of magnitude by lowering the ionic strength of the medium from 300 to 20 mM of any monovalent cation (6).

Second, problems arising from handling ChTX must be considered. Since the easiest way to separate bound from free ligand is by using filtration techniques, the filters employed must have specific characteristics, or be treated accordingly to minimize binding of the positively charged ChTX. It has been found that GF/C glass fiber filters presoaked in 0.3% (w/v) polyethylenimine provide a low binding support if high ionic strength buffer is used to quench the binding reaction. In addition, the characteristics of the test tubes in which the binding reaction is carried out are important. Since optimal binding conditions employ low ionic strength media, glass tubes should be avoided because toxin will adhere to these surfaces. Polystyrene tubes (12 × 75 mm) can routinely be used but, given the low toxin concentrations employed in the studies, 0.1% (v/v) bovine serum albumin should be added to the reaction medium, otherwise toxin will also be adsorbed onto the surface of these tubes.

Finally, the last consideration is the source of receptor. Because ChTX is known to block two different types of K^+ channels (i.e., $P_{K,Ca}$ and $P_{K,V}$), it is important to select a tissue in which either, but not both, of these channels is present. $P_{K,Ca}$ is very abundant in various smooth muscle tissues, and methods to prepare highly purified sarcolemmal membrane vesicles from these sources are available (15, 16). It is known that a ChTX-sensitive $P_{K,V}$ is present in rat brain, and purified synaptic plasma membrane vesicles derived from this source can easily be obtained (16). Using sarcolemmal membrane vesicles prepared from either bovine aortic smooth muscle, or rat brain synaptic plasma membrane vesicles, high-affinity binding sites for ^{125}I-labeled ChTX have been identified in both tissues. The pharmacological characteristics of these binding sites suggest that they represent $P_{K,Ca}$ in smooth muscle (14), whereas they are associated with $P_{K,V}$ in brain (17).

Given the scope of this article, we will focus on the characterization of ChTX-binding sites in brain.

When rat brain synaptic plasma membrane vesicles are incubated with increasing concentrations of ^{125}I-labeled ChTX at 22°C in a medium consisting of 50 mM NaCl, 20 mM Tris-HCl, pH 7.4, until equilibrium is established, there is concentration-dependent association of toxin with the membranes (Fig. 2A). The nonspecific binding component, determined in the presence of excess native ChTX, varies linearly with ^{125}I-labeled ChTX concentration. Specific binding, determined as the difference between total and nonspecific association, is a saturable function of ^{125}I-labeled ChTX concentration. A Scatchard analysis of these data (Fig. 2B) indicates the presence of a single class of binding sites for ^{125}I-labeled ChTX that under defined experimental conditions displays an affinity (K_d) of 29 pM, and a maximum density (B_{max}) of 0.3 pmol/mg protein. It is noteworthy that these binding sites are easily observed because the specific binding component, at a K_d concentration of ligand, represents 90% of total binding. This binding reaction is a reversible bimolecular association of toxin with its receptor as demonstrated by measuring the kinetics of toxin association and dissociation (17). Another feature determined in these studies is the observation that the association rate con-

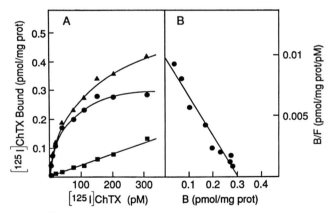

FIG. 2   Binding of ^{125}I-labeled ChTX to rat brain synaptic plasma membrane vesicles. (A) Membrane vesicles were incubated with increasing concentrations of ^{125}I-labeled ChTX at 22°C until equilibrium was achieved, in the absence (total binding; ▲), or presence (nonspecific binding; ■), of 10 nM ChTX. Specific binding (●) was assessed from the difference between total and nonspecific ligand binding. (B) Specific binding data from (A) are presented in the form of a Scatchard representation. [Reprinted with permission from Vazquez *et al.*, *J. Biol. Chem.* (1990) **265**, 15,564–15,571 (17).]

stant for ChTX, 6.8×10^8 M^{-1} sec^{-1}, is a value greater than the diffusion control rate expected for a small peptide. This is further evidence for the existence of an electrostatic interaction between ChTX and the ChTX receptor.

To ascertain the pharmacological characteristics of the ChTX receptor in brain, several compounds known to interact with different types of K$^+$ channels were tested for their ability to modulate the binding reaction. Native ChTX completely displaces ^{125}I-labeled ChTX from its receptor with a K_i value of 8–10 pM (Fig. 3) as measured under the same ionic strength conditions as those of Fig. 2. Thus, iodination of Tyr$_{36}$ results in about a threefold loss in ligand affinity. In addition, both α-dendrotoxin and noxiustoxin com-

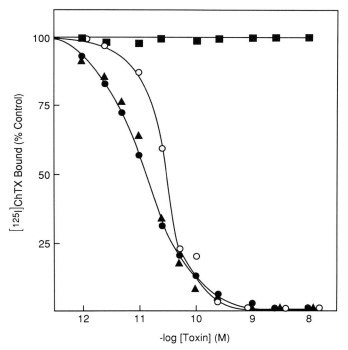

FIG. 3   Effect of toxins on ^{125}I-labeled ChTX binding to rat brain synaptic plasma membrane vesicles. Membrane vesicles were incubated with 12 pM ^{125}I-labeled ChTX in the absence or presence of increasing concentrations of either ChTX ($\bullet$), noxiustoxin ($\blacktriangle$), α-dendrotoxin ($\bigcirc$), or iberiotoxin ($\blacksquare$). The incubation medium consisted of 50 mM NaCl, 20 mM Tris-HCl, pH 7.4, and incubations were carried out at room temperature. Specific binding data in each case are presented relative to an untreated control.

pletely inhibit toxin binding with K_i values of 20 and 8 pM, respectively. In marked contrast, iberiotoxin has no affect on ChTX binding in brain at concentrations up to 100 nM. Since α-dendrotoxin (11) and noxiustoxin (18) are known to block $P_{K,V}$, whereas iberiotoxin is a selective inhibitor of $P_{K,Ca}$ (19), the ChTX-binding site identified in rat brain synaptic plasma membrane vesicles must be functionally associated with an inactivating, voltage-dependent K^+ channel. A similar conclusion has been obtained from binding studies with ^{125}I-labeled ChTX and intact human peripheral T lymphocytes (20). In this system, ChTX-binding sites display the characteristic properties expected of the $P_{K,V}$ that represents more than 90% of the outward current in whole-cell clamp experiments. The reason why ^{125}I-labeled ChTX is unable to identify $P_{K,Ca}$ sites in brain remains unknown. It is possible that the density of these channels in rat brain synaptic plasma membrane vesicles is low compared to $P_{K,V}$. Alternatively, rat brain $P_{K,Ca}$ channels may not recognize the monoiodotyrosine adduct of ChTX. It has been observed that iodination of toxin alters its structure because there is a 10-fold loss in binding affinity for $P_{K,Ca}$ in smooth muscle. Thus, if $P_{K,Ca}$ in brain is more sensitive to conformational differences between iodinated and native toxin than the smooth muscle channel, it may not be feasible to use ^{125}I-labeled ChTX to study $P_{K,Ca}$ in brain.

In addition to toxins, a number of different metal ions such as Ba^{2+}, Cs^+, and Ca^{2+}, as well as organic cations such as tetraethylammonium ion and tetrabutylammonium ion, are known to inhibit different K^+ channels by distinct mechanisms. When these ions are tested for their ability to modulate ^{125}I-labeled ChTX binding to rat brain membranes, a variety of effects are observed. Whereas Ba^{2+}, Cs^+, Ca^{2+}, and tetrabutylammonium ion all produce concentration-dependent inhibition of toxin-binding activity, tetraethylammonium ion has no effect on the interaction of ChTX in brain (Fig. 4A). Such lack of effect of tetraethylammonium ion in brain is in marked contrast to its effects in vascular smooth muscle, where this agent is a potent inhibitor of ChTX binding to sites associated with $P_{K,Ca}$. Perhaps the most interesting effect of ions is observed when ChTX binding is monitored in brain in the presence of either K^+ or Na^+. At low concentrations (below 20 mM), these ions stimulate ChTX binding before producing complete inhibition of binding as their concentration is increased (Fig. 4B). Lithium ion, on the other hand, causes only inhibition of ChTX binding. The data shown in Fig. 4B have been described by a mathematical model that accounts for the dual effects of the ions (17). According to this model, enhancement of ChTX binding produced by low concentrations of ions is the result of either two K^+ or a single Na^+ binding to the ChTX receptor. In addition, the dissociation constants calculated for K^+ and Na^+ (ca. 0.1 and 2.0 mM, respectively) indicate that the affinity of K^+ is at least 10-fold greater than that of Na^+. On the

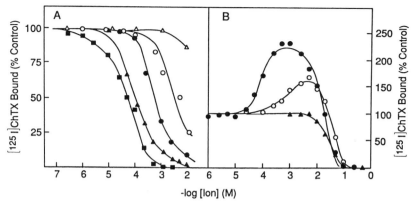

FIG. 4   Effect of ions on ^{125}I-labeled ChTX binding to rat brain synaptic plasma membrane vesicles. (A) Membrane vesicles were incubated with 12 pM ^{125}I-labeled ChTX in 50 mM NaCl, 20 mM Tris-HCl, pH 7.4, in the absence or presence of increasing concentrations of either BaCl$_2$ (■), CsCl (▲), CaCl$_2$ (●), tetrabutylammonium ion (○), or tetraethylammonium ion (△). (B) Membrane vesicles in 20 mM Tris-HCl, pH 7.4, were incubated with 12 pM ^{125}I-labeled ChTX in the absence or presence of increasing concentrations of either KCl (●), NaCl (○), or LiCl (▲). In both (A) and (B), incubations were carried out at room temperature and specific binding data are presented relative to an untreated control in each case. [Reprinted with permission from Vazquez *et al.*, *J. Biol. Chem.* (1990) **265**, 15,564–15,571 (17).]

other hand, the inhibitory effect caused by all three ions at high millimolar concentrations most likely represents an ionic strength effect on toxin binding (see above).

Although the molecular composition of the rat brain ChTX receptor is unknown, several possibilities can be considered. Three different rat brain cDNA clones that express voltage-dependent K$^+$ channels in *Xenopus* oocytes have been reported to be sensitive to ChTX. Two of these clones, RCK$_3$ (3) and K$_V$3 (18), are essentially identical, differing only by a single amino acid in their predicted sequences. Although K$_V$3 has been shown to be blocked with high affinity by noxiustoxin, neither RCK$_3$ nor K$_V$3 display any sensitivity toward inhibition by α-dendrotoxin. On the other hand, RCK$_5$ displays a moderate sensitivity toward both ChTX and α-dendrotoxin, but there are no reports on the effects of noxiustoxin on this channel (3). Given these data, it is difficult to identify which if any of the individual K$^+$ channel clones from rat brain represent the ChTX receptor. Perhaps ChTX binding in brain occurs to a receptor that is formed from several different subunits, with each subunit displaying a distinctive pharmacological profile. Assembly of these subunits could produce a K^+ channel with unique pharmacological and biophysical properties.

References

1. G. Gimenez-Gallego, M. A. Navia, J. P. Reuben, G. M. Katz, G. J. Kaczorowski, and M. L. Garcia, *Proc. Natl. Acad. Sci. U.S.A.* **85,** 3329 (1988).
2. C. Miller, E. Moczydlowski, R. Latorre, and M. Phillips, *Nature (London)* **313,** 316 (1985).
3. W. Stuhmer, J. F. Ruppersberg, K. H. Schroter, B. Sakmann, M. Stocker, K. P. Giese, A. Perschke, A. Baumann, and O. Pongs, *EMBO J.* **8,** 3235 (1989).
4. M. Price, S. C. Lee, and C. Deutsch, *Proc. Natl. Acad. Sci. U.S.A.* **86,** 19171 (1989).
5. C. Oliva, K. Folander, and J. S. Smith, *Biophys. J.* **59,** 450a (1991).
6. C. Anderson, R. MacKinnon, C. Smith, and C. Miller, *J. Gen. Physiol.* **91,** 317 (1988).
7. R. MacKinnon and C. Miller, *J. Gen. Physiol.* **91,** 335 (1988).
8. H. H. Valdivia, J. S. Smith, B. M. Martin, R. Coronado, and L. D. Possani, *FEBS Lett.* **2,** 280 (1988).
9. K. Lucchesi, A. Ravindran, H. Young, and E. Moczydlowski, *J. Membr. Biol.* **109,** 269 (1989).
10. P. N. Strong, S. W. Weir, D. J. Beech, P. Heistand, and H. P. Kocher, *Br. J. Pharmacol.* **98,** 817 (1989).
11. H. Schweitz, J.-N. Bidard, P. Maes, and M. Lazdunski, *Biochemistry* **28,** 9708 (1989).
12. E. E. Sugg, M. L. Garcia, J. P. Reuben, A. A. Patchett, and G. J. Kaczorowski, *J. Biol. Chem.* **265,** 18,745 (1990).
13. P. Lambert, H. Kuroda, N. Chino, T. X. Watanabe, T. Kimura, and S. Sakakibara, *Biochem. Biophys. Res. Commun.* **170,** 684 (1990).
14. J. Vazquez, P. Feigenbaum, G. Katz, V. F. King, J. P. Reuben, L. Roy-Contancin, R. S. Slaughter, G. J. Kaczorowski, and M. L. Garcia, *J. Biol. Chem.* **264,** 20,902 (1989).
15. R. S. Slaughter, A. F. Welton, and D. W. Morgan, *Biochim. Biophys. Acta* **904,** 92 (1987).
16. R. S. Slaughter, J. L. Shevell, J. P. Felix, M. L. Garcia, and G. J. Kaczorowski, *Biochemistry* **28,** 3995 (1989).
17. J. Vazquez, P. Feigenbaum, V. F. King, G. J. Kaczorowski, and M. L. Garcia, *J. Biol. Chem.* **265,** 15,564 (1990).
18. R. Swanson, J. Marshall, J. S. Smith, J. B. Williams, M. B. Boyle, K. Folander, C. J. Luneau, J. Antanavage, C. Oliva, S. A. Buhrow, C. Bennett, R. B. Stein, and L. K. Kaczmarek, *Neuron* **4,** 929 (1990).
19. A. Galvez, G. Gimenez-Gallego, J. P. Reuben, L. Roy-Contancin, P. Feigenbaum, G. J. Kaczorowski, and M. L. Garcia, *J. Biol. Chem.* **265,** 11,083 (1990).
20. C. Deutsch, M. Price, S. C. Lee, V. F. King, and M. L. Garcia, *J. Biol. Chem.* **266,** 3668 (1991).

[11] Ciguatoxin: A Tool for Research on Sodium-Dependent Mechanisms

Jordi Molgo, Evelyne Benoit, Joan X. Comella, and
Anne-Marie Legrand

A wide variety of potent toxins isolated from marine organisms has drawn the attention of neurobiologists because of their specific pharmacological actions on excitable membranes and physiological processes (for recent reviews, see Refs. 1–4). Although the effects of many of these toxins, i.e., tetrodotoxin, saxitoxin, palytoxin, sea anemone toxins, maitotoxin, and conotoxins, are well characterized on excitation, secretion, and synaptic signaling mechanisms, the actions of other neurotoxins like ciguatoxin, reviewed by Legrand and Bagnis (5), are less well known mainly due to difficulties in obtaining enough quantities of purified toxin.

Ciguatoxin (CTX) is the principal ichthyotoxin involved in a complex human food poisoning known as ciguatera, characterized mainly by neurological, gastrointestinal, and, in the most severe cases, cardiovascular disorders (6–10). At present, ciguatera constitutes one of the largest scale seafood toxicities associated with the consumption of many species of tropical and subtropical fishes. The examination of the feeding behavior of ciguatoxic fish revealed that despite the variety of feeding habits, all poisonous herbivorous and carnivorous fish acquired the toxicity from their diet and transferred it to other fish through the marine food chain and ultimately to humans (8, 11–14). It is worth noting that CTX is apparently harmless to ciguateric fish although present in their flesh and viscera. This has been explained by an evolved partitioning or sequestering mechanism that prevents the toxin from acting on its target acceptors (15).

The source of CTX was discovered only in 1977, when collaborative studies between the Bagnis (Tahiti) and Yasumoto (Japan) groups revealed the presence of the toxin, or closely related compounds, in dinoflagellate-rich samples of algae and toxic detritus collected on coral beds of the Gambier Islands in French Polynesia (16, 17). The collected dinoflagellate was then identified as belonging to a new genus and was named *Gambierdiscus toxicus* (18). Although the wild species of this dinoflagellate produces under natural conditions both CTX and the well-known maitotoxin (19), cultured cells still provided maitotoxin but failed to produce more than traces of the CTX-like compound (20, 21).

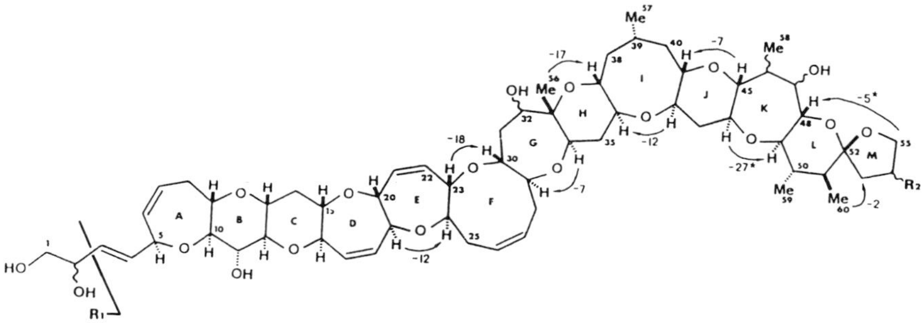

FIG. 1   Structure of ciguatoxin (**1**) and gambiertoxin 4b (**2**). **1**, R_2 = OH; **2**, R_1 =
$\overset{1}{CH_2} = CH^-$; R_2 = H. (From Ref. 27.)

In the present chapter, after a brief documentation regarding the structure of CTX, we shall review experiments, performed mainly in our laboratories, which have given further insight into the basis of CTX action on excitable membranes and neurotransmitter release.

Chemical Characterization of Ciguatoxin

Although CTX is more concentrated in large carnivorous fish, its extraction, purification, and chemical characterization have been a long and tedious process, because toxic fish contain only very small amounts of toxin [~0.2–0.5 parts per billion (ppb)].

Ciguatoxin is a complex lipid-soluble compound that was first purified in Hawaii by Scheuer and co-workers (22) from the red snapper *Lutjanus bohar,* the shark *Carchahinus menisorrha,* and the moray eel *Gymnothorax javanicus.* In subsequent studies, the toxin was crystallized and, based on ${}^1H$ nuclear magnetic resonance data, was presumed to be a polyether having a molecular weight of 1111.7 (23–25). Finally, a collaboration between Yasumoto's group (Japan) and Legrand's group (Tahiti) provided the chemical structure elucidation of CTX by sophisticated spectral analysis of a small (0.35 mg), highly purified sample of toxin (26). Ciguatoxin was disclosed to have a brevetoxin-like polyether structure comprising 13 contiguous ether rings with a primary alcohol at 1 terminal of the molecule and a molecular formula of $C_{60}H_{86}O_{19}$ (27, 28) (Fig. 1). In addition, it was shown that the main toxic compound extracted from the dinoflagellate *Gambierdiscus toxicus,* named gambiertoxin 4b, possesses a ladder-shaped skeleton identical to that of CTX extracted from the moray eel, but with fewer oxidized terminal groups (28) (Fig. 1). This suggests that gambiertoxin 4b may undergo some structural changes through passages in the herbivorous and carnivorous fish along the marine food chain. Thus, CTX can be considered as the oxidized form in the carnivorous fish of the food-borne dinoflagellate toxin. Therefore this can explain the various reported types of toxins implicated in ciguatera fish poisoning (8, 13, 14). Most of the experimental work carried out with CTX has been performed with toxic samples extracted from the moray eel *Gymnothorax javanicus.*

Action of Ciguatoxin on Excitable Membranes

Effects on Myelinated Nerve Fibers

The effects of external application of CTX (0.2 and 1 nM) were studied under current-clamp and voltage-clamp conditions, according to the method of Nonner (29), on the nodal membrane of frog single isolated myelinated nerve fibers (30). Under voltage-clamp conditions, CTX modified neither linear leakage and capacitative currents nor K$^+$ currents but altered Na$^+$ current. In the presence of the toxin, a fraction of the Na$^+$ current failed to inactivate during long-lasting depolarizations (Fig. 2b) and was activated and reversed at membrane potentials about 30 mV more negative than CTX-unmodified or control Na$^+$ current. This fraction of the Na$^+$ current that did not inactivate was quantitatively independent of the concentrations of toxin tested, but was larger when the holding potential was made less negative, i.e., about 10 and 30% at -120 and -70 mV, respectively. Under current-clamp conditions, as a consequence of the specific CTX-induced modification of the fraction of Na$^+$ current that is activated at the normal resting membrane potential (-70 mV) and which fails to inactivate, the nodal membrane was depolarized and spontaneous action potentials could be recorded, as shown in Fig. 2f. The effects of CTX on resting membrane potential and Na$^+$ current were completely suppressed by the addition of 300 nM tetrodotoxin (TTX) to the external medium or by washing out CTX with control solution.

The action of CTX on the Na$^+$ current shares some similarities with that of other lipid-soluble toxins such as brevetoxins and alkaloids, including batrachotoxin, veratridine, aconitine, and grayanotoxin, all of which partially or totally block Na$^+$ current inactivation (Fig. 2c) and largely shift the potential dependence of activation of the modified Na$^+$ current toward more negative values (for recent reviews, see Refs. 2, 3, 31, and 32). Thus these toxins, like CTX, induce persistent activation of the Na$^+$ current at the resting membrane potential at which Na$^+$ channels are normally closed, which in turn causes membrane depolarization. However, in contrast to CTX and brevetoxins, alkaloids hardly produce repetitive firing, but

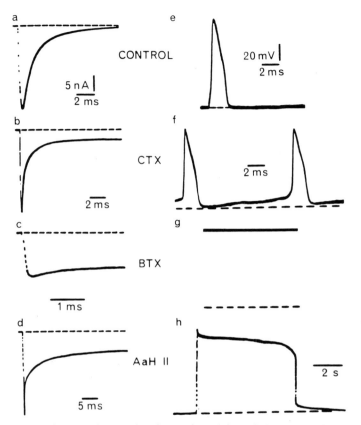

FIG. 2   Effects of 1 nM ciguatoxin (CTX) (b and f) and the comparison with those of 10 μM batrachotoxin (BTX) (c and g) and 70 nM scorpion *Androctonus australis Hector* toxin II (AaH II) (d and h) on Na$^+$ current (a–d) and membrane potential (e–h) in single frog myelinated nerve fibers. The Na$^+$ current was recorded during depolarization to either 0 mV (a,b,d) or -20 mV (c). The action potentials were evoked with 0.5-msec depolarizing stimulus (e and h) while in (f) in the absence of stimulation. Note that in (g) no action potential could be elicited due to the large membrane depolarization. Interrupted lines indicate either the zero current level (a–d) or the holding potential (-70 mV) level (e–h). The nodal membrane was superfused with Ringer's solution in the presence (a–d) or in the absence (e–h) of 10 mM tetraethylammonium. [For more experimental details, see Refs. 29 and 32 and J.-M. Dubois, M. F. Schneider, and B. I. Khodorov, *J. Gen. Physiol.* **81,** 829 (1983).]

consistently cause inhibition of action potentials as the result of their membrane-depolarizing effect (Fig. 2g). Other toxins, such as scorpion α-toxins and sea anemone toxins, specifically slow down and/or produce incomplete Na^+ current inactivation (Fig. 2d) but, in contrast to the above toxins, do not produce a significant shift of the potential dependence of activation of the modified Na^+ current (see Refs. 2 and 3). Consequently, such toxins hardly induce membrane depolarization but increase the duration of action potentials (Fig. 2h). It thus appears that the various toxins that similarly affect Na^+ current inactivation can stimulate (CTX and brevetoxins), slow down (scorpion α-toxins and sea anemone toxins), or inhibit (alkaloids) nerve conduction. These in some way different effects may be due to quantitative rather than qualitative differences in toxin-induced modifications of Na^+ current (see Refs. 30 and 33). It can be noted that another class of scorpion toxins, including scorpion β- and γ-toxins, which does not notably affect Na^+ current inactivation, causes repetitive firing by shifting the potential dependence of Na^+ current activation toward more negative values (see Refs. 2 and 31).

In addition to the effects of CTX on myelinated nerve fibers described above, the toxin has been reported to depolarize neuronal cells (34), to induce TTX-sensitive membrane depolarization and repetitive action potentials in neuroblastoma cells (35), and to enhance and prolong the supernormal period of nerves (15, 36). All these effects are believed to stem from the ability of CTX to increase Na^+ influx through voltage-dependent Na^+ channels.

Effects on Skeletal Muscle Fibers

Partially purified CTX was previously reported to enhance the rate constant for Na^+ entry and to induce a maintained depolarization in frog muscle fibers (37, 38). This depolarization did not occur in muscle fibers exposed to CTX in an Na^+-free medium but promptly appeared on subsequent addition of Na^+. Furthermore, it was shown that the depolarization could be reversed or prevented by 1–3 μM TTX. These results have been basically confirmed using highly purified CTX in frog skeletal muscle fibers (39).

In frog neuromuscular preparations, CTX (1–2.5 nM) caused either sponta- neous or repetitive muscle action potentials at rates varying from a few hertz to tens of hertz (39). Figure 3b shows an example of such trains of action potentials recorded at extrajunctional sites of a muscle fiber in response to a single nerve stimulus. Analysis of the time course of action potentials during the repetitive firing revealed that their repolarizing phase was prolonged at the time their amplitude and rise time remained unchanged (Fig. 3a). The effects of CTX here reported have some similarities with those previously

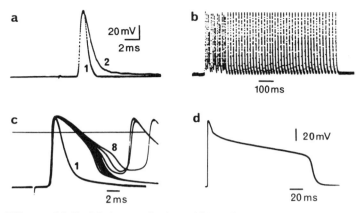

FIG. 3   Effects of 2.5 n*M* ciguatoxin (a and b) and 10 µ*M* sea anemone *Anemonia sulcata* toxin II (c and d) on indirectly elicited action potentials recorded at extrajunctional sites of frog skeletal muscle fibers. (a) Action potential recorded in response to a single nerve stimulus (1) superimposed on a spontaneous action potential (2) recorded during a train, as shown in (b). (b) Train of repetitive action potentials in response to a single nerve stimulus. Note that repetitive action potentials appear at a faster rate at the beginning of the train. (c) Recordings obtained before (1) and after ATX-II action (eight superimposed tracings). In (c), the horizontal line represents the zero-potential level. Note the repetitive responses appearing on the falling phase of action potentials and the increase in duration with the sequence of stimulation (8). (d) Action potential recorded in the presence of ATX-II, in which the falling phase has been replaced by a long-lasting plateau. (For more experimental details, see Refs. 39 and 40.)

obtained with the sea anemone *Anemonia sulcata* toxin II (ATX-II) (40). However, as shown in Fig. 3c and d, in contrast to ATX-II, action potentials with a long plateau were never detected in the presence of CTX. This supports the view that the mode of action of these two toxins on the muscle membrane is different.

Ciguatoxin (1–2.5 n*M*), when applied to isolated mouse or frog skeletal neuromuscular preparations, within seconds induced uncoordinated contractions of the muscle fibers. The contractile activity was also detected, but with less intensity, after blocking postsynaptic acetylcholine receptors with 60 µ*M* (+)-tubocurarine and could be completely suppressed either by TTX (1 µ*M*) or by uncoupling the excitation–contraction process with formamide (39). These results suggest that both pre- and postsynaptic actions are involved in the contractile effects of CTX.

Effects on Atrial Cells

Studies performed on isolated guinea pig atrial cells (41), using the patch-clamp technique in the whole-cell configuration, showed that CTX (5.4 to 18 nM) modified the Na$^+$ current in a manner somewhat similar to the node of Ranvier. In the presence of the toxin, the Na$^+$ current activated and reversed at membrane potentials 10 to 40 mV more negative than under control conditions, and a small but sustained Na$^+$ inward current appeared at holding potentials close to the resting membrane potential. However, in contrast to the results obtained on the node of Ranvier, CTX induced an increase in the duration of action potentials and the cell membrane was not or only slightly depolarized by the toxin. These effects could be reversed by the addition of 1 μM TTX to the external medium. It is worth noting that in the same preparation, CTX at concentrations as low as 1.2 nM was reported to produce a marked depolarization of the membrane and a decrease of the amplitude of action potentials (42, 43).

In guinea pig atria, as in papillary muscles, CTX has been shown to induce a TTX-sensitive increase in the contactile force (41, 42, 44). Although all studies agree with these results for low concentrations of CTX (up to 1.2 nM), the effects of higher doses of toxin (over 2.4 nM) remain controversial because either a positive (41) or a negative (43) inotropic action in guinea pig cardiac cells was reported. Until now, there was no explanation for such a discrepancy. In rat and rabbit isolated atria, the application of CTX always caused biphasic responses due to negative and positive inotropic effects (45, 46). It should be noticed that CTX has also been shown to stimulate smooth muscle contractility in the guinea pig vas deferens (47) and ileum (48), whereas the toxin inhibited contractile activity in guinea pig taenia cecum (49) and rat jejunum (50).

The contractile effects of CTX on the various types of muscles (skeletal, cardiac, and smooth) have been explained by a direct action on muscle Na$^+$ channels or by an indirect action on Na$^+$ channels of the nerves supplying the muscles, or by both.

Ciguatoxin Acceptor Site Associated with the Na$^+$ Channel Protein

Five distinct acceptor sites associated with Na$^+$ channels of excitable membranes that bind low-molecular-weight natural toxins with high affinity and specificity were known before purified CTX was available. Based on the independence of toxin binding as well as toxin action, these sites were

TABLE I   Toxin-Identified Binding Sites Associated with Na^+ Channel Protein

Receptor site	Toxin	Main origin	Chemical nature	Electrophysiological effects on axonal membranes
1	Tetrodotoxin	Puffer fish, *Tetraodontidae*	Heterocycle	Block of current and inhibition of action potential
	Saxitoxin	Dinoflagellate, *Gonyaulax catenella*	Heterocycle	
	μ-Conotoxins	Snail, *Conus geographus*	Protein	
2	Batrachotoxin	Frog, *Phyllobates aurotaenia*	Alkaloid	Inhibition of inactivation, negative shift of potential dependence of activation and inhibition of action potential
	Veratridine	Plant, *Veratrum album*	Alkaloid	
	Aconitine	Plant, *Aconitum napellus*	Alkaloid	
	Grayanotoxin	Plant, *Ericaceae*	Alkaloid	
3	Scorpion α-toxins	Scorpions, *Androctonus, Buthus Leiurus*	Protein	Inhibition of inactivation and prolongation of action potential
	Sea anemone toxins	Sea anemone, *Anemonia*	Protein	
4	Scorpion β-toxins	Scorpion, *Centruroides*	Protein	Negative shift of potential dependence of activation and repetitive firing
	Scorpion γ-toxins	Scorpion, *Tityus*	Protein	
5	Brevetoxins	Dinoflagellate, *Gymnodinium breve*	Polyether	Inhibition of inactivation, negative shift of potential dependence of activation and repetitive firing
	Ciguatoxin	Dinoflagellate, *Gambierdiscus toxicus*	Polyether	

classified as presented in Table I (for recent reviews, see Refs. 2, 31, and 32). Site 1 binds TTX, saxitoxin, and μ-conotoxin and the occupancy at this site blocks the passage of ions; site 2 exhibits an affinity for alkaloids; site 3 is known to bind scorpion α-toxins and sea anemone toxins; site 4 binds scorpion β- and γ-toxins and site 5 is the binding site for brevetoxins.

According to $^{22}Na^+$ flux measurements and binding experiments involving competition of CTX with a variety of other labeled Na^+ channel toxins, the CTX-acceptor site associated with the Na^+ channel has been identified. Bidard *et al.* (35) demonstrated an enhancement of the $^{22}Na^+$ influx through the voltage-sensitive Na^+ channels of neuroblastoma cells and rat skeletal myoblasts when CTX was used in synergy with veratridine, batrachotoxin, sea anemone, or scorpion α- and γ-toxins. In addition, these authors reported that the concentration dependence of TTX inhibition of CTX action on the net accumulation of radiolabeled γ-aminobutyric acid by brain synaptosomes was independent of CTX concentration. Therefore, CTX cannot obviously associate with the respective acceptors for these four classes of toxins, i.e., sites 1 to 4 (see Table I). Several lines of evidence lead to the confirmation of this conclusion. First, CTX was shown to have no effect on the binding of radiolabeled TTX, sea anemone toxin, and scorpion α- and γ-toxins to their acceptor sites in rat brain membranes. Second, CTX was reported to increase the binding of radiolabeled batrachotoxin to the Na^+ channel protein in synaptosomes (35, 51, 52). Finally, CTX was demonstrated to inhibit competitively the binding of tritiated brevetoxins to rat brain membranes (51, 52). The whole set of results strongly supports the notion that CTX and brevetoxins share a common acceptor site on the neuronal voltage-dependent Na^+ channel protein (Table I).

Action of Ciguatoxin on Neurotransmitter Release

Effects on Norepinephrine, γ-Aminobutyric Acid, and Dopamine Release

Partially purified CTX was reported to cause a dose-dependent release of norepinephrine from the adrenergic nerve terminals supplying the isolated guinea pig vas deferens (53). Such an action was almost completely abolished by previous treatment with TTX, suggesting that CTX causes an increase in Na^+ permeability through TTX-sensitive Na^+ channels of adrenergic terminals.

Purified CTX has also been shown to increase dose dependently the rate of release of ^3H-labeled γ-aminobutyric acid and $[^3H]$dopamine from rat brain synaptosomes. The CTX-elicited release was sensitive to blockade by TTX but was unaffected by Ca^{2+} channel antagonists such as nitrendipine and D-600 (35). The stimulation of neurotransmitter release of CTX and its inhibition by TTX are similar to those previously observed with veratridine or with sea anemone toxins (54). Since CTX was reported to have no action on the activity of the Na^+, K^+-ATPase, it was suggested that the enhancement of neurotransmitter release may be due to the depolarization caused by the activation of voltage-dependent Na^+ channels of the synaptosomal membrane (35).

Effects on Evoked and Spontaneous Quantal Acetylcholine Release

At frog neuromuscular preparations equilibrated in solutions containing high Mg^{2+}/low Ca^{2+} concentrations, to reduce quantal transmitter release, the addition of CTX (1.5 nM) first increased about twofold the mean quantal content of end-plate potentials (EPPs) evoked by nerve stimulation, subse-

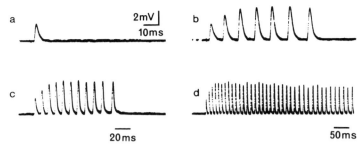

FIG. 4   End-plate potentials evoked by a single nerve stimulus before (a) and after (b–d) the addition of 1.7 nM ciguatoxin to the normal Ringer's solution containing 3.5 μM (+)-tubocurarine. Note that in (b), (c), and (d) the repetitive EPPs exhibited some facilitation with respect to the first EPP in each train. The recordings were obtained at a single junction of a frog neuromuscular preparation treated with formamide to uncouple excitation to contraction. (For more experimental details, see Ref. 39.)

quently reduced, and finally blocked irreversibly transmitter release. Extensive washing of the preparation with a CTX-free solution did not reverse the blockade of quantal release (39). As shown in Fig. 4, CTX (1–2 nM) induced transient trains of repetitive EPPs in response to a single nerve stimulus in junctions equilibrated in a normal Ringer's solution containing 4 μM (+)-tubocurarine. These trains of EPPs, which are due to the repetitive release of transmitter, were usually short lived (1–3 min) (39).

Several drugs and toxins, which affect presynaptic K^+ or Na^+ channels, induce repetitive EPPs at the neuromuscular junction (55–57). However, the repetitive firing of the motor nerves produced by these agents did not attain the high frequency observed with CTX.

It is likely that the facilitatory effect of CTX is not due to an enhanced phasic Ca^{2+} entry, during the presynaptic action potential, but to an increase in intraterminal Ca^{2+} due to Na^+ entry (see below). The reduction and blockade of evoked transmitter release are most likely due to the depolarization of the terminals, which may reduce the driving force for Ca^{2+} entry. The blockade of evoked transmitter release cannot be explained by the depletion of transmitter stores in the nerve terminal. Because at the time stimulation failed to elicit EPPs, spontaneous quantal release was markedly increased.

CTX (1.5–2.5 nM) increased the spontaneous quantal release of acetylcholine from motor nerve terminals measured electrophysiologically as an increase in miniature end-plate potential (MEPP) frequency (39). Typical recordings obtained at frog neuromuscular junctions are shown in Fig. 5. This effect also occurred in neuromuscular preparations bathed in a nominally

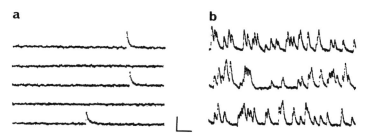

FIG. 5   Miniature end-plate potentials recorded in the same junction of a frog neuro-muscular preparation just before (a) and after (b) the addition of 2.5 nM ciguatoxin to the control Ringer's solution. Vertical calibration is 1 mV, horizontal calibration is 50 msec (a) and 20 msec (b). (For more experimental details, see Ref. 39.)

Ca^{2+}-free solution supplemented with 1 mM EGTA. These results ruled out the possibility that CTX enhanced CA^{2+} influx through voltage-sensitive Ca^{2+} channels of the nerve terminal, in contrast to the structurally related lipid-soluble brevetoxin T-17 and the hydrosoluble maitotoxin whose stimulant effects on spontaneous MEPPs depended on Ca^{2+} entry into the nerve endings (58, 59).

Tetrodotoxin (1 μM) was found not only to prevent, but also to inhibit, once developed, the effect of CTX (2.5 nM) on MEPP frequency (39). These results strongly suggest that an increased permeability of the nerve terminal to Na^+ is responsible for the enhancement of spontaneous quantal release caused by CTX. It is worth noting that in motor nerve terminals the effect of TTX was more easily reversible than that of CTX, as evidenced by experiments in which both toxins were applied together and then removed from the medium (39, 60). No reversal of CTX action was observed under those conditions even after extensive washing of the preparation. Interactions with TTX similar to those reported for CTX have been previously described for ATX-II (61).

It is likely that CTX enhances the probability of opening TTX-sensitive Na^+ channels of the motor nerve terminal at the resting membrane potential, causing thereby a sustained Na^+ entry that may produce an increase of intraterminal sodium concentration. In various secretory systems it is well documented that increases of intracellular Na^+ concentration may mobilize intracellular stores of Ca^{2+} (62–64). In this context, it is interesting, as reported by Gusovsky et al. (65), that sodium influx can stimulate phosphatidylinositol systems, which are capable of mobilizing Ca^{2+} from internal stores.

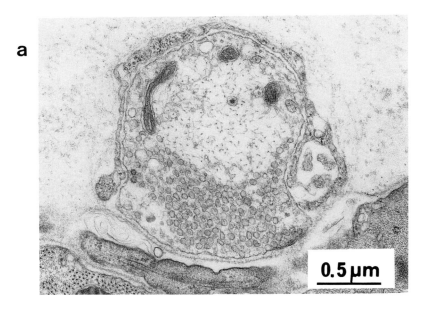

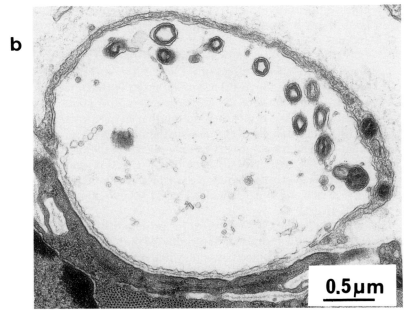

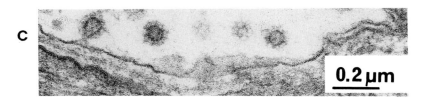

Effects on Motor Nerve Terminal Ultrastructure

In an attempt to correlate the pharmacological actions of CTX with morphological changes at the subcellular level of motor endings, the ultrastructure of frog motor nerve terminals was investigated.

The ultrastructural analysis of junctions exposed for 1–3 hr to CTX (2.5 nM) revealed that CTX caused a marked reduction in the number of small, clear, synaptic vesicles and large, dense-core vesicles per nerve terminal cross-section (Fig. 6). The depletion occurred either in a nominally Ca^{2+}-free solution containing 1 mM EGTA or in standard Ringer's solution containing 2 mM Ca^{2+}. Concomitant with the depletion of clear and dense synaptic vesicles was an increase in the number of coated vesicles that were associated either with elements of the endoplasmic reticulum or with cisternae-like double membranes. In addition, the area of cross-sectioned nerve terminal profiles was dramatically increased following CTX exposure. The depletion of synaptic vesicles seems to be related to the CTX-induced high-intensity quantal transmitter release, since no depletion of synaptic vesicles was observed when TTX (1 μM) was applied together with CTX (2.5 nM) either in a normal medium or in Ca^{2+}-free medium. Under these conditions, CTX did not stimulate quantal transmitter release despite its binding to the Na^+ channel protein of the nerve terminal. The depletion of clear synaptic vesicles caused by CTX seems to be due to an alteration of the synaptic vesicle recycling process caused by enhanced Na^+ entry into the terminal (60).

Effects on Na^+-Dependent Ca^{2+} Mobilization in Nerve Cells

The possibility that CTX may cause release of Ca^{2+} from intracellular stores was directly investigated in cultured mouse neuroblastoma × rat glioma NG108-15 hybrid cells using the calcium-sensitive fluorescent probe Fura-2 (66). Ciguatoxin was found to consistently increase cytoplasmic Ca^{2+} levels when tested in cells bathed in a Ca^{2+}-free medium supplemented with 1mM EGTA (60). In contrast, when cells were previously exposed to 1 μM TTX,

---

FIG. 6   Ultrastructure of cross-sectioned motor nerve terminals from frog neuromuscular junctions treated for 3 hr either with 2.5 nM CTX and 1 μM TTX (a) or with CTX only (b). Notice in (a) the normal appearance of the terminal, while in (b) the nerve terminal is swollen and almost completely devoid of synaptic vesicles; mitochondria exhibit signs of internal disruption. Notice in (c) the presence of coated vesicles in relation to the prejunctional membrane after CTX treatment.

subsequent addition of 2.5 nM CTX did not modify the cytoplasmic Ca^{2+} concentration. Because TTX prevented CTX effects on Ca^{2+} mobilization, it is likely that CTX-induced Na^+ entry may be the trigger for Ca^{2+} release from intracellular stores. The potential source for the putative CTX-induced release of intraterminal Ca^{2+} by Na^+ is not known. Studies examining the possibility that CTX-induced Ca^{2+} mobilization may be mediated by second messengers are now in progress.

In conclusion, research on CTX has expanded significantly over the last 15 years in large part due to the identification of the benthic dinoflagellate responsible for toxin production, a discovery that has been followed by the chemical characterization of CTX and some information on its actions at the cellular level. Clearly, CTX is a unique and extremely potent substance that provides an important tool for research on sodium channels and sodium-dependent mechanisms. Further work is needed to clarify the functional domains of the complex structure of CTX involved in the binding and underlying its action on the Na^+ channel protein. This brief survey indicates that several major key aspects of the subcellular and molecular actions of CTX remain to be elucidated, offering interesting possibilities for further fruitful research.

Acknowledgments

Supported in part by Direction de Recherches Etudes et Techniques, Association Française contre les Myopathies and the French Polynesian Government. The authors wish to thank Dr. J.-M. Dubois for many helpful comments. This chapter is dedicated to Dr. R. Bagnis for pioneer studies and multiple contributions to the field of ciguatera.

References

1. P. N. Kaul and P. Daftari, *Annu. Rev. Pharmacol. Toxicol.* **26,** 117 (1986).
2. G. Strichartz, T. Rando, and G. K. Wang, *Annu. Rev. Neurosci.* **10,** 237 (1987).
3. C. H. Wu and T. Narahashi, *Annu. Rev. Pharmacol. Toxicol.* **28,** 141 (1988).
4. A. Harvey, *Int. Rev. Neurobiol.* **32,** 201 (1990).
5. A.-M. Legrand and R. Bagnis, *in* "Seafood Toxins" (E. P. Ragelis, ed.), p. 217. Am. Chem. Soc., Washington, D.C., 1984.
6. R. Bagnis, T. Kuberski, and S. Laugier, *Am. J. Trop. Med. Hyg.* **28,** 1067 (1979).
7. D. N. Lawrence, M. B. Enriquez, R. M. Lumish, and A. Maceo, *JAMA, J. Am. Med. Assoc.* **244,** 254 (1980).
8. N. W. Withers, *Annu. Rev. Med.* **33,** 97 (1982).
9. Y. Hokama and J. T. Miyahara, *J. Toxicol. Toxin Rev.* **5,** 25 (1986).

10. N. C. Gillespie, R. J. Lewis, J. H. Pearn, A. T. C. Bowre, M. J. Holmes, I. B. Bowre, and W. J. Shields, *Med. J. Aust.* **145,** 584 (1986).

11. J. E. Randall, *Bull. Mar. Sci. Gulf Caribb.* **8,** 236 (1958).

12. M. J. Cooper, *Pac. Sci.* **18,** 411 (1964).

13. R. Bagnis, *Ann. Inst. Oceanogr. (Paris)* **57,** 5 (1981).

14. D. M. Anderson and P. S. Lobel, *Biol. Bull. (Woods Hole, Mass.)* **172,** 89 (1987).

15. A. E. Flowers, M. Capra, and J. Cameron, *in* "Progress in Venom and Toxin Research" (P. Gopalakrishnakone and C. K. Tan, eds.), p. 418. Natl. Univ. of Singapore, Singapore, 1988.

16. R. Bagnis, S. Chanteau, and T. Yasumoto, *C. R. Hebd. Seances Acad. Sci., Ser. D* **285,** 105 (1977).

17. T. I. Yasumoto, I. Nakajima, R. Bagnis, and R. Adachi, *Nippon Suisan Gakkaishi* **43,** 1021 (1977).

18. R. Adachi and Y. Fukuyo, *Nippon Suisan Gakkaishi* **45,** 67 (1978).

19. F. Gusovsky and J. W. Daly, *Biochem. Pharmacol.* **39,** 1633 (1990).

20. M. Durand, *Toxicon* **24,** 1153 (1987).

21. M. Durand-Clement, *Biol. Bull. (Woods Hole, Mass.)* **172,** 108 (1987).

22. P. J. Scheuer, W. Takahashi, J. Tsutsumi, and T. Yoshida, *Science* **155,** 1267 (1967).

23. K. Tachibana, Ph.D. thesis. Univ. of Hawaii, Honolulu, Hawaii, 1980.

24. M. Nukina, L. M. Koyanagi, and P. J. Scheuer, *Toxicon* **22,** 169 (1984).

25. K. Tachibana, M. Nukina, Y. G. Joh, and P. J. Scheuer, *Biol. Bull. (Woods Hole, Mass.)* **172,** 122 (1987).

26. A.-M. Legrand, M. Litaudon, J. N. Genthon, R. Bagnis, and T. Yasumoto, *J. Appl. Phycol.* **1,** 183 (1989).

27. M. Murata, A.-M. Legrand, Y. Ishibashi, and T. Yasumoto, *J. Am. Chem. Soc.* **111,** 8929 (1989).

28. M. Murata, A.-M. Legrand, Y. Ishibashi, M. Fukui, and T. Yasumoto, *J. Am. Chem. Soc.* **112,** 4380 (1990).

29. W. Nonner, *Pfluegers Arch. Gesamte Physiol.* **309,** 176 (1969).

30. E. Benoit, A.-M. Legrand, and J.-M. Dubois. *Toxicon* **24,** 357 (1986).

31. W. A. Catterall, *ISI Atlas Sci.: Pharmacol.* **2,** 190 (1988).

32. D. G. Baden, *FASEB J.* **3,** 1807 (1989).

33. E. Benoit and J.-M. Dubois, *J. Physiol. (London)* **383,** 93 (1987).

34. L. L. Boyarsky and M. D. Rayner, *Proc. Soc. Exp. Biol. Med.* **134,** 322 (1970).

35. J.-N. Bidard, H. P. M. Vijverberg, C. Frelin, E. Chungue, A.-M. Legrand, R. Bagnis, and M. Lazdunski, *J. Biol. Chem.* **259,** 8353 (1984).

36. M. F. Capra and J. Cameron, *Proc. Int. Coral Reef Congr., 5th* **4,** 457 (1985).

37. M. D. Rayner, *Fed. Proc., Fed. Am. Soc. Exp. Biol.* **31,** 1139 (1972).

38. M. D. Rayner and T. I. Kosaki, *Fed. Proc., Fed. Am. Soc. Exp. Biol.* **29,** 548 (1970).

39. J. Molgo, J. X. Comella, and A.-M. Legrand, *Br. J. Pharmacol.* **99,** 695 (1990).

40. A. R. Khan, M. Lemeignan, and J. Molgo, *Toxicon* **24,** 373 (1986).

41. A. Seino, M. Kobayashi, K. Momose, T. Yasumoto, and Y. Ohizumi, *Br. J. Pharmacol.* **95,** 876 (1988).

42. R. J. Lewis and R. Endean, *Naunyn-Schmiedeberg's Arch Pharmacol.* **334**, 313 (1986).
43. R. J. Lewis, *Toxicon* **26**, 639 (1988).
44. J. T. Miyahara, C. K. Akau, and T. Tasumoto, *Res. Commun. Chem. Pathol. Pharmacol.* **25**, 177 (1979).
45. H. Ohshika, *Toxicon* **9**, 337 (1971).
46. A.-M. Legrand and R. Bagnis, *Toxicon* **22**, 471 (1984).
47. Y. Ohizumi, S. Shibata, and T. Tachibana, *J. Pharmacol. Exp. Ther.* **217**, 475 (1981).
48. R. J. Lewis and R. Endean, *J. Pharmacol. Exp. Ther.* **228**, 756 (1984).
49. J. T. Miyahara and S. Shibata, *Fed. Proc., Fed. Am. Soc. Exp. Biol.* **35**, 842 (1976).
50. D. M. Miller, R. W. Dickey, and D. R. Tindall, *Fed. Proc., Fed. Am. Soc. Exp. Biol.* **41**, 1561 (1982).
51. A. Lombet, J.-N. Bidard, and M. Lazdunski, *FEBS Lett.* **219**, 355 (1987).
52. C. Frelin, M. Durand-Clement, J.-N. Bidard, and M. Lazdunski, *in* "Natural Toxins from Aquatic and Marine Environments" (S. Hall, ed.), p. 192. Am. Chem. Soc., Washington, D.C., 1990.
53. Y. Ohizumi, *Biol. Bull. (Woods, Hole, Mass.)* **172**, 132 (1987).
54. J. P. Abita, R. Chicheportiche, H. Schweitz, and M. Lazdunski, *Biochemistry* **16**, 1838 (1977).
55. J. Molgo, *in* "Advances in the Biosciences" (P. Lechat, S. Thesleff, and W. C. Bowman *et al.*, eds.), p. 95. Pergamon, Oxford, England, 1982.
56. A. J. Anderson and A. L. Harvey, *Br. J. Pharmacol.* **93**, 215 (1988).
57. J. Molgo and A. Mallart, *Pfluegers Arch. Gesamte Physiol.* **405**, 349 (1985).
58. W. D. Atchison, V. S. Luke, T. Narahashi, and S. M. Vogel, *Br. J. Pharmacol.* **89**, 731 (1986).
59. Y. I. Kim, I. S. Login, and T. Yasumoto, *Brain Res.* **346**, 357 (1985).
60. J. Molgo, J. X. Comella, T. Shimahara, and A.-M. Legrand. *Ann. N.Y. Acad. Sci.* (in press) (1991).
61. J. Molgo, M. Lemeignan, and F. Tazieff-Depierre, *Toxicon* **25**, 441 (1986).
62. A. D. Lowe, B. P. Richardson, P. Taylor, and P. Donatsch, *Nature (London)* **260**, 337 (1976).
63. R. Rahamimoff, A. Lev-Tov, and H. Meiri, *J. Exp. Biol.* **89**, 5 (1980).
64. R. Melinek, A. Lev-Tov, H. Meiri, S. D. Erulkar, and R. Rahamimoff, *Isr. J. Med. Sci.* **18**, 37 (1982).
65. F. Gusovsky, E. B. Hollingsworth, and J. W. Daly, *Proc. Natl. Acad. Sci. U.S.A.* **83**, 3003 (1986).
66. G. Grynkiewicz, M. Poenie, and R. Y. Tsien, *J. Biol. Chem.* **260**, 3440 (1985).

[12] Purification and Radiolabeling of *Clostridium botulinum* Type F Neurotoxin

Clifford C. Shone, Howard S. Tranter, and
Frances C. G. Alexander

Introduction

Botulism, a frequently fatal disease affecting both humans and animals, is caused by any one of seven antigenically different neurotoxins (types A–G) produced by various strains of the bacterium *Clostridium botulinum* (1, 2). Botulinum F neurotoxin, a typical representative of this family of potent neuroparalytic agents, is a protein of molecular mass approximately 155 kDa consisting of heavy (ca. 105 kDa) and light (ca. 55 kDa) subunits linked by a disulfide bridge (3, 4). The primary site of action of all the botulinum neurotoxins is the neuromuscular junction where, following a binding step in which toxin molecules interact with acceptor sites on the presynaptic nerve surface, they enter the nerve ending and block the calcium-dependent release of neurotransmitter. Not all the botulinum neurotoxins appear to recognize the same type of acceptor molecule on the presynaptic nerve surface (4, 5) and once inside the nerve ending not all the toxin types appear to block the transmitter release process by the same mechanism (6). The potential of the botulinum neurotoxins to provide several probes with which to study the poorly understood process of calcium-mediated transmitter release, together with the growing clinical applications of these toxins, make them worthy of intensive study.

In comparison with botulinum type A, B, and E neurotoxins, type F neurotoxin has been little studied primarily because strains of *C. botulinum* type F are relatively poor producers of toxin, making purification difficult. A small-scale purification procedure for type F neurotoxin was first developed by Yang and Sugiyama in 1975 (3) but until recently a procedure (4) for producing sufficient quantities of neurotoxin to allow a detailed characterization of the structure and action of the toxin has not been available. Type F neurotoxin is secreted from the bacterium in the form of a protein complex of molecular weight ca. 235 kDa (M complex) in which the neurotoxin is associated with a nontoxic protein of similar molecular size (7). The M complex is stable at pH values below 6.5, but above pH 7.5 the two proteins dissociate. This pH-dependent dissociation of the neurotoxin complex, which is also a feature of the toxin complexes of other botulinum types, has been exploited in the purification of several of the botulinum neurotoxins (8), including type F as described below.

Safety

Botulinum type F neurotoxin is an extremely potent neuroparalytic agent with a human lethal dose on the order of a few micrograms and, unlike botulinum toxins A–E, a vaccine to type F neurotoxin is presently not widely available. Considerable care should therefore be exercised both during the growth of the organism and purification of the toxin. Manipulations of bacterial culture and solutions of toxin should be performed under contained conditions, ideally in a class III microbiological safety cabinet. Centrifugation steps should be carried out only in well-sealed centrifuge tubes contained within a sealed rotor. As far as possible nonbreakable plasticware should be used in place of glassware.

Growth of *Clostridium botulinum* Type F

Strain Selection and Maintenance

Although several different bacterial strains and culture conditions have been used to prepare small quantities of botulinum type F toxin, the Langeland strain (9) of *C. botulinum* type F has been most widely used because of the high yields of toxin obtained during growth (3, 10). Data from this laboratory concur with these findings. Measurements of toxin production by a number of isolates of *C. botulinum* type F grown in a variety of media have shown the *C. botulinum,* Langeland strain to produce the highest levels of toxin: in the appropriate media, toxin concentrations of 5×10^4 to 2×10^5 mouse lethal dose 50% (MLD_{50}) per milliliter were consistently produced by this strain.

Viable stock cultures of all types of *C. botulinum* can be maintained for several years in cooked meat medium (Oxoid, Columbia, MD) at 4°C. However, under these conditions the toxin-producing ability of many strains appears to decrease with prolonged storage. It is advisable, therefore, to store stock cultures at $-70°C$ or in liquid nitrogen. Following initial growth in cooked meat medium at 30°C for 24 hr, cultures are stored in 2- or 5-ml cryovials as 1.8- or 3-ml aliquots, each containing 10% (v/v) glycerol.

Growth Media

The growth of *C. botulinum* type F is normally carried out in complex culture media since such media have been reported to produce approximately 10-fold higher levels of toxin than that obtained with the presently available chemically defined media (11). For the routine procedure of type F botulinum toxin, two growth media have been selected.

Medium 1: Brain–Heart Infusion (BHI Medium) (12)

This medium consists of brain–heart infusion broth, 37.0 g/liter (Oxoid); yeast extract, 5 g/liter (Oxoid); cysteine hydrochloride, 0.5 g/liter. To this 10 ml/liter of a 0.5 mg/ml hemin solution and 1 ml/liter of a vitamin K solution [0.1% (v/v) in 95% ethanol] are added and the medium adjusted to pH 7.0 with 10 M HCl before autoclaving. Immediately before inoculation the medium is supplemented with 1% (w/v) glucose.

Medium 2: NZ Case Plus (NZCP Medium)

Comparable yields of type F toxin can also be achieved in a simple medium that does not contain animal protein. This medium consists of 40 g/liter NZ case plus (Sheffield Products, Norwich, NY) and 1 g/liter cysteine hydrochloride, sterilized by autoclaving. The medium is supplemented with 1% (w/v) glucose immediately before inoculation.

Small amounts of media (up to 200 ml) are prepared in screw-capped bottles and are presteamed for 30 min and cooled to 30°C prior to the addition of glucose. All larger volumes of media are used as soon as possible after preparation.

Fermentation

Medium-Scale Fermentation

For this, *C. botulinum* type F, Langeland strain, is grown in a contained fermenter (13) consisting of 40 liters of growth medium in two 25-liter glass vessels. Stock culture is removed from liquid nitrogen, thawed, and 1 ml used to inoculate 20 ml of cooked meat medium. This culture is incubated anaerobically at 30°C for 24 hr and 4-ml portions removed to inoculate four 200-ml amounts of growth medium. These cultures are grown anaerobically at 30°C for 22 hr before they are used to inoculate two-liter vented seed bottles, each containing 1 liter of growth medium. After incubation at 30°C for 20 hr these cultures are then used to inoculate the fermenter vessels. During fermentation the temperature is maintained at 30°C and the agitation rate at 50 rpm. Nitrogen (2 liters/min) is flushed through the growth medium prior to inoculation and during growth of the culture. Although production of types A and B botulinum toxins can be enhanced by a nitrogen overlay rather than by sparging during fermentation (14), a similar effect during fermentation of *C. botulinum* type F was not observed.

At the end of fermentation the culture is acidified to pH 3.5 by the addition of 3 *M* H₂SO₄. The culture is stirred at 200 rpm during the addition of acid to ensure efficient mixing and the resulting precipitate recovered by centrifugation at 40,000 rpm, using a continuous-flow centrifuge (Carl Padberg, Zentrifugenbau GmbH) mounted inside a class III microbiological safety cabinet (13).

Large-Scale Fermentation

The production of large amounts of toxin from *C. botulinum* type F can be carried out in a high containment 225-liter (150-liter working volume) fermenter (L. H. Fermentation Ltd, UK) (15). Two 3-ml vials of stock culture are removed from liquid nitrogen, thawed, and used to inoculate 200 ml of growth medium in a screw-capped bottle. This primary seed is incubated anaerobically at 30°C for 22 hr and used to inoculate 1 liter of growth medium in a 2-liter vented glass bottle (secondary seed). This is grown for a further 10 hr at 30°C before 350 ml is used to inoculate three 5-liter vented glass aspirators, each containing 3.5 liters of medium. This tertiary seed is grown at 30°C for 10 hr before it is used to inoculate the 225-liter fermenter.

The fermentation parameters are scaled up as closely as possible to those used in the medium-scale fermentations. The temperature is maintained at 30°C and the agitation rate at 60–85 rpm, respectively. Nitrogen gas is sparged through the culture, usually for the first 8–10 hr only, at a rate of 40 liters/min. At the end of fermentation the culture is acidified by pumping 3 *M* H₂SO₄ into the fermenter until the pH falls to 3.0–3.2. The acidified culture is harvested from the fermenter by tangential flow filtration using a Millipore (Bedford, MA) Pellicon system fitted with four cassettes containing 0.45-μm Durapore membranes (Millipore). The concentrated slurry resulting from this operation is harvested by centrifugation using an H6000A rotor at 5000 rpm in a Sorvall RC5B centrifuge.

Acidified paste containing botulinum toxin can be stored in this form at 4°C for several months without significant loss of activity.

Growth Characteristics

Growth of the Langeland strain of *C. botulinum* type F in supplemented brain–heart infusion medium is exponential for the first 8–10 hr, reaching a

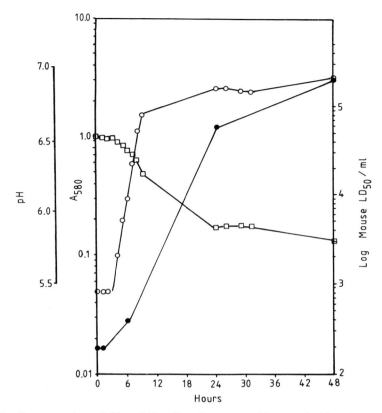

FIG. 1   Fermentation of *Clostridium botulinum* type F: growth (absorbance at 580 nm) (○), toxin production (●), and change in culture pH (□) during fermentation of *C. botulinum* type F, Langeland strain. The medium was supplemented brain–heart infusion broth containing 1% (w/v) glucose. Fermentation was carried out at 30°C with an agitation rate of 50 rpm and nitrogen sparging (2 liters/min).

maximum absorbance (580 nm) after 24 hr of growth (Fig. 1). During the initial growth phase the pH drops rapidly to pH 5.8 by 24 hr and does not alter for the duration of the fermentation. The toxin levels increase initially during the growth phase to reach 7×10^4 MLD$_{50}$/ml after 24 hr. Toxin appears to accumulate after a further 24-hr incubation, despite no changes in the absorbance (580 nm) or pH, to reach a maximum $1-2 \times 10^5$ MLD$_{50}$/ml after 48 hr. Continued incubation after this time does not appear to increase toxin production. Maximum levels of toxin are produced in the absence of cell lysis, which indicates that autolysis is not the mechanism by which this toxin is released.

Growth and toxin production by the Langeland strain in NZ case plus medium occurs more rapidly. Maximum levels of toxin are produced after 24 hr of fermentation but type F toxin does not appear to be stable in this medium beyond this time.

Purification of Botulinum Type F Neurotoxin

The purification procedure for botulinum type F neurotoxin takes advantage of the different chromatographic properties of neurotoxin in its free and complexed form; at pH values between 5.5 and 6.0 the neurotoxin, in its complex form, is not retained by cation-exchange columns while the free neurotoxin is strongly adsorbed. A similar strategy has also been successfully employed in the purification of type E neurotoxin (8). During the first column stage type F neurotoxin, in its M complex form, is fractionated on an anion-exchange column at pH 5.8. The neurotoxin complex is then dissociated by raising the pH to 8.5 and fractionated on a second anion-exchange column. Finally, the neurotoxin in its free form is chromatographed on a cation-exchange column at pH 5.5. During this stage the neurotoxin is virtually the only protein retained by the column, with the bulk of the contaminating proteins eluting in the wash fraction.

The procedure outlined below describes the purification of botulinum type F neurotoxin, commencing with the acid-precipitated toxin obtained from a total of 150–160 liters of bacterial culture obtained using BHI growth medium. Column chromatography steps are performed at room temperature.

Buffers Required

Extraction buffer: 4 liters of sodium phosphate buffer (0.2 M, pH 6.0); 500 ml sodium hydroxide (2 M)

First column stage buffers

Dialysis and equilibration buffer: 30 liters of Bis-Tris-HCl buffer (0.05 M, pH 5.8)

Elution buffers: 2 liters of Bis-Tris-HCl buffer (0.05 M, pH 5.8) containing 0.15 M NaCl; 2 liters of Bis-Tris-HCl buffer containing 1 M NaCl

Second column stage buffers

Dialysis and equilibration buffer: 15 liters of triethanolamine buffer (0.05 M, pH 8.5) containing 0.05 M NaCl

Elution buffers: 1 liter of triethanolamine buffer (0.05 M, pH 8.5, containing 0.15 M NaCl; 1 liter of triethanolamine buffer (0.05 M, pH 8.5) containing 1 M NaCl

Third column stage buffers

Dialysis and equilibration buffer: 6 liters of sodium succinate buffer (0.05 M, pH 5.5)

Elution buffers: 500 ml of succinate buffer (0.05 M, pH 5.5); 500 ml of succinate buffer (0.05 M, pH 5.5) containing 0.3 M NaCl

Storage buffer: 2 liters of Tris-HCl buffer (0.1 M, pH 8.0) containing 0.1 M NaCl

Assay Procedure

At present the only methods available for the routine assessment of the biological activity of botulinum type F neurotoxin are acute toxicity tests performed in mice (16). Toxin samples are serially diluted in sodium phosphate buffer (0.07 M, pH 6.5) containing 0.2% (w/v) gelatin. Portions of the diluted toxin (2 ml) are then injected (intraperitoneally) into groups of four mice (0.5 ml/animal) and deaths monitored over a period of 4 days. The MLD_{50}/ml is estimated from the toxin dilution that killed half the animals in the group over the 4-day period.

Purification Procedure

1. The precipitate obtained from 150 liters of acidified culture is resuspended in 1400 ml of sodium phosphate buffer (0.2 M, pH 6.0). Depending on the consistency of the acid-precipitated toxin it may be necessary to employ gentle homogenization at this stage to break up any lumps. A stomacher-type homogenizer (Seward Laboratories, London, UK) is ideal for this purpose. Portions of the toxin solution are placed in double-layered stomacher bags and homogenized for 2–3 min, turning the bags through 180° at least once during the process. If another homogenization technique is employed, care should be taken to avoid excessive frothing of the toxin solution. After homogenization, the toxin is transferred to a plastic 5-liter beaker and the solution stirred rapidly. Sodium hydroxide (2 M) is added slowly (in 20-ml portions) to the stirred toxin solution and the pH measured a few minutes after each addition. When the pH reaches pH 5.5, the sodium hydroxide solution is added more slowly until the pH of the solution is between 6.0 and 6.1. During this stage the toxin solution should be stirred quickly enough to ensure the rapid mixing of the sodium hydroxide solution; it is essential to avoid localized rises in pH significantly above pH 6. The solution is stirred for a further 50 min and then centrifuged at 30,000 g for 40 min. The supernatant fluid, which contains the toxin, is carefully decanted and stored at 4°C.

2. The resulting pellets are then resuspended in 1400 ml of sodium phosphate buffer (0.2 M, pH 6.0) and the extraction procedure repeated as described in step 1. During the second extraction it is not necessary to adjust the pH of the solution.

3. The supernatant fluids obtained from steps 1 and 2 are combined and ribonuclease A (25 mg/ml in 0.2 M phosphate buffer, pH 6.0; Sigma, St. Louis, MO) added to a final concentration of 0.1 mg/ml. The mixture is then transferred to a plastic container and incubated for 90 min at 37°C.

4. The toxin is precipitated by slowly adding solid ammonium sulfate to 60% saturation (390 g/liter) to a rapidly stirred solution. After all the ammonium sulfate has been added the mixture is stirred for a further 30 min and then centrifuged at 30,000 g for 30 min at 4°C. The supernatant fluid is carefully removed and the toxin precipitate redissolved in 700 ml of Bis-Tris-HCl buffer (0.05 M, pH 5.8). The suspension is stirred for 10 min to break up any undissolved lumps, then the solution is transferred to several dialysis sacs (4-cm diameter) and dialyzed for 16–24 hr against 10 liters of Bis-Tris-HCl buffer (0.05 M, pH 5.8) at 4°C. After this period the dialysis sacs are transferred into fresh buffer and the dialysis continued for a further 16–24 hr.

5. A column (11.2-cm diameter × 7 cm; 700-cm^3 volume) is packed with Sepharose Q (Pharmacia, Piscataway, NJ), taking care to ensure the column is precisely level during the packing procedure, and then the Sepharose Q is equilibrated with 5 liters of Bis-Tris-HCl buffer (0.05 M, pH 5.8). The dialyzed toxin solution is centrifuged at 30,000 g for 60 min; then the supernatant fluid is removed, taking care not to disturb the pellet of insoluble material. The toxin solution is applied at a flow rate of 50 ml/min to the Sepharose Q and, after all the toxin has been applied, the column is washed with a further 1100 ml of the Bis-Tris-HCl buffer. Toxin is eluted with Bis-Tris-HCl buffer (0.05 M, pH 5.8) containing 0.15 M NaCl. The type F toxin peak is eluted in a volume of approximately 700 ml, beginning after 500 ml of the salt buffer has passed through the column. After the toxin fraction has been eluted the remaining bound protein may be eluted from the column with Bis-Tris-HCl buffer (0.05 M, pH 5.8) containing 1 M NaCl.

6. The eluted toxin is dialyzed against 10 liters of triethanolamine buffer (0.05 M, pH 8.5) containing 0.05 M NaCl for 16–24 hr at 4°C, then applied at a flow rate of 50 ml/min to a column (5-cm diameter × 8 cm) of Sepharose Q previously equilibrated with 1.5 liters of the triethanolamine buffer. After loading, the column is washed with a further 600 ml of triethanolamine buffer (0.05 M, pH 8.5) containing 0.05 M NaCl and then the type F toxin is eluted with triethanolamine buffer (0.05 M, pH 8.5) containing 0.15 M NaCl. The protein peak containing the toxin, which begins to elute after approximately 80–100 ml of the latter buffer has passed through the column, is collected.

7. The toxin fraction (ca. 250–400 ml) is dialyzed against 5 liters of succinate buffer (0.05 M, pH 5.5) for 16–24 hr at 4°C. Should any precipitation occur during the dialysis step, then the solution should be clarified by centrifugation at 30,000 g for 20 min at 4°C. The toxin is applied at a flow rate of 5 ml/min to a column (1.6-cm diameter × 5 cm) of Sepharose S previously equilibrated with the succinate buffer. The column is washed with a further 50 ml of succinate buffer (0.05 M, pH 5.5) and eluted with a 200-ml linear gradient from 0 to 0.3 M NaCl in the succinate buffer. The flow rate is 5 ml/min and 3-ml fractions are collected. Type F neurotoxin is the first major protein peak to eluate after application of the salt gradient (eluting in approximately 100 mM NaCl).

8. The major neurotoxin fractions obtained in step 7 are pooled and dialyzed against Tris-HCl buffer (0.1 M, pH 8.0) containing 0.1 M NaCl, aliquoted, and stored at −25°C.

Commencing with 150 liters of brain–heart infusion medium the above procedure generally yields between 60 and 110 mg of purified botulinum type F neurotoxin. Sodium dodecyl sulfate (SDS)-polyacrylamide gel electrophoresis of various fractions obtained during the purification procedure is shown in Fig. 2 and a summary of typical purification yields given in Table I.

Comments on Purification Procedure

The final Sepharose S chromatography step represents the critical step of the procedure, in which the bulk of the contaminating proteins is removed from the neurotoxin (Fig. 2). During this step very little protein other than the type F neurotoxin is retained by the column. Botulinum type F neurotoxin has a fairly low solubility at pH 5.5 and to minimize losses at the final column stage it is important that the volume of the Sepharose S column be no larger than necessary (ca. 1-ml column volume/15 liters of initial culture volume). Also, in view of the large sample volume (250–400 ml) and relatively small column volume at this stage, the use of prepacked, high-resolution (10-μm bead size) columns should be avoided because these are easily clogged.

Storage of the purified neurotoxin (>1 mg/ml) for any length of time in the pH 5.5 succinate buffer should be avoided because some precipitation can occur over a period of several days at 4°C.

The medium used to grow *C. botulinum* type F has a considerable effect on the nature of the nontoxic proteins produced by the bacterium. This is illustrated by Fig. 3, which compares two chromatographic profiles representing the final column stage of the procedure (stage 7), obtained from two purification runs using different bacterial growth media. During the final

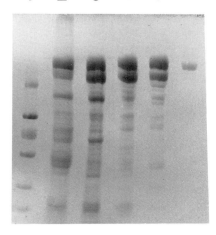

FIG. 2   SDS-polyacrylamide gel electrophoresis of samples of botulinum type F neurotoxin during purification. Electrophoresis was performed on 4–30% gradient gels (PAA 4/30; Pharmacia) as described previously (4). Samples are as follow: lane 1, molecular weight ($\times$ 10^{-3}) markers (from top to bottom, 94, 67, 43, 30, 20, and 14.4); lane 2, combined sodium phosphate buffer extracts from steps 1 and 2; lane 3, resuspended ammonium sulfate precipitate; lane 4, 0.15 M NaCl fraction obtained from Sepharose Q (pH 5.8); lane 5, 0.15 M NaCl fraction obtained from Sepharose Q (pH 8.5); lane 6, purified botulinum type F neurotoxin obtained from Sepharose S (pH 5.5). All samples were electrophoresed under nonreducing conditions.

column stage of a procedure in which brain–heart infusion growth medium has been used (Fig. 3A), type F neurotoxin is virtually the only protein to bind to the column. In contrast, when NZCP medium is used, additional protein bands are observed that elute at higher salt concentration relative to the neurotoxin band (Fig. 3B). The choice of growth medium also has a significant effect on the yield of purified neurotoxin: yields of between 20 and 45% were obtained when BHI medium was used, whereas consistently lower yields (5–10%) were obtained with the NZCP medium. It is recommended, therefore, unless it is essential to avoid using a medium containing protein of animal origin, that BHI medium be used for the growth of *C. botulinum* type F.

The suitability of the above procedure for the purification of type F neurotoxin from strains other the *C. botulinum* type F, Langeland strain has presently not been assessed.

TABLE I   Purification of Botulinum Type F Neurotoxin

Purification stage	Volume (ml)	Protein (mg/ml)	Toxicity (LD_{50})		Yield (%)	
			Total	Specific	Stage	Overall
Resuspended acidified culture	2030	nd[a]	8.1×10^9	nd	100	100
Combined phosphate buffer extract	2750	8.2	4.7×10^9	2.1×10^5	58	58
Resuspended $(NH_4)_2SO_4$ precipitate	1095	8.2	3.8×10^9	4.3×10^5	81	47
Sepharose Q (pH 5.8), 0.15 M NaCl elute	725	7.7	3.3×10^9	5.9×10^5	87	41
Sepharose Q (pH 8.5), 0.15 M NaCl elute	250	11	2.5×10^9	9.1×10^5	76	31
Sepharose S (pH 5.5), neurotoxin peak	50	2	1.8×10^9	1.8×10^7	72	22

[a] nd, Not determined.

Properties of Botulinum Type F Neurotoxin

The above purification method generally yields neurotoxin greater than 95% pure with a specific toxicity in mice between 1.5 and $2 \times 10^7 \, LD_{50}$/mg protein. On SDS-PAGE under nonreducing conditions the neurotoxin appears as a major protein band of approximately 155 K with minor impurity bands visible at approximately 180 K, 95 K, and 70 K (Fig. 2). In the presence of 50 mM dithiothreitol the neurotoxin appears as two protein bands of 105 K and 55 K, corresponding to the heavy and light subunits, respectively, of the neurotoxin.

Radiolabeling of Botulinum Type F Neurotoxin

The scope of studies aimed at characterizing the botulinal neural acceptors and intracellular site of action is greatly broadened by the availability of radiolabeled botulinum neurotoxin. Botulinum type F neurotoxin may be ^{125}I-labeled to a high specific radioactivity activity with retention of biological

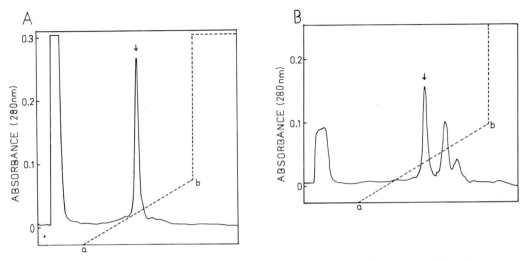

FIG. 3   Elution profiles (absorbance at 280 nm) of botulinum type F fractions separated by ion-exchange chromatography. Portions (1 ml) of the triethanolamine (0.05
M, pH 8.5)/0.15 M NaCl fraction obtained from Sepharose Q columns (stage 6) were
dialyzed against succinate buffer (0.05 M, pH 5.5) and applied to a column of Mono
S (HR 5/5; Pharmacia) equilibrated with the succinate buffer. Proteins were eluted
with a linear, 20-ml, 0–0.3 M NaCl gradient in the succinate buffer. (A) Elution profile
obtained using brain–heart infusion growth medium. (B) Elution profile obtained
using NZCP medium. The dashed lines (a–––b) indicate the theoretical NaCl gradient
from 0 to 0.3 M NaCl. The arrows ($\downarrow$) show the protein peak corresponding to
botulinum type F neurotoxin.

activity using a chloramine-T method. This procedure is a slight modification
of that initially developed for the radioiodination of botulinum type A neurotoxin (17) and may also be used to radiolabel botulinum type A, B, and E
neurotoxins.

Buffers and Reagents Required

Gel filtration and dialysis buffer: 1 liter of HEPES buffer (0.05 M,
pH 7.5) containing 0.2 M NaCl (HEPES/NaCl buffer)
Iodination reagents:
Iodine-125, carrier free, 5 mCi (100 mCi/ml) in NaOH solution,
pH 7–11

Chloramine-T (0.88 mM) in HEPES/NaCl buffer (freshly prepared before use)

Tyrosine (1 mg/ml) in HEPES/NaCl buffer (warm to 50°C to dissolve)

Safety

The millicurie quantities of volatile ^{125}I together with the high concentrations of botulinum neurotoxin used in the procedure pose a significant safety hazard. It is recommended that the iodination procedure be conducted in a class III (13) microbiological safety cabinet vented externally.

Iodination Procedure

If a 5-mCi lot of ^{125}I is to be used, the iodination reaction is most conveniently performed in the small glass vial containing the isotope, which should be centrifuged briefly (200 g for 2 min) before use.

1. To 50 μl of ^{125}I, 100 μl of type F neurotoxin (1–5 mg/ml) in HEPES/NaCl buffer (or in 0.1 M Tris-HCl, pH 8.0, containing 0.1 M NaCl) is carefully added. To this solution 50 μl of 0.88 mM chloramine-T solution is introduced, gently mixed, and incubated for 1 min at 22°C. The reaction is then stopped by the addition of 50 μl tyrosine (1 mg/ml).

2. The iodinated neurotoxin is then immediately applied to a column (1.5 × 5 cm) of Sephadex G-25 (PD10 column, Pharmacia) previously equilibrated with 50 ml of the HEPES/NaCl buffer. After allowing the toxin solution to almost completely flow onto the column, 4 drops of the HEPES/NaCl is carefully added and this volume allowed to run onto the column. The column is then eluted with HEPES/NaCl buffer at a flow rate of between 0.15 and 0.2 ml/min and 35 fractions (7 drops/fraction) are collected.

3. Portions (3 μl) of fractions 10–30 are removed and their radioactivity determined. The four fractions displaying the highest radioactivity are then combined. If the original concentration of the type F neurotoxin was less than 2 mg/ml it is advisable to add a suitable carrier protein at this stage. After a portion of the iodinated toxin has been removed for protein determination, ovalbumin is added to a final concentration of 1 mg/ml from a 10 mg/ml solution in HEPES/NaCl buffer.

4. The ^{125}I-labeled type F neurotoxin is dialyzed twice against HEPES/NaCl buffer (250 ml each time) for 16 hr at 4°C to remove the small proportion of free [125]I.

Comments on Iodination Procedure

The above procedure generally yields ^{125}I-labeled botulinum type F neurotoxin (ca. 0.7–1 mCi total) with a specific radioactivity between 600 and 1400 Ci/mmol and retention of >70% of the original specific toxicity (4). Stored at 4°C the radiolabeled neurotoxin retains its biological activity for up to 14 days: neurotoxin labeled to a high specific radioactivity (>1200 Ci/mmol) is usually less stable than that labeled to a lower specific radioactivity (<800 Ci/mmol). Botulinum type F neurotoxin labeled by the above method may be used in a wide variety of binding studies at toxin concentrations as low as 0.2 nM.

Acknowledgment

This work was supported in part by Contract No. DAMD 17-87-R-0092 from the U.S. Army Medical Research and Development Command.

References

1. L. L. Simpson, *Pharmacol. Rev.* **33,** 155 (1981).
2. C. C. Shone, *in* "Natural Toxicants in Foods" (D. H. Watson, ed.), p. 11. Ellis Horwood, Chichester, England, 1987.
3. K. H. Yang and H. Sugiyama, *Appl. Microbiol.* **29,** 598 (1975).
4. J. D. F. Wadsworth, M. Desai, H. S. Tranter, H. J. King, P. Hambleton, J. Melling, J. O. Dolly, and C. C. Shone, *Biochem. J.* **268,** 123 (1990).
5. J. D. Black and J. O. Dolly, *J. Cell Biol.* **103,** 521 (1986).
6. L. C. Sellin, S. Thesleff, and B. R. DasGupta, *Acta Physiol. Scand.* **119,** 127 (1983).
7. I. Ohishi and G. Sakaguchi, *Appl. Microbiol.* **29,** 444 (1975).
8. J. J. Schmidt and L. S. Siegel, *Anal. Biochem.* **156,** 213 (1986).
9. V. Moeller and I. Schiebel, *Acta Pathol. Microbiol. Scand.* **48,** 80 (1960).
10. I. Ohishi and G. Sakaguchi, *Appl. Microbiol.* **28,** 923 (1974).
11. D. A. Boroff and B. R. DasGupta, *in* "Microbial Toxins" (S. Kadis, T. C. Montie, and S. J. Ajl, eds.), Vol. IIA, p. 1. Academic Press, New York, 1971.
12. L. V. Holdeman, E. P. Cato, and W. E. C. Moore (eds.), "Anaerobe Laboratory Manual," 4th Ed., p. 144. Va. Polytech. Inst., Blacksberg, Virginia, 1977.
13. J. Melling and K. Allner, *in* "Essays in Applied Microbiology" (J. R. Norris and M. H. Richmond, eds.), p. 11/1. Wiley, London, 1981.
14. L. S. Siegel, *in* "Biomedical Aspects of Botulism" (G. E. Lewis, Jr., ed.), p. 121. Academic Press, New York, 1981.

15. P. Hambleton, J. B. Griffiths, D. R. Cameron, and J. Melling, *J. Chem. Tech. Biotechnol.* **50,** 167 (1991).
16. C. Lamanna, W. I. Jenson, and D. J. Bross, *Am. J. Hyg.* **62,** 21 (1955).
17. R. S. Williams, C. K. Tse, J. O. Dolly, P. Hambleton, and J. Melling, *Eur. J. Biochem.* **131,** 437 (1983).

[13] Retrograde Tracing with Cholera Toxin B–Gold or with Immunocytochemically Detected Cholera Toxin B in Central Nervous System

Ida J. Llewellyn-Smith, Jane B. Minson, and
Paul M. Pilowsky

Horseradish peroxidase (HRP) coupled to cholera toxin was shown to be a sensitive retrograde tracer by Trojanowski and co-workers in the early 1980s (1). Because the B subunit of cholera toxin (CTB) lacks the toxic effects of the intact toxin molecule but still binds to neurons and is retrogradely transported, CTB is now routinely used instead of cholera toxin. The advantage of CTB–HRP as a retrograde tracer lies in its ability to reveal distal dendrites, giving labeled neurons a Golgi-like appearance (see, e.g., Refs. 2 and 3). This property is not shared by other retrograde tracers (for example, unconjugated HRP, wheat germ agglutinin–HRP, or wheat germ agglutinin–apoHRP–gold), which localize in lysosomes and therefore label only neuronal cell bodies and proximal dendrites. Nevertheless, CTB–HRP has some disadvantages. Since high concentrations of glutaraldehyde are needed for the optimal demonstration of peroxidase activity, the use of CTB–HRP is incompatible with immunocytochemistry for fixation-sensitive antigens. Furthermore, the reaction product of tetramethylbenzidine, the most sensitive chromogen for detecting the peroxidase activity of CTB–HRP, is difficult to stabilize (4). In contrast, unconjugated CTB, demonstrated with anti-CTB antibodies (5, 6) also labels cell bodies and proximal and distal dendrites, but can be detected after fixation with a wide variety of fixatives (7; see below). This tolerance for a range of fixatives makes unconjugated CTB eminently suitable for studies on the neurochemistry of inputs to retrogradely labeled neurons, where light fixation may be required for demonstrating some neurotransmitters (for example, serotonin) and heavy fixation for others [for example, γ-aminobutyric acid (GABA)]. In addition, we have recently discovered that retrograde transport of CTB can reveal axons as well as dendrites (8; see below), opening up the possibility of defining the neurotransmitter content of synapses on the output as well as the input processes of retrogradely labeled neurons. Furthermore, unconjugated CTB is also anterogradely transported (5, 7).

Methods in Neurosciences, Volume 8

CTB linked to colloidal gold particles (CTB–gold) (9) has proved to be another powerful retrograde tracer. CTB–gold is revealed for light microscopy by silver intensification; for electron microscopy, it is visible with or without silver intensification. CTB–gold is particularly useful for examining the neurotransmitter content of retrogradely labeled neurons (see, e.g., Ref. 10). Retrogradely transported silver-intensified gold particles, which are localized in lysosomes in neuronal somata and proximal dendrites, are distinguishable from the peroxidase reaction product used to demonstrate immunoreactivity for neurotransmitters or neurotransmitter-synthesizing enzymes. Furthermore, CTB–gold is insensitive to fixation conditions and so can be used in combination with immunocytochemistry for any antigen.

The purpose of this chapter is to document techniques we use to study central neurons retrogradely labeled with CTB–gold or unconjugated CTB. Included are methods for making CTB–gold, for injecting CTB–gold and unconjugated CTB, for detecting these two tracers at both light and electron microscope levels, and for combining their demonstration with immunocytochemistry for neurotransmitters or their synthetic enzymes. All steps in these methods are carried out at room temperature unless otherwise stated. For perfusions, ''4% formaldehyde'' means either a 10% (v/v) solution of analytical reagent-grade formaldehyde solution [e.g., Univar, stabilized over 10% (v/v) methanol] or a 4% (w/v) solution of paraformaldehyde (see Ref. 11). Except during processing for electron microscopy, vibratome sections are always incubated and washed on a shaker with continuous gentle agitation.

Preparation of Cholera Toxin B Conjugated to Colloidal Gold

Colloidal gold particles can be prepared by any one of a number of methods. For making small gold particles (7 and 15 nm), we use the method of Slot and Geuze (12) and for larger gold particles (20–21 nm), the method of Frens (13). We calculate the mean diameter of the colloidal gold particles with a standard statistical package from measurements on electron micrographs of gold particles spread on poly (L-lysine)-coated butvar-coated mesh grids. The method of Horisberger and Rosset (14) is used to link CTB to colloidal gold.

1. Dissolve CTB (lyophylized; List Biological Laboratories, Campbell, CA) in distilled water to give a concentration of 1 mg/ml (0.1%, w/v).
2. Adjust the pH of 50 ml of gold sol to 7.6 with 0.2 M K_2CO_3.
3. Determine by titration the amount of CTB that is required to stabilize the gold particles: add decreasing quantities of 0.1% CTB to 200-μl aliquots of gold sol. Check the stability of the complex by adding 10% NaCl solution to a final concentration of 1%.

4. Add the appropriate amount of CTB to the 50 ml of gold and stir for 30 min.
5. Add 1% (w/v) polyethylene glycol (M_r 20,000) to the CTB–gold complex to give a final concentration of 0.05%.
6. Centrifuge at 20,000 rpm for 45 min at 4°C to pellet CTB–gold. Resuspend in distilled water at 1/100 of original volume. Dilute 1 : 1 with physiological saline for injection. Resuspended pellets can be pooled and centrifuged again to concentrate further.

CTB conjugated to 7-nm gold particles is now commecially available in lyophilized form (14a).

Injection of CTB–Gold and Unconjugated CTB

CTB–gold is pressure-injected. It gives smaller, more discrete injection sites than either HRP-based tracers or CTB applied in a similar way. This is an advantage because neuronal projections can be traced much more accurately from small injections sites than from large ones. The size of the gold particle to which CTB is conjugated will determine the size of the injection site, if similar volumes of gold conjugate are injected. CTB linked to small gold particles will give bigger injection sites than CTB linked to large gold particles (for more details, see Ref. 9).

Unconjugated CTB (List Biological Laboratories) can be either pressure injected or applied iontophoretically. With pressure, injection sites can be very large, similar in size to pressure injection sites of equivalent volumes of, for example, wheat germ agglutinin–HRP. Recently, iontophoretic injection of CTB has been shown to produce small, well-localized injection sites with little associated cellular damage. [Refer to Luppi and co-workers (7) for a more detailed description of iontophoretic application of CTB.] These small iontophoretic injection sites allow for a more precise definition of nerve pathways than the large pressure injection sites.

Experimentally defined transport times suggest that both CTB–gold and unconjugated CTB are carried by fast axonal transport. Both reach target neurons in similar times to HRP or wheat germ agglutinin–HRP.

Detection of Retrogradely Transported CTB–Gold

For both light microscopic (LM) and electron microscopic (EM) studies, we detect retrogradely transported CTB–gold with commercially available silver intensification kits: the Sigma silver enhancer kit (Sigma, St. Louis, MO; Cat.

No. SE-100) or the Amersham (formerly Janssen) IntenSE kits (Amersham, Arlington Heights, IL; Cat. No. RPN 491 or RPN 492). Although CTB–gold can be detected by EM without intensification, the advantage of silver intensification for EM is that retrogradely labeled neurons can be selected by LM for subsequent ultrastructural study (Fig. 1A). We also usually gold tone our sections. After silver intensification and gold toning, material often contains more retrogradely labeled neurons with heavier deposits than after silver intensification alone by bright-field microscopy. For EM, gold toning is essential for preserving silver deposits through osmication. Gold toning does not significantly affect either ultrastructural integrity (Fig. 1B) or subsequent immunocytochemistry for neurotransmitter-related markers (Fig. 6). We use the following protocol routinely for demonstrating retrogradely transported CTB–gold in rat brain or spinal cord.

1. Anesthetize the animal and perfuse transcardially with heparin (1000–5000 IU) followed by oxygenated Dulbecco's modified Eagle's/Ham's F12 (DMEM/F12) tissue culture medium (Sigma, Cat. No. D-8900; 200 ml in rats, 1 liter in rabbits).

2. Perfuse with fixative made up in 0.1 M sodium phosphate buffer, pH 7.4 (1 liter in rats; 2 liters in rabbits). Perfusions are carried out at a pressure of 80–100 mmHg. Remove the brain or spinal cord and postfix by immersion in the same fixative. [*Note:* We obtain good retrograde labeling with all of the following fixatives: 4% (v/v) formaldehyde; 4% (v/v) formaldehyde, 0.05% (v/v) glutaraldehyde, 0.2% (w/v) picric acid; 1% (v/v) glutaraldehyde, 1% (v/v) formaldehyde; 2.5% (v/v) glutaraldehyde; 2.5% (v/v) glutaraldehyde, 1% (v/v) formaldehyde; 5% (v/v) glutaraldehyde.]

3. Wash tissue with buffer and cut vibratome sections (50 μm for LM; 70 μm for EM) *into distilled water.* [*Note:* Care must be taken to prevent contamination of the silver intensification solution with phosphate ions because even minute traces can cause the enhancer to precipitate. Consequently, we avoid the use of phosphate buffer until after the sections have been intensified and gold toned.]

4. Wash sections in 50% (v/v) ethanol in distilled water. For LM, sections are washed for at least 30 min regardless of fixative. For EM, sections fixed with 0.1% (v/v) glutaraldehyde or less are washed for 10 min and sections fixed with 1% (v/v) or more glutaraldehyde are washed for 30 min. [*Notes:* (1) Ethanol treatment makes membranes permeable so that other permeants, such as Triton X-100, are unnecessary. Furthermore, ethanol washing allows antibodies to penetrate completely through vibratome sections without significantly compromising their ultrastructural preservation (15, 16; see also Figs. 1B, 4, and 6). (2) This step can be omitted if sections are not to be processed for immunocytochemistry.]

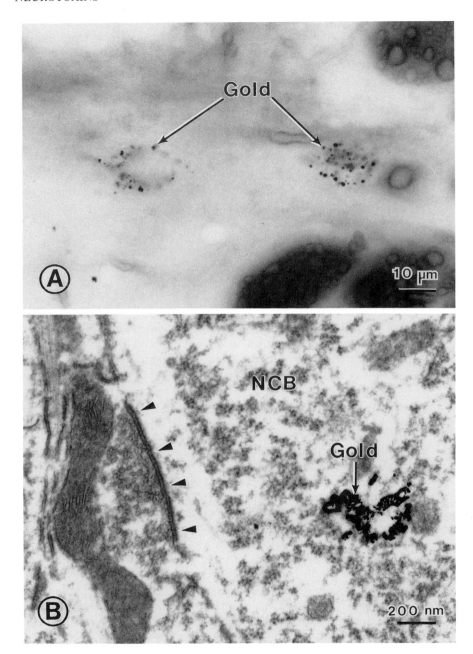

5. Wash sections three times in distilled water (30 min each time). [*Notes:* (1) With the Amersham kit, sections can be washed three times (20 min each) in citrate–acetate buffer, pH 5.5 (50 ml 0.2 M citric acid plus 50 ml 0.2 M ammonium acetate, pH adjusted to 5.5 with 25% ammonia solution), if it is desirable to limit the exposure of the section to hypoosmotic solutions. With the Sigma kit, citrate–acetate buffer speeds up the silver intensification reaction to unacceptably rapid rates. (2) When transferred from 50% ethanol to water or buffer, the sections will float. Swirl them immediately so that they sink.]

6. Immediately before use, prepare the silver intensification solution according to the manufacturer's instructions. [*Note:* The enhancer solution precipitates with time.]

7. Silver intensify the sections. With the Sigma kit, incubate the sections three times (5 min each). With the Amersham kit, incubate the sections twice (20 min each). [*Notes:* (1) For each incubation, make up fresh silver intensification solution immediately before use. (2) The development steps may be increased or decreased in number or shortened or lengthened if there is a high background of silver particles over the surfaces of the sections or if the silver deposits in the retrogradely labeled neurons are small and faint.]

Steps 8–12 are gold-toning steps and may be omitted for LM. If sections are not gold toned, wash briefly in doubly distilled water and skip to step 13.

8. Wash sections three times in distilled water (10 min each).

9. Incubate sections in 0.05% tetrachloroauric acid (gold chloride; w/v) in doubly distilled water *in the dark* for 10 min.

10. Wash sections three times, in the dark, in doubly distilled water (10 min each time).

11. Incubate sections in 0.2% oxalic acid (w/v) in doubly distilled water *in the dark* at 4°C for 2 min.

12. Wash sections three times in doubly distilled water (5 min each time) in the dark.

FIG. 1 Retrograde labeling with CTB–gold. (A) Light micrograph of two rat sympathetic preganglionic neurons. CTB–gold (Gold) is transported from the superior cervical ganglion. (Fixative, 1% formaldehyde, 1% glutaraldehyde; silver intensification, gold toning, and EM processing.) (B) Electron micrograph of a synapse (arrowheads) on the cell body (NCB) of a rat sympathetic preganglionic neuron. CTB–gold (Gold) was transported from the superior cervical ganglion. (Fixative, 5% glutaraldehyde; silver intensification, gold toning, and EM processing.)

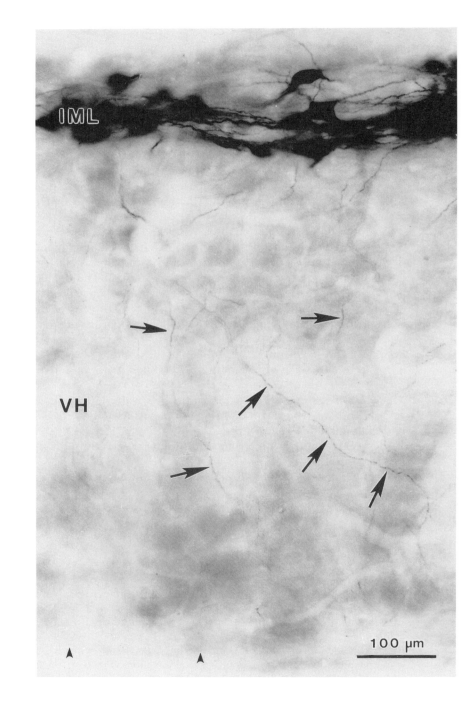

13. Fix sections in 2.5% (w/v) sodium thiosulfate in doubly distilled water for 5 min.

14. Wash briefly in doubly distilled water or in doubly distilled water followed by buffer or phosphate-buffered saline.

Sections containing neurons labeled with CTB–gold can be stained subsequently with neutral red or cresyl violet and mounted for LM. Alternatively, they can be used for LM or EM preembedding immunocytochemistry with any standard peroxidase–antiperoxidase or avidin–biotin–peroxidase technique (see Figs. 5 and 6) or for postembedding immunocytochemistry. This procedure is recommended for studies on (1) the neurotransmitter content of retrogradely labeled neurons by LM and EM and (2) neurotransmitter content of synapses onto retrogradely labeled neurons by EM (if synapses appear to occur on cell bodies and proximal dendrites).

Immunocytochemical Detection of Retrogradely Transported CTB

CTB immunoreactivity has been shown to be sensitive to fixation parameters (7). In our experience, the level of CTB immunoreactivity that can be detected in retrogradely labeled neurons is affected both by the concentration of glutaraldehyde in the fixative and by the amount of time that CTB-containing neurons are exposed to glutaraldehyde. Using rat sympathetic preganglionic neurons retrogradely labeled with CTB from the superior cervical ganglion as our test system, we have found that many cell bodies, dendrites, and axons are revealed by immunocytochemistry for CTB after perfusion with 4% formaldehyde and postfixation times of several days. A similar result is obtained after perfusion with 4% formaldehyde, 0.05% glutaraldehyde, 0.2% picric acid and 4 hr of postfixation or with 1% glutaraldehyde, 1% formaldehyde and 2 hr of postfixation (Fig. 2). However, overnight postfixation at 4°C with either fixative decreases the number of cell bodies, dendrites, and axons that can be detected. Furthermore, the decrease in labeling is greater in tissue fixed with 1% glutaraldehyde, 1% formaldehyde than in tissue fixed with 4%

FIG. 2 Retrograde labeling with unconjugated CTB detected immunocytochemically: light micrograph of rat sympathetic preganglionic neurons. Unconjugated CTB was transported from the superior cervical ganglion. Parasagittal section is through the intermediolateral cell column (IML) and ventral horn (VH). Large arrows, CTB-immunoreactive axons; small arrowheads, ventral boundary of the ventral horn. (Fixative, 4% formaldehyde, 0.05% glutaraldehyde, 0.2% picric acid.)

formaldehyde, 0.05% glutaraldehyde, 0.2% picric acid. Spinal cords fixed with 2.5% glutaraldehyde and postfixed for only 45 min contain very few retrogradely labeled nerve cell bodies with filled proximal dendrites (Fig. 3). Another indicator of glutaraldehyde sensitivity is our finding that the dilution of anti-CTB antiserum that is required for optimally revealing neurons retrogradely labeled with CTB drops from 1:200,000 for tissue fixed with 4% formaldehyde to 1:50,000 for tissue fixed with 1% glutaraldehyde, 1% formaldehyde.

The following immunocytochemical protocol gives good staining of retrogradely labeled sympathetic preganglionic neurons in rat thoracic spinal cord and bulbospinal medullary neurons for either LM or EM. It can be adapted for other brain regions and other species. The choice of fixative and postfixation parameters will be determined by subsequent processing of the tissue. For example, rats for EM are perfused with 4% formaldehyde, 0.05% glutaraldehyde, 0.2% picric acid if we plan to localize another fixation-sensitive antigen in the same sections as CTB or with 2.5% glutaraldehyde if we plan to do postembedding staining for GABA on ultrathin sections (I. J. Llewellyn-Smith and A. Rustioni, unpublished observations, 1991).

1. Anesthetize, heparinize, and perfuse with tissue culture medium as under Detection of Retrogradely Transported CTB-Gold, above.

2. Perfuse with fixative made up in 0.1 M sodium phosphate buffer, pH 7.4 (1 liter for rats, 2 liters for rabbits). Remove the brain or spinal cord. If necessary, do a preliminary dissection to give fixative good access to the area of interest (for examples, see below) and postfix by immersion. The following are our routine procedures for perfusing and postfixing spinal cords.

4% formaldehyde: Intact spinal cord should be postfixed at least overnight at room temperature. [*Note:* Longer postfixation times of up to several days do not significantly affect CTB immunoreactivity.]

4% formaldehyde, 0.05% glutaraldehyde, 0.2% picric acid: Divide spinal cord in half dorsoventrally along the midline or into segments. Postfix 4 hr at room temperature with agitation (e.g., on a shaker).

1% formaldehyde, 1% glutaraldehyde: Divide spinal cord in half dorsoventrally along the midline or into segments. Postfix 2 hr at room temperature with agitation.

2.5% glutaraldehyde: Divide spinal cord in half dorsoventrally along the midline or into segments and postfix 45 min at room temperature with agitation.

3. Wash *briefly* with buffer and cut vibratome sections (50 μm for LM; 70 μm for EM).

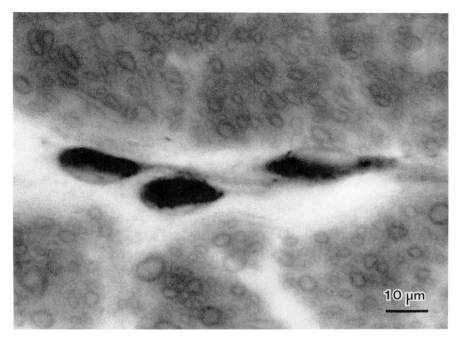

FIG. 3 Retrograde labeling with unconjugated CTB detected immunocytochemi-cally: light micrograph of three rat sympathetic preganglionic neurons. Unconjugated CTB was transported from the superior cervical ganglion. (Fixative, 2.5% glutaralde-hyde; EM processing.)

4. To improve antibody penetration, wash the sections in 50% ethanol in distilled water *immediately* after they are cut, using similar wash times as under step 5 of Detection of Retrogradely Transported CTB–Gold, above.

5. Wash sections briefly in 0.1 M sodium phosphate buffer, pH 7.4, until they sink. Wash briefly in another change of 0.1 M sodium phosphate buffer, pH 7.4.

6. Preincubate sections for at least 30 min in 10% (v/v) normal serum in 10 mM Tris, 0.05% thimerosal (Sigma, Cat. No. T-5125), 10 mM sodium phosphate buffer, pH 7.4, (TPBS). [*Note:* Normal serum should come from the species in which the second antibody was raised. For example, if the second antibody is biotinylated donkey anti-sheep immunoglobulin, normal donkey (or horse) serum should be used.]

7. Incubate sections in anti-CTB antiserum (List Biological Labora-tories) diluted with TPBS containing 10% normal serum. Sections for LM

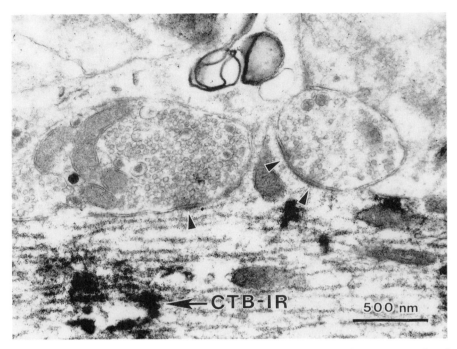

FIG. 4 Retrograde labeling with unconjugated CTB detected immunocytochemically: electron micrograph of two synapses (arrowheads) on the axon of a rabbit sympathetic preganglionic neuron. The axon has regularly arranged microtubules and contains peroxidase reaction product, which indicates CTB immunoreactivity (CTB-IR). Unconjugated CTB was transported from the stellate ganglion.

are in primary antibody for at least 24 hr; sections for EM, for 2–4 days. [*Note:* When detecting CTB immunoreactivity in sympathetic preganglionic neurons with a nickel-intensified diaminobenzidine reaction, we use the following dilution of anti-CTB: 1:200,000 for sections from tissue fixed with 4% formaldehyde, 1:100,000 for tissue fixed with 4% formaldehyde, 0.05% glutaraldehyde, 0.2% picric acid, 1:50,000 for sections fixed with 1% formaldehyde, 1% glutaraldehyde or 1:25,000 for sections fixed with 2.5% glutaraldehyde.]

8. Wash sections three times in TPBS (10 min each for LM; 30 min each for EM).

9. Incubate sections in biotinylated anti-goat IgG in TPBS containing 1% normal serum (overnight for LM; 24 hr for EM).

10. Wash sections as in step 9.

11. Incubate section in a 1:1000 or 1:1500 dilution of Extravidin (Sigma, Cat. No. E-2886) in TPBS (4–6 hr for LM; overnight for EM). [*Note:* ABC reagent (Vector Laboratories; Burlingame, CA) and avidin–HRP (Sigma) also work well.]

12. Wash sections as in step 9.

13. Do a peroxidase reaction (see Peroxidase Reactions, below) to reveal the retrogradely transported CTB.

Sections containing neurons retrogradely labeled with unconjugated CTB can be mounted for LM or they can be double labeled using LM or EM preembedding immunocytochemical techniques. They can also be embedded in resin for postembedding immunocytochemistry at LM or EM levels.

This procedure is recommended for studies on (1) the morphology of retrogradely labeled neurons by LM and EM, (2) neurotransmitter-identified inputs onto retrogradely labeled neurons by LM and EM (sequential preembedding antibody labeling), and (3) postembedding staining to identify neurotransmitter content of inputs onto retrogradely labeled neurons by LM and EM.

Immunocytochemistry after Localization of CTB–Gold or Unconjugated CTB

For immunocytochemistry, it is desirable to treat vibratome sections to help the penetration of immunoreagents. For LM studies, we either wash our sections with 50% (v/v) ethanol (step 5 of Detection of Retrogradely Transported CTB–Gold, above) or include a detergent, Triton X-100, in our protocol. If Triton is used, precede step 1 below with two 10-min washes in TPBS containing 0.1–0.3% (v/v) Triton and include 0.1–0.3% Triton in the diluent for the immunoreagents. For EM studies, Triton treatment is not an option because the detergent solubilizes cell membranes. Consequently, for ultrastructural studies, we always wash sections with alcohol.

1. Preincubate sections for at least 30 min in 10% normal serum in TPBS. [*Note:* omit this step if unconjugated CTB has been localized first.]

2. Incubate sections in primary antibody diluted with TPBS containing 10% normal serum (LM sections, for 24 hr; EM sections, for 2–4 days). (*Note:* titrate primary antibody to give the maximum number of immunoreactive neurons and/or fibers combined with the lowest achievable level of background staining. Changes in incubation time or in fixative or chromogen used for the peroxidase reactions will all affect the concentration of primary antibody that will give the optimal result.)

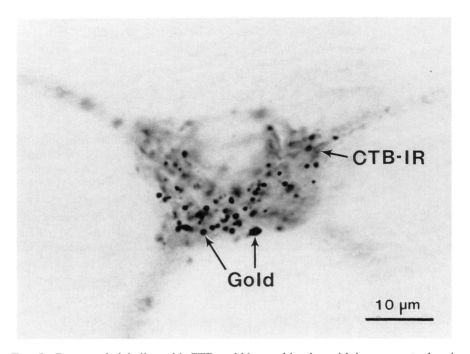

FIG. 5   Retrograde labeling with CTB–gold in combination with immunocytochemical detection of an antigen: light micrograph of a rabbit sympathetic preganglionic neuron. CTB–gold was transported from the superior cervical ganglion. CTB was detected immunocytochemically. Gold particles (Gold) occur in the cell body and proximal dendrites. CTB immunoreactivity (CTB-IR) is clumped around the nucleus and spreads through proximal into distal dendrites. This result indicates that the colloidal gold is decoupled from CTB intraneuronally, with gold particles remaining in lysosomes and CTB dispersing throughout the cytoplasm.

FIG. 6   Retrograde labeling with CTB–gold in combination with immunocytochemical detection of an antigen. (A) Electron micrograph of the cell body (NCB) of a rat sympathetic preganglionic neuron. CTB–gold was transported from the superior cervical ganglion. Enkephalin was detected immunocytochemically. Arrows B and C indicate the features that are shown at higher power in Figs. 6B and C. (B) Electron micrograph of a synapse (arrowheads) by an enkephalin-immunoreactive bouton, which is marked by electron-dense peroxidase reaction product, on the retrogradely labeled neuron. (C) Electron micrograph of a lysosome (L) that contains gold particles (arrows), which have been silver intensified and gold toned.

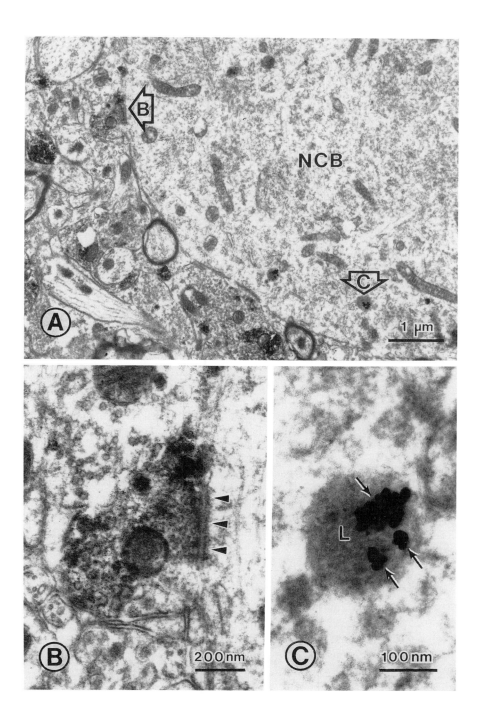

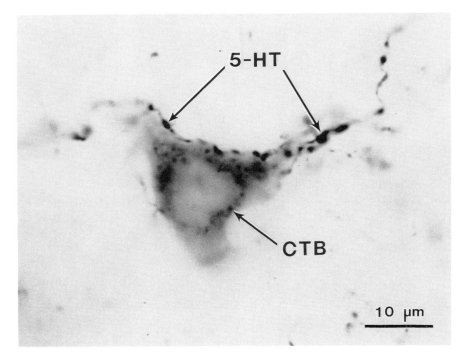

FIG. 7   Retrograde labeling with unconjugated CTB detected immunocytochemically in combination with immunocytochemical detection of another antigen: light micrograph of a rat sympathetic preganglionic neuron. Unconjugated CTB was transported from the stellate ganglion. CTB immunoreactivity (CTB) was detected with an amberbrown peroxidase reaction product (imidazole-intensified DAB). Serotonin immunoreactivity (5-HT) was detected with a black peroxidase reaction product (nickel-intensified DAB). The serotonin fiber contacts the retrogradely labeled neuron at several places.

3. Wash sections three times in TPBS (for LM, 10 min each; for EM, 30 min each).

4. Incubate sections in biotinylated secondary antibody in TPBS containing 1% normal serum (overnight for LM; 24 hr for EM).

5. Wash sections as in step 3.

6. Incubate section in a 1 : 1000 or 1 : 1500 dilution of Extravidin in TPBS (or in ABC reagent or avidin–HRP) made up in TPBS (4–6 hr for LM; overnight for EM).

7. Wash sections as in step 3.

8. Do a peroxidase reaction (see Peroxidase Reactions, below) to reveal

the location of the antigen. A chromogen that gives a reaction product of a different color to the one for revealing CTB immunoreactivity should be used.

Peroxidase Reactions

When doing peroxidase reactions with chromogens other than tetramethylbenzidine, we use glucose oxidase to generate peroxide (17). We find that this gives a better signal-to-noise ratio than exogenously supplied peroxide. However, reaction times with glucose oxidase can be much longer than with added peroxide. Furthermore, with glucose oxidase, reaction product is often not visible by LM until at least 3–4 min into the reaction. The following stock solutions are required for the glucose oxidase generation of peroxide and are used in all the peroxidase reactions described below:

NH_4Cl (0.4%, w/v) in distilled water
D-Glucose (20%, w/v) in distilled water containing 0.05% sodium azide [*Note:* store at 4°C.]
Glucose oxidase solution (Sigma, Cat. No. G-6891) [*Note:* store at 4°C; active for at least a year].

After any of the following peroxidase reactions, sections can be mounted onto subbed glass slides for LM or processed for EM (see Processing Vibratome Sections Containing Retrogradely Labeled Neurons for Electron Microscopy, below).

Imidazole-Intensified Diaminobenzidine

This procedure is adapted from Straus (18). Imidazole-intensified diaminobenzidine gives an amber-brown amorphous reaction product by LM, an amorphous electron-dense reaction product by EM.

Warning: 3,3′-Diaminobenzidine (DAB) is a potential carcinogen. Wear gloves while handling. After reaction, DAB should be disposed of carefully. We deactivate DAB with chlorine bleach and bleach all glassware and disposable items that have come in contact with it.

Diaminobenzidine reaction product is stable in commonly used buffers and organic solvents.

Stock Solutions

> 3,3'-Diaminobenzidine tetrahydrochloride (5 mg/ml) in 100 mM Tris-HCl, pH 7.6. [*Note:* store frozen at $-15°C$ for up to 1 year without loss of activity]
> Imidazole (1 M) in distilled water:
>   [*Note:* store at 4°C]
> Tris-HCl (100 mM), pH 7.6

Preparation of Preincubation Solution
To 1 ml 5 mg/ml DAB:

1. Add 4 ml Tris-HCl, pH 7.6.
2. Add 100 μl 1 M imidazole.
3. Add 100 μl 0.4% NH_4Cl.
4. Add 100 μl 20% glucose.
5. Make up to 10 ml with distilled water.

Protocol

1. Incubate sections in freshly prepared preincubation solution for 10 min with agitation.
2. To make reaction mix, add 1 μl glucose oxidase to each milliliter of preincubation solution.
3. Remove preincubation solution from sections and add freshly prepared reaction mix. React for up to 30 min with agitation. [*Note:* If reaction product is too weak, make up fresh reaction mix, add sections to fresh mix, and react another up to 30 min.]
4. Remove reaction mix and wash sections in buffer several times.

Nickel-Intensified Diaminobenzidine

Nickel-intensified diaminobenzidine gives a black amorphous reaction product by LM; an amorphous electron-dense reaction product by EM. [*Notes:* (1) In our hands, nickel-intensified diaminobenzidine reactions are more sensitive than imidazole-intensified diaminobenzidine reactions. (2) The reaction products of imidazole-intensified and nickel-intensified diaminobenzidine reactions are not distinguishable at EM.]

Stock Solutions

Nickel ammonium sulfate (ammonium nickel sulfate), 1% (w/v) in distilled water

Sodium phosphate buffer (0.2 M), pH 7.4

Preparation of Preincubation Solution

1. Dissolve 10 mg of DAB in 10 ml of 0.2 M phosphate buffer. [*Notes:* DAB can be stored preweighed and tightly covered at $-15°C$. Alternatively, 10-mg DAB tablets (Sigma, Cat. No. D-5905) can be used. If DAB tablets are used, this solution should be passed through a disposable filter.]
2. Add 200 μl 0.4% NH_4Cl.
3. Add 200 μl 20% glucose.
4. Slowly add 800 μl 1% nickel ammonium sulfate.
5. Make up to 20 ml with distilled water.

Protocol

1. Wash sections twice (10 min each) in 0.1 M phosphate buffer, pH 7.4, or wash sections three times (10 min each) in nickel phosphate buffer (4 ml of 1% nickel ammonium sulfate plus 50 ml of 0.2 M phosphate buffer, pH 7.4 plus 46 ml of distilled water).
2. Incubate sections in freshly prepared preincubation solution for 10 min with agitation.
3. To make reaction mix, add 1 μl glucose oxidase to each milliliter of preincubation solution.
4. Remove preincubation solution and add freshly prepared reaction mix to sections. React for up to 30 min with agitation.
5. Remove reaction mix and wash sections several times in 0.1 M phosphate buffer, pH 7.4.

Benzidine Dihydrochloride

This procedure is adapted from Levey *et al.* (19). Benzidine dihydrochloride gives a blue-black crystalline reaction product by LM; a crystalline electron-dense reaction product by EM.

Warning: Benzidine dihydrochloride (BDHC) is a proven carcinogen. Weigh out BDHC on a balance reserved for toxic chemicals and wear a mask and gloves. Do all steps in a fume hood that can be easily cleaned of spills with bleach. Wear gloves throughout procedure. Dispose of BDHC by deactivation with chlorine bleach. Bleach all glassware and disposable items that have come in contact with BDHC.

In our hands, benzidine dihydrochloride reactions are somewhat less sensitive than imidazole-intensified diaminobenzidine reactions.

The reaction product from benzidine dihydrochloride is stable only in solutions of low ionic strength and is soluble in ethanol.

Stock Solutions

> Sodium phosphate buffer (0.2 M), pH 6.8: Stock solution should be prepared by adding 24.5 ml of 0.2 M Na_2HPO_4 to 25.5 ml of 0.2 M NaH_2PO_4 to give correct ionic strength
>
> Sodium phosphate buffer (10 mM), pH 6.8: Stock solution should be prepared by diluting 1 part 0.2 M sodium phosphate buffer, pH 6.8, with 19 parts distilled water

Preparation of Preincubation Solution

1. Dissolve 5 mg BDHC in 47.5 ml of distilled water. [*Note:* BDHC can be stored at $-15°C$ preweighed, tightly covered, and carefully protected against spilling.]
2. Filter through filter paper.
3. Add 2.5 ml of 0.2 M phosphate buffer, pH 6.8.
4. Add 2.5 mg of sodium nitroprusside.
5. Stir to dissolve.
6. Add 0.5 ml of 0.4% NH_4Cl.
7. Add 0.5 ml of 20% D-glucose.

Protocol

1. Wash sections thoroughly five times (5 min each) in 10 mM phosphate buffer, pH 6.8.
2. Incubate sections in freshly prepared BDHC preincubation solution for 10 min with agitation.
3. To make reaction mix, add 1 μl glucose oxidase to each milliliter of BDHC preincubation solution.
4. Remove preincubation solution and add freshly prepared reaction mix to sections. React for up to 30 min with agitation.
5. Remove reaction mix and wash sections extensively in 10 mM phosphate buffer, pH 6.8. [*Note:* For LM, mount sections directly from 10 mM phosphate buffer, pH 6.8, onto subbed glass slides.]

Choice of Chromogen

The choice of chromogen for a peroxidase reaction will depend on the experiment being conducted. For determining by LM whether a neuron retrogradely labeled with CTB–gold contains another antigen, the homogeneous brown product from an imidazole-intensified DAB reaction is easy to distinguish from the black punctate silver-intensified gold deposits (Fig. 5). For identifying by EM the neurotransmitter content of synapses on CTB–gold-labeled neurons (Fig. 6), either an imidazole-intensified DAB or a nickel-intensified DAB reaction can be used because both have the same appearance at EM. For studies of neuronal morphology after retrograde transport of unconjugated CTB, a nickel–DAB reaction, which fills the cytoplasm homogeneously but is more sensitive than imidazole–DAB, gives a better picture of cell shape (Fig. 2). When immunocytochemistry for CTB and a neurotransmitter are done on the same section for LM, it is generally preferable to have retrogradely labeled neurons brown and nerve fibers black. We use BDHC for double preembedding antibody labeling at the EM level because its crystalline reaction product is clearly distinguishable from the amorphous reaction products of imidazole–DAB or nickel–DAB. We find BDHC good for labeling cell bodies but not for terminals (see also Ref. 19). Because the blue crystalline reaction product of BDHC is stable only at low ionic strength, antigens in nerve fibers are revealed with imidazole–DAB or nickel–DAB *before* BDHC is used to show CTB immunoreactivity. The tissue is then either mounted on subbed glass slides or immediately processed for electron microscopy.

Processing Vibratome Sections Containing Retrogradely Labeled Neurons for Electron Microscopy

We use the following protocol for EM processing of vibratome sections that contain neurons labeled with CTB–gold or neurons labeled with CTB revealed with a diaminobenzidine reaction. A modified and shortened procedure is used for processing CTB-labeled neurons reacted with BDHC since BDHC reaction product is soluble in 0.1 M phosphate buffer and in ethanol. Instructions in parentheses indicate changes for processing BDHC-reacted sections.

1. Sodium phosphate buffer (0.1 M), pH 7.4: at least three times, 10 min each. (Omit.)
2. OsO_4 (0.5%, w/v) in 0.1 M sodium phosphate buffer, pH 7.4 (1% OsO_4, 10 mM sodium phosphate buffer, pH 6.8): 1 hr floating.

3. Distilled water: four times, 5 min each, floating. (Omit.)
4. Aqueous uranyl acetate (2%, w/v): 20 min flat plus 10 min floating. (Omit.)

[*Note:* "flat" in steps 4–10 implies that the sections are sandwiched between the lid and bottom of a Petri dish or between a slide and a coverslip. If sections are kept flat during dehydration, they will remain flat when they are embedded.]

5. Distilled water: twice, 5 min each, floating. (Omit.)
6. Ethanol (50%): 5 min flat plus 10 min floating. (Omit.)
7. Ethanol (70%): 5 min flat plus 10 min floating. (Two minutes flat plus 3 min floating.)
8. Ethanol (90%): 5 min flat plus 10 min floating. (Two minutes flat plus 3 min floating.)
9. Ethanol (95%): 5 min flat plus 10 min floating. (Two minutes flat plus 3 min floating.)
10. Dry absolute ethanol: 5 min flat plus 10 min floating. (Two minutes flat plus 3 min floating.)
11. Dry absolute ethanol: three times, 15 min each, floating. (Twice, 5 min floating.)
12. Propylene oxide: twice, 5 min each, floating. (Once, 2 min floating, plus once, 3 min floating.)
13. Propylene oxide : Durcupan (1 : 1): at least 45 min. (Thirty minutes.)

[*Note:* Other resins, such as Araldite or TAAB embedding resin, can be used with this protocol.]

14. Durcupan: 10 min, 60°C, then overnight at room temperature.
15. Flat embed on slides.

Acknowledgments

This work was supported by the National Health and Medical Research Council of Australia, the National Heart Foundation of Australia, and the Flinders Medical Centre Research Foundation. Adrian Wright, Rachael Coffey, and Kathy Branch provided expert technical assistance. We thank Dr. Aldo Rustioni and Dr. Richard Weinberg for helpful comments on the manuscript.

References

1. J. Q. Trojanowski, J. O. Gonatas, and N. K. Gonatas, *Brain Res.* **231,** 33 (1982).
2. G. Ju, S. Liu, and J. Tao, *Neuroscience* **19,** 803 (1986).
3. S. J. Bacon and A. D. Smith, *J. Auton. Nerv. Syst.* **24,** 97 (1988).
4. D. B. Rye, C. B. Saper, and B. H. Wainer, *J. Histochem. Cytochem.* **32,** 1145 (1984).
5. H. Ericson and A. Blomqvist, *J. Neurosci. Methods* **24,** 225 (1988).
6. P.-H. Luppi, K. Sakai, D. Salvert, P. Fort, and M. Jouvet, *Brain Res.* **402,** 339 (1987).
7. P.-H. Luppi, P. Fort, and M. Jouvet, *Brain Res.* **534,** 209 (1990).
8. I. J. Llewellyn-Smith, P. M. Pilowsky, J. B. Minson, and J. P. Chalmers, manuscript in preparation (1991).
9. I. J. Llewellyn-Smith, J. B. Minson, A. P. Wright, and A. J. Hodgson, *J. Comp. Neurol.* **294,** 179 (1990).
10. J. Minson, I. Llewellyn-Smith, A. Neville, P. Somogyi, and J. Chalmers, *J. Auton. Nerv. Syst.* **30,** 209 (1990).
11. I. J. Llewellyn-Smith, M. Costa, and J. B. Furness, *J. Histochem. Cytochem.* **33,** 857 (1985).
12. J. W. Slot and H. J. Geuze, *Eur. J. Cell Biol.* **38,** 87 (1985).
13. G. Frens, *Nature (London)* **241,** 20 (1973).
14. M. Horisberger and J. Rosset, *J. Histochem. Cytochem.* **25,** 295 (1977).
14a. Available from Gilt Products, Department of Medicine, Flinders University, South Australia. (International Fax: 61-8-204-5268.)
15. I. J. Llewellyn-Smith, J. B. Minson, D. A. Morilak, J. R. Oliver, and J. P. Chalmers, *Neurosci. Lett.* **108,** 243 (1990).
16. P. M. Pilowsky, D. de Castro, I. J. Llewellyn-Smith, J. Lipski, and M. Voss, *Neuroscience* **10,** 1091 (1990).
17. B. J. Oldfield, A. Hou-Yu, and A.-J. Silverman, *J. Histochem. Cytochem.* **31,** 1145 (1983).
18. W. Straus, *J. Histochem. Cytochem.* **30,** 491 (1982).
19. A. I. Levey, J. P. Bolam, D. B. Rye, A. E. Hallanger, R. M. Demuth, M.-M. Mesulam, and B. H. Wainer, *J. Histochem. Cytochem.* **34,** 1449 (1986).

[14] ω-Conotoxin: Calcium Currents and Neurosecretion

Ken Takeda and Jean J. Nordmann

Introduction

Many reviews on the molecular structure and biology of peptide neurotoxins from predatory cone snails (*Conus*) have appeared (1–4), as is also the case for voltage-dependent calcium channels (5–11). Our purpose here is to describe the use of ω-conotoxin GVIA (ω-conotoxin or ω-CgTX) in analyzing the relationship between the activation of presynaptic calcium channels and the secretory response of neurons and other neuroendocrine cell types.

Because of the small size of nerve terminals [with a few notable exceptions (12–15)], direct electrophysiological investigations of presynaptic calcium channels involved in neurosecretion are exceedingly difficult to carry out, even using patch-clamp methodology (16, 17). Moreover, while dihydropyridine antagonists have been shown to inhibit strongly the voltage-dependent calcium currents in a variety of cardiac, skeletal, and smooth muscle preparations (for reviews, see Refs. 18–20), relatively few reports exist where blocking actions of dihydropyridines on calcium-dependent neurotransmitter release are convincingly described (21). The dihydropyridine insensitivity of different secretory processes is commonly inferred as evidence that the calcium channels mediating calcium entry into nerve terminals are different from those in muscle cells. Thus, following the initial description of the presynaptic blocking actions of ω-conotoxin (22), it was thought that this toxin would represent a powerful means of characterizing calcium channels in nerve terminals and their eventual role in the processes responsible for the secretion of neurotransmitters.

A discussion is also presented as to the utility of ω-conotoxin as a specific pharmacological tool in discriminating different subclasses of calcium channels. Two major conclusions arise: (1) ω-conotoxin blocks certain subtypes of calcium channels in a less specific manner than has been commonly held, and therefore, (2) its use in functional studies of neurosecretion does not easily allow a clear classification of calcium channels underlying stimulus–secretion coupling.

Methods in Neurosciences, Volume 8

ω-Conotoxin

Predatory cone snails (*Conus*) inject venom to capture their prey. The major pharmacologically active components in crude venom are all small peptides, 10–30 amino acids in length, containing many disulfide bonds. These peptides are unusual in that they are made up of relatively small numbers of amino acids, and their tertiary conformational stability arises because of the disulfide bonds (1–3). A common effect of these peptides in vertebrates is paralysis. The presence of many different peptide neurotoxins in crude venom, each having discrete targets (which include the nicotinic acetylcholine receptor at the neuromuscular junction, the voltage-dependent sodium channel in skeletal muscle, and the presynaptic calcium channel), represents a unique evolutionary strategy developed by the *Conus* snails. One such neurotoxin is ω-conotoxin GVIA (G for *geographus* and VIA for fraction VIA; often abbreviated as ω-CgTX), a 27-amino acid peptide isolated from *Conus geographus,* a fish-hunting cone snail. A review of the characteristics of the ω-conotoxin receptor appears elsewhere in this volume (23).

Historically, much interest was generated by the initial report (22) describing the irreversible blocking effects of ω-conotoxin on nerve-evoked transmitter release at the frog neuromuscular junction and on the calcium current component of the action potential in neurons from chick dorsal root ganglia. A suggestion was that ω-conotoxin might act to decrease presynaptic calcium entry, perhaps by "interfering directly with Ca^{2+} channels" (22). Because, in the presence of ω-conotoxin, direct electrical stimulation of the postsynaptic muscle fibers caused contraction, it was apparent that calcium channels present in skeletal muscle were unaffected by the toxin, thus indicating a certain heterogeneity in the characteristics of calcium channels and in their localization. It was also noted by the same authors that the mechanism of action of ω-conotoxin was distinct from other known peptide neurotoxins such as botulinum toxin, β-bungarotoxin and α-latrotoxin, all of which also have presynaptic effects.

Electrophysiological Analysis of Calcium Channels

At about the same time, it was proposed that voltage-dependent calcium channels could be classified into different subgroups (24–28). Various names have been given to the different calcium channel subtypes (e.g., T for transient low-threshold, N for neither T nor L, and L for long lasting; HVA and LVA for high- and low-voltage-activated; FD and SD for fast- and slow-deactivating). Detailed reviews of the properties of these calcium channel classes can be found elsewhere (5–11, 29). Although it is now clear that the criteria allowing division into three (or more) versus two channel subclasses are less straightforward than originally described (see, e.g., Refs. 6 and 30–32), we give below a brief description of some of the characteristics that were used initially to distinguish between the various calcium channel subtypes.

A first distinction was activation threshold: it was shown that small step depolarizations of the plasma membrane (to -60 or -50 mV) from a hyperpolarized resting potential (e.g., -90 mV) caused activation of a transient, rapidly inactivating calcium current that has been classified as T type for transient or LVA, for low voltage activated, or low threshold [or I_{fast}, in cardiac cells (33)]. The whole-cell T-type calcium current was of small amplitude, often seen as a slight shoulder when the peak current–voltage relationship was plotted. Maximum T-type current was observed around -40 mV. On greater depolarization from a -90-mV holding potential, another class of calcium currents was evoked, with an activation threshold between -40 and -20 mV and maximal current at about 0 mV (high voltage activated or HVA; also high threshold). A prominent feature of the whole-cell, high voltage-activated calcium current is its relatively sustained, noninactivating time course during step depolarization (compared to T-type currents). In cardiac cells, this type of calcium current has been called I_{slow} or I_{si} [for slow inward (33)]. As discussed below, some workers have proposed that in fact there are two types of high voltage-activated calcium currents: N (for neither T nor L) and L (for long lasting).

A second clear distinction was the behavior of macroscopic calcium channel tail currents as a function of the initial holding potential. Tail currents arise from channels opened by brief step depolarizations closing on repolarization back to the resting potential. When calcium channels were activated from a hyperpolarized holding potential (e.g., -90 mV), tail currents having a biphasic decay time course were observed, with a fast time constant in the submillisecond range and a slower time constant of several milliseconds (24, 34, 35). When more depolarized holding potentials (~ -40 mV) were used (which cause steady-state inactivation of T- and N-type Ca^{2+} channels; see below), tail current decay was rapid and monophasic. It was shown that the slow-deactivating (SD) tail currents were associated with low voltage-activated (LVA, or T-type) calcium channels and that the fast-deactivating (FD) tail currents were associated with high voltage-activated (HVA, or N- and/or L-type) calcium channels.

A third criterion was the difference in decay time courses for high voltage-activated calcium channels during a test pulse as a function of holding potential. For step depolarization to 0 mV or so, little or no inactivation of whole-cell calcium current was seen for depolarized holding potentials (e.g., -40 mV), whereas for the same test pulse both a decaying and a sustained component were seen from a hyperpolarized holding potential (e.g., −90 mV). It was proposed that L-type channels give rise to the sustained current and that N-type channels are responsible for the decaying component. The steady state inactivation of N-type calcium channels by maintained depolarization was thus postulated to be much more pronounced than for L-type calcium channels. Note that relatively depolarized holding potentials also result in steady state inactivation of T-type calcium channels.

This difference in decay time course is perhaps the most difficult to demonstrate in an unambiguous fashion, especially at the whole-cell current level. During step depolarization, calcium channels inactivate in both a voltage-dependent and an internal calcium-dependent manner (for a review, see Ref. 36). However, the relative contribution of these two inactivation mechanisms is different for different cell types. For example, cardiac L-type channels show perhaps the most pronounced voltage-dependent inactivation, with many neuronal N- and L-type channels having much less or no voltage-dependent inactivation (5). On the other hand, the decay time course of neuronal high voltage-activated calcium channels is much more sensitive to internal calcium concentration. Furthermore, because barium is often used as a charge carrier instead of calcium, and barium does not replace internal calcium in producing calcium-dependent inactivation, the rate of inactivation of calcium versus barium currents differs widely. Thus, L-type currents are quite sustained or noninactivating when barium is the permeant cation, but are much less so when calcium is used, especially in cardiac cells (5). Moreover, as has been widely pointed out, the decay time course of calcium currents of especially the N and L subclasses is the most variable parameter between different cell types: decay time constants for neuronal N-type currents range from 25 to several hundred milliseconds, while the rate of inactivation of cardiac L-type channels can vary 10-fold (for reviews, see Refs. 5, 6, and 8). These considerations emphasize the possible ambiguity in identifying distinct N- versus L-type calcium channel subclasses, especially when only macroscopic current decay is used as the sole distinguishing criterion.

Fourth, it is at the single-channel level that the strongest data have been obtained for the classification of calcium channels into three subtypes: L-type channels have a large single-channel conductance, ranging from around 20 to 30 pS, while T-type channels have a tiny single-channel conductance of about 8 pS, and N-type channels have an intermediate single-channel conductance of about 15 pS (but for another view, see Ref. 32). These values vary depending on cell type and it should be mentioned that the data are obtained invariably using isotonic ($\sim$100 mM) external barium solutions (which undoubtedly influence the membrane surface charge potential) and cell-attached patches [for incompletely understood reasons, single-channel calcium currents usually "wash out" (disappear) very quickly from cell-free patches]. It is of interest to note that the averaged kinetic behavior of a single conductance class of channels [for example the 13-pS, N-type channels in chick dorsal root ganglion neurons (30)] can vary dramatically from cell to cell, suggesting perhaps that two kinds (inactivating and sustained) of N-type currents exist. A minimal conclusion is that the inactivation behavior of N-type channels varies widely. Ion selectivity differs between channel subgroups: for example, cardiac T-type channels are about equiselective for calcium and barium, whereas barium is about twice as permeable as calcium through L-type channels. A similar ion selectivity was found for calcium currents in chick dorsal root ganglion neurons (for a review, see Ref. 10).

Fifth, the pharmacology of calcium channel antagonists differs between the different channel subgroups, although in some cases these differences are not sufficiently clear-cut enough to permit unequivocal classification of channel subclasses by the blockers used. Inorganic divalent cation blockers like cadmium or nickel have been particularly useful: low concentrations ($\sim$50 μM) of nickel almost completely block T-type channels, leaving high voltage-activated calcium channel currents largely unaffected, while the inverse situation holds for low concentrations ($\sim$50 μM) of cadmium. Although a complete analysis of the diverse effects of dihydropyridines is far beyond the scope of this chapter (for reviews, see Refs. 18–20), a general conclusion is that antagonists like nifedipine or nitrendipine in the micromolar or less range antagonize L-type channels more potently than N- or T-type channels, while agonists like BAY K 8644 are similarly more effective in potentiating L-type compared to N- or T-type channels (although exceptions do exist, with neuronal high voltage-activated channels being notably much less sensitive than their counterparts in cardiac or smooth muscle). A fairly similar situation holds for verapamil and its methoxy derivative D600, with L-type channels being blocked more potently than T-type channels by these two agents. T-type calcium channels have recently been found to be inhibited by amiloride (37).

Caution should be used in correlating or comparing electrophysiological descriptions of dihydropyridine effects between different species and different cell types (even when from the same species) with their effects in functional studies. This is also especially so when functional parameters (like neurosecretion or contraction) are tested using dihydropyridines with a view to classifying the channel subtype responsible for the calcium dependence of the studied process. An often remarked on discrepancy is the difference between effective dihydropyridine concentrations in electrophysiological measurements compared to functional studies (and to dissociation constants obtained from binding experiments), with the former often being 10- to 100-fold greater than the latter. The reasons for these differences are not immediately obvious. In addition, not all dihydropyridine derivatives are equipotent in different systems, and consideration should be given to testing more than one derivative before drawing conclusions. Finally, the voltage dependence of dihydropyridine action (38) means that the resting membrane potential (which is zero in binding studies done on membrane fragments and is often unknown in functional studies) becomes a critical determinant of dihydropyridine effectiveness.

Electrophysiological Analysis of ω-Conotoxin Action

Based on this background, electrophysiological characterization of ω-conotoxin was carried out with the hope that it would be perhaps a selective inhibitor of presynaptic calcium channels. A first clear result was that the different calcium channel currents from skeletal, cardiac, and smooth muscles in a variety of different species were unaffected by ω-conotoxin (39), although recently it was reported that 10 μM ω-conotoxin produced a persistent block of calcium current in cultured neonatal rat ventricular myocytes (40). On the other hand, high voltage-activated calcium currents from various neuronal, neuroendocrine, and some endocrine cells were almost completely inhibited by ω-conotoxin in an irreversible manner, while low voltage-activated, T-type calcium currents were unaffected or, at best, only weakly antagonized (for reviews, see Refs. 5, 6, and 39). The effective toxin concentrations for block of calcium currents were in the 1 to 10 μM range, which is in marked contrast to the nanomolar K_d values obtained in binding studies (23). As is the case for the dihydropyridines, the reasons for this discrepancy are also not immediately obvious. From a technical point of view, it should be remembered that the ω-conotoxin GVIA used in most of the studies described hereafter was purified from crude snail venom, and thus may contain variable amounts of contaminants. Although in some studies, no large differences were seen between the actions of purified and totally synthetic ω-conotoxin, in others, apparently conflicting results might be explained by the use of purified versus synthetic toxin (for a review, see Ref. 6). Because ω-conotoxin is very basic in nature, high concentrations of divalent cations antagonize toxin binding, and thus comparison between different observations first requires consideration of the ionic composition of the incubating solutions used. This latter constraint unfortunately precludes the use of ω-conotoxin in measurement of single-channel calcium currents, where 100 mM barium is the usual divalent cation concentration (cf. Refs. 30 and 39).

Effects of ω-Conotoxin on Calcium Currents from Sympathetic Neurons

A first report (41) demonstrated that calcium currents from cultured chick dorsal root ganglion neurons were blocked completely by micromolar concentrations of ω-conotoxin. The onset of blocking action was time dependent, being more rapid for higher ω-conotoxin concentrations. Essentially no recovery was seen, although this was for a relatively short period (after which whole-cell calcium currents usually "run down"). However, the calcium current component of intracellularly recorded action potentials was blocked for several hours following ω-conotoxin washout, while after overnight incubation in toxin-free medium the calcium current component was again apparent. It might be, as was suggested, that this recovery represents dissociation of ω-conotoxin from its binding site or, for example, insertion of newly synthesized calcium channels into the cell membrane. A more complete analysis in cultured chick dorsal root ganglion neurons (39, 42) was in general agreement with these results. Both N- and L-type currents were persistently blocked by 10 μM ω-conotoxin. The block was rapid in onset, being 90% complete after a 1-min application of toxin. It was suggested that there may be a very small component of L-type current that was toxin resistant. Neither the kinetics of activation nor of inactivation of calcium currents were apparently altered by submaximally effective toxin concentrations. Additionally, it was reported that T-type current was not inhibited or only transiently so in a minor fashion (39, 42). A quite similar situation was reported for N- and L-type current inhibition in rat sympathetic neurons (39, 43). Interestingly, in chick dorsal root ganglion neurons, it was demonstrated (44) that ω-conotoxin was incapable of blocking sodium current through calcium channels, which is observed with low (less than micromolar) external calcium concentrations. This observation was taken as evidence favoring the idea that a regulatory site of high affinity for calcium, when occupied by calcium, prevents sodium permeation through the calcium channel (cf. Ref. 10).

In isolated neurons from frog dorsal root ganglia, synthetic ω-conotoxin suppressed the high-threshold calcium current in a time- and concentration-dependent manner, with 10 μM being required for complete block (45). In a more detailed analysis of calcium currents in isolated neurons from bullfrog paravertebral ganglia, it was concluded that N-type channels were largely predominant, with no T-type and a very minor contribution from L-type calcium channels (46). In this preparation, 100 nM ω-conotoxin gave rise to ~80% block of calcium current, with a slow onset.

However, there exists substantial disagreement as to the degree and specificity of block for N- and L-type currents, and also as to the irreversibility of block. For example, in chick dorsal root ganglion neurons, N-type currents were completely and irreversibly blocked by 10 μM ω-conotoxin in only 50% of the cells studied ($n = 59$ cells in total), while in the other 50%, a small, toxin-resistant, dihydropyridine-sensitive L-type current component was found (47). Both from macroscopic current and from single-calcium channel current recordings (30, 47) it was concluded, in contrast to other reports (39, 42), that ω-conotoxin was at best only a partial and reversible blocker of L-type channels. Moreover, the same authors (47) observed a reversible, 30%

decrease in T-type currents. In a detailed study of cultured neurons from rat superior cervical ganglia and in PC-12 cells, it was convincingly demonstrated that dihydropyridine-sensitive, L-type calcium channels were ω-conotoxin insensitive (32). It was also shown by the same authors that dihydropyridine-insensitive N-type calcium currents were composed of two components: inactivating and noninactivating. Moreover, a fraction of the N-type current was only partially and reversibly blocked by ω-conotoxin (32). Similar results were reported in adult rat dorsal root ganglion neurons, where complete block of high voltage-activated currents was seen in only 10% of the cells studied, while in the other 90%, an average inhibition of 72% was found with micromolar ω-conotoxin (48). Essentially the same observations were made in a human neuroblastoma cell line, with only 85% of high voltage-activated current being blocked in 50% of the cells by 6 μM ω-conotoxin (31). The toxin-resistant component in both cell types was sensitive to dihydropyridines. A somewhat different situation was described in another human neuroblastoma cell line (49), with two kinetically distinct N-like currents being blocked by ~90% with 1 μM ω-conotoxin. However, in these cells, dihydropyridines were completely ineffective. In F-11 cells (which are a hybrid rat dorsal root ganglion × neuroblastoma cell line), 81% of sustained, high voltage-activated currents and 27% of transient high voltage-activated currents were blocked by 10 μM ω-conotoxin (50). It was concluded in this study that both sustained and transient current components were likely to be composed of two different channel classes.

In summary, it seems clear that whole-cell calcium currents cannot be reliably separated using only voltage-dependent, macroscopic kinetic criteria. Moreover, the demonstration (30–32, 48, 50) of an ω-conotoxin-insensitive fraction of N-type calcium current suggests the existence of two separate classes of N-type calcium channels. Indeed, both sustained and transient components of dihydropyridine-insensitive, N-type currents were observed in these studies. Further, dihydropyridine-sensitive L-type current was found to be ω-conotoxin resistant (30, 32, 47), leaving unconfirmed other reports describing irreversible ω-conotoxin block of sustained calcium current. As has been pointed out (31, 32, 48, 50), the classification of calcium channels into subtypes based on activation–inactivation kinetics and holding potential sensitivity (9–11, 27, 28) appears somewhat inadequate, and it was suggested that a pharmacological dissection using ω-conotoxin and dihydropyridine derivatives might provide a more reliable means of defining multiple high voltage-activated calcium currents.

Effects of ω-Conotoxin on Calcium Currents from Central Neurons

In acutely isolated hippocampal CA1 pyramidal cells from the rat, 1 μM synthetic ω-conotoxin blocked N- and L-type currents by 16 and 46%, respectively (51). A somewhat similar result was reported for cultured rat hippocampal neurons, with persistent block in some cells and others being toxin insensitive (39). In rat locus coeruleus neurons studied in brain slices, 0.1 μM ω-conotoxin was reported to increase the spike threshold of calcium action potentials and to decrease their firing frequency (52). Interestingly, barium currents expressed in *Xenopus* oocytes after injection of total mRNA from rat brain were insensitive to both ω-conotoxin and dihydropyridines, while being inhibited by 50% by 6 μM cadmium (53). These slowly inactivating calcium currents were clearly different in pharmacology compared to those expressed in the same system after injection of mRNA from rat heart (54), again emphasizing differences between neuronal and muscle calcium channels.

Effects of ω-Conotoxin on Presynaptic Calcium Currents

Extracellularly recorded calcium currents from motor nerve terminals at the mouse neuromuscular junction were blocked by verapamil, but not by micromolar amounts of ω-conotoxin (55). It was concluded by these authors that the presynaptic calcium channels here were unlike other L-type (and, presumably, N-type) channels present in neuronal somata. Using the same technique, calcium currents from lizard motor nerve terminals were reported to be blocked by 3.5 μM ω-conotoxin, 50 μM cadmium and nifedipine, while nickel was ineffective at concentrations <100 μM (56). No evidence was found for multiple classes of presynaptic calcium currents [unlike in mouse (55, 57)], and it was concluded that only L-type channels were present at lizard neuromuscular junctions. In another presynaptic nerve terminal, the chick ciliary ganglion calyx, both N- and L-type "whole-terminal" calcium currents were blocked by 10 μM ω-conotoxin (58). Interestingly, in contrast to these recordings from ciliary ganglion slice preparations, only presynaptic L-type calcium currents were observed after acute enzymatic dissociation of this ganglion (15). Perhaps N-type calcium channels were lost following enzyme treatment, or another possibility is that N-type calcium channels are localized to the most distal portion of the nerves and not in the nerve terminals themselves. In nerve terminals isolated from the rat neurohypophysis (14), both N- and L-type calcium channels were characterized (59).

Effects of ω-Conotoxin on Calcium Currents from Invertebrate Neurons

Interestingly, in two invertebrate preparations, no blocking action of ω-conotoxin was observable: high-threshold calcium current from *Aplysia* bag cell neurons was unaffected by 10 μM ω-conotoxin (39) and, similarly, the calcium current in an identified giant, central neuron from an African snail was insensitive to up to 50 μM synthetic ω-conotoxin (60).

Effects of ω-Conotoxin on Calcium Currents from Other Cell Types

In GH_3 cells (a clonal cell line derived from a rat pituitary tumor), synthetic ω-conotoxin (2 μM) was shown to block L-type calcium current (61) and not T-type current [unlike an earlier study by the same authors (62) in which 50 nM toxin was reported to block T-type current carried by 50 mM barium]. In bovine chromaffin cells, a maximal block of about 50% of both decaying and sustained calcium currents elicited from -90- and -40-mV holding potentials was observed for ω-conotoxin concentrations between 0.3 and 25 μM (63). For these cells, it was concluded that a significant fraction of calcium current was insensitive to ω-conotoxin, somewhat at odds with usual descriptions of chromaffin cells possessing only L-type channels. It will be of much interest to know whether "facilitation" calcium currents (64) induced by large depolarizations or by dopaminergic D_1 receptor stimulation and subsequent kinase A activation in these cells are ω-conotoxin sensitive, as these "latent L-type" channels are dihydropyridine sensitive (64).

Advantages of the Patch-Clamp Technique

From a methodological point of view, it should be noted that the patch-clamp technique (16, 17) presents powerful advantages, with perhaps the most striking feature being the increased resolution in current amplitude to the picoampere (10^{-12} A) range, sufficient to allow current through a single open ion channel to be measured. Single-channel recording allows dissection of macroscopic whole-cell current into the following: n, the number of channels available; $P(o)$, the probability that a channel is open (which in fact is determined by two measurable components, the frequency of channel opening and τ, the mean channel open time); and γ, the single-channel conductance (which is the elementary single-channel current amplitude normalized by the driving force). As well, the noninvasive, tight-seal nature of whole-cell recording allows small cells to be studied (to a limiting diameter of about 5 μm), without the inevitable leakage conductances associated with intracellular microelectrode measurements. Temporal resolution is also greatly enhanced by the reduced capacitance and low access resistance characteristic of patch-recording pipettes, unlike high-resistance intracellular microelectrodes. This is a critical condition for resolving, for example, fast-deactivating calcium channel tail currents, which have decay time constants in the submillisecond range (24). Clearly, with patch-clamp methodology, ionic current measurement under technically correct voltage control (both spatially and temporally) has become accessible and possible in a much larger number of applications. Control of the ionic composition of the solutions bathing both membrane faces, an immediate consequence of most patch-recording configurations, is essential for accurate biophysical description of, for instance, single-channel conductance, ion selectivity, and mechanisms of open channel block. The study of the regulatory actions of intracellular messengers (like calcium, ATP, or cyclic AMP) and effectors (like protein kinases or GTP-binding proteins) in ionic channel function (for a review, see Ref. 11) is also greatly facilitated by the relatively easy access to the intracellular membrane surface afforded by the patch-clamp technique. As well, the use of single cells obviates the technical limitations associated with, for example, electrical coupling or extracellular ion accumulation, which often arise when multicellular preparations are used. Finally, the recent extension of patch-clamp methods to tissue slices (65) promises to open new vistas. It is thus obvious that the patch-clamp technique has revolutionized membrane physiology and must be the *de facto* method of choice for most kinds of electrophysiological studies at the cellular level.

Effects of ω-Conotoxin at the Neuromuscular Junction

As already mentioned above, it has been shown that ω-conotoxin blocks transmitter release at the frog and bullfrog neuromuscular junction and it was inferred that the calcium channels responsible for calcium entry during activation of the secretory mechanism were blocked (22). ω-Conotoxin (40 nM–2 μM) decreased the end-plate potential amplitude by up to 90%. This was due to a decrease in quantal content and not to a smaller quantal size (66, 67). Whereas ω-conotoxin blocks transmission at amphibian neuromuscular junctions and in the electric organ of *Torpedo* (68), almost no effect of ω-conotoxin was seen at the neuromuscular junction of mouse (67) or rat (69). For example, electrically evoked neurotransmitter release from rat phrenic nerve terminals was not inhibited by ω-conotoxin (69), while on the other hand quantal content was increased by BAY K 8644 at the frog neuromuscular junction (70). Does this lack of effect of ω-conotoxin indicate the absence of a subclass of calcium channels in peripheral nerve terminals of higher vertebrates? As mentioned above, ω-conotoxin had no effect on presynaptic calcium currents at the mouse neuromuscular junction (55), but was active at the lizard neuromuscular junction (56) and at the chick ciliary ganglion nerve terminal (58). Alternatively, does ω-conotoxin bind only to certain calcium channels of one (or a few) subclass(es)? We shall try to answer these questions in the final part of this chapter. But from the above one can conclude, at least at the neuromuscular junction, that the potency of ω-conotoxin depends on the species studied.

Effects of ω-Conotoxin on Autonomic Nerve Terminals

The potency of ω-conotoxin in inhibiting neurotransmission at different autonomic neuroeffector junctions has been investigated in vertebrates such as rat, guinea pig, mouse, and rat (71–74). Two major conclusions can be drawn. Firstly, similar to the skeletal neuromuscular junction, the potency of ω-conotoxin block of neurotransmission depends on the animal considered. Second, within the same species the toxin has a different potency depending on the nerve endings studied. For instance, in the vas deferens preparation, ω-conotoxin inhibited to a similar extent the response to field stimulation in both rat and guinea pig (73). However, in the isolated urinary bladder preparation, ω-conotoxin blocked only 25% of the response in rat, whereas in guinea pig the inhibition was ~75% (73). Finally, the same authors found that the relaxation of the rat duodenum evoked by field stimulation was totally resistant to ω-conotoxin. In another study (71), the perivascular nerves of isolated tail arteries from rat were stimulated with field pulses and as little as $10 \, \text{n}M$ ω-conotoxin totally inhibited the neurogenically mediated contractions as well as the release of prelabeled noradrenaline. Inhibition of neurogenically mediated contractions of rat mesenteric arteries by nanomolar amounts of ω-conotoxin has also been described (75). Similar findings were reported for neurally mediated contractions in the rat (76) and guinea pig (77) ileum. Intracellularly recorded excitatory postsynaptic potentials (EPSPs) in submucosal neurons from guinea pig isolated ileum were blocked reversibly by micromolar amounts of ω-conotoxin (78). Further, comprehensive studies of various autonomic noradrenergic and cholinergic neuroeffector junctions showed a clear inhibitory effect of ω-conotoxin on neurotransmission (72, 74, 77). However, in rat parasympathetic neurons in culture, ω-conotoxin, up to a concentration of $1 \, \mu M$, had no effect on synaptic transmission (79). This has also been shown for neurotransmission between cultured sympathetic neurons from the guinea pig vas deferens (80). One possible explanation of these latter two results is that ω-conotoxin-sensitive calcium channels in these cell types might be lost following enzymatic dissociation or that during cell culture certain factors are required for continued expression of such channels.

Effects of ω-Conotoxin on Neurons in Culture

The effects of ω-conotoxin on neurons in culture have been studied mostly in somata isolated from the striatum and the hippocampus and in sympathetic neurons (81, 82). On depolarization of sympathetic neurons, calcium currents having a biphasic decay are observed and 10 μM ω-conotoxin blocks ~70% of both the peak and late inward currents (83). Furthermore, in these neurons the potassium-induced increase in cytoplasmic calcium concentration, as measured by the fluorescent probe Fura-2, was blocked by 50% by ω-conotoxin. Note that nitrendipine also inhibited by ~50% this increase in internal calcium. Interestingly, it was shown in the same study that ω-conotoxin decreased by ~70% the release of prelabeled [^{3}H]noradrenaline whereas nitrendipine had no effect. In another study (82), ω-conotoxin had no significant effect on the increase in internal calcium induced by potassium depolarization of striatal neurons, whereas the response to the same stimulus in hippocampal neurons was inhibited by ~80%. These results are puzzling, because in a recent study on striatal neurons it was shown that the potassium-induced, calcium-dependent release of endogenous γ-aminobutyric acid (GABA) was inhibited 55% by both ω-conotoxin and nifedipine (81). It appears that there may be a large discrepancy between the effects of ω-conotoxin on the increase in cytoplasmic calcium resulting from activation of calcium channels and on the secretory process.

Effects of ω-Conotoxin in Brain Slices

The effects of ω-conotoxin on the release of prelabeled neurotransmitter in brain slices from rabbit, rat, guinea pig, and human have been investigated (84–87). Although there was a large variability in the concentrations of ω-conotoxin reported to inhibit the release of noradrenaline, 5-hydroxytryptamine (5-HT), and acetylcholine, the data clearly demonstrate that ω-conotoxin decreases the depolarization-induced release of these molecules. Studies on hippocampal slices from guinea pig (88), rabbit (89), and rat (90, 91) have shown that both EPSPs and IPSPs (excitatory and inhibitory postsynaptic potentials) resulting from stimulation of nerve endings and release of labeled neurotransmitter were inhibited by ω-conotoxin. Note that the release of 5-HT was decreased by 30 to 48% whereas the EPSPs and the IPSPs were inhibited by 69 and 84%, respectively. Note also that in one study (84) the dihydropyridine agonist S-202-791 had no effect in rabbit hippocampal slices, whereas in another study (91), BAY K 8644 potentiated the effect of depolarization and this effect was insensitive to ω-conotoxin in this same preparation. Synaptic transmission between mossy fibers and CA3 neurons was decreased 70% by ω-conotoxin (88). In slices from the striatum, different authors (92–94) reported that the release of either prelabeled or endogenous neurotransmitter was reduced by ω-conotoxin. Whereas ω-conotoxin was usually effective when release was stimulated both electrically and by potassium-induced depolarization, the effect of dihydropyridines observed by some authors occurred only for potassium stimulation. In summary, the majority of the studies on slices from different areas of the brain show that ω-conotoxin inhibits depolarization-induced neurotransmitter release to a variable degree (30 to 80%).

Effects of ω-Conotoxin on Brain Synaptosomes

Synaptosomes are pinched off nerve endings obtained after, for example, homogenization of the brain. They contain synaptic vesicles and release of different neurotransmitters can thus be studied *in vitro*. Furthermore, by use of fluorescent indicators, it is possible to correlate the rise in cytoplasmic calcium concentration and the rate of transmitter release that follows depolarization of the nerve terminals. In a large number of studies, ω-conotoxin inhibited potassium-induced ^{45}Ca uptake to varying degrees. For example, in frog and chicken synaptosomes this uptake was almost completely blocked (22, 93, 95–98), whereas in the rat, only partial inhibition (30–50%) was observed (82, 97, 99, 100). Similarly, in the chicken the release of endogenous or prelabeled neurotransmitters was blocked by 70% (95), whereas in the rat decreases from a few percent up to 60% of the secretory activity have been reported (82, 86, 101). Thus, again we see that the effect of ω-conotoxin on calcium uptake and on release of neurotransmitters depends on the species used and the experimental paradigm employed to elicit the measured responses.

Effects of ω-Conotoxin on Neurosecretory Nerve Terminals

Recently, a new preparation of nerve endings has been developed (14). This involves the homogenization of the neural lobe, which contains only nerve endings that originate from cell bodies located in the hypothalamus. The size of these nerve endings [up to 12 μM in diameter (102)] makes them a very useful preparation for the study of mechanisms involved in stimulus-secretion coupling. Studies on the effects of ω-conotoxin on calcium entry into these neurohypophyseal nerve terminals have produced conflicting results. Using Fura-2 measurement of cytoplasmic calcium concentration in single nerve terminals, no effects of ω-conotoxin at concentrations as high as 0.3 μM were seen (103), while in populations of nerve endings, inhibition of both rises in internal calcium and neuropeptide release was described (104). Similarly, no effects were seen on neurohypophyseal "whole-terminal" calcium currents with up to 2 μM ω-conotoxin, in the absence of bovine serum albumin (BSA) (104a). However, if 0.1% (v/v) BSA was added to the medium and had access to the entire surface of the isolated nerve terminal, then the same concentration of ω-conotoxin inhibited both the L- and N-type calcium current components (59) by 80% (104a). Presumably, this increased efficiency of ω-conotoxin is due to BSA binding to nonspecific sites, thus perhaps maximizing the effective toxin concentration. Note that in the work of Dayanithi *et al.* (104) the concentration of ω-conotoxin that inhibited 50% of the depolarization-evoked neurosecretion was very close to the K_d for the toxin-binding site in this preparation. Furthermore, the same authors showed that these neurosecretory nerve terminals had about seven times more binding sites for ω-conotoxin than for dihydropyridines. Although nicardipine and nitrendipine inhibited potassium-induced release of vasopressin by 80%, a mixture of dihydropyridines and ω-conotoxin did not completely abolish the secretory process. Similar results were recently observed following electrical and potassium-induced stimulation of the whole neural lobe from rat (105), and from a rodent that lives in a semidesert climate (106). As well, in the *Xenopus* neurohypophysis, an ω-conotoxin-sensitive, dihydropyridine-insensitive calcium influx was demonstrated using optical recording of changes in membrane voltage and light scattering (107). In summary, here we clearly see that a component of the calcium influx as well as part of the neurosecretory process cannot be blocked by either ω-conotoxin or dihydropyridines.

Effects of ω-Conotoxin on Synaptosomes Isolated from Electroplax

The potassium-induced secretion from synaptosomes of the ray electric organ (*Ommata discopyge*) has been shown to be largely inhibited by ω-conotoxin (108, 109). For example, ATP, which is contained in synaptic vesicles and is coreleased, can be used as a measure of the secretory activity from synaptosomes. This release was blocked by 75% in the presence of 40 μM ω-conotoxin, as also was depolarization-induced ^{45}Ca uptake. It is of interest to note that in one study (108), the K_d for toxin binding was 3 μM, whereas half-inhibition of release and calcium uptake was observed for concentrations of 5 and 3 μM, respectively. As in this preparation, dihydropyridines had no effect on the release of ATP; these results suggest that, in the electroplax of *O. discopyge*, N-type calcium channels are responsible for the activation of the secretory process. This suggestion is supported by the observation that calcium currents expressed in *Xenopus* oocytes after injection of mRNA isolated from *Torpedo* electric lobe were blocked by ω-conotoxin, but not by dihydropyridines (110).

Effects of ω-Conotoxin on Chromaffin Cells

Bovine chromaffin cells in culture, on either potassium-induced depolarization or nicotinic cholinergic activation, release primarily adrenaline and noradrenaline. This release is not blocked by ω-conotoxin but, interestingly, depolarization-induced increases in cytoplasmic calcium are partially inhibited. Different groups have shown that an elevation of the external potassium concentration triggers a transient increase in internal calcium. This transient is followed by a plateau that is abolished if dihydropyridines are present in the incubating medium. Although some authors (111, 112) have found no effects of ω-conotoxin on the rise of internal calcium, others have observed an inhibition of this transient by the toxin, both in bovine chromaffin cells (113) and in PC-12 cells [a pheochromocytoma cell line (114)]. The small or absent effect of ω-conotoxin on both calcium influx and secretion is puzzling because the number of toxin-binding sites is about four times greater than the number of dihydropyridine-binding sites in these cells (112). Nevertheless, it has been repeatedly demonstrated in bovine chromaffin cells that dihydropyridine antagonists effectively block potassium-induced calcium uptake and catecholamine secretion and that dihydropyridine agonists cause appropriate potentiation of these two processes (115), although voltage-dependent calcium currents in these cells are not particularly sensitive or are insensitive to dihydropyridines. This puzzling discrepancy might be in part explained by assuming that most directly measured calcium current flows through N-type channels, and that "facilitation" calcium channels (64), which can be activated by kinase A stimulation (64) and which are dihydropyridine-sensitive, are perhaps latent under standard electrophysiological recording conditions.

Effects of ω-Conotoxin on Endocrine Cells

Although somewhat beyond the scope of this chapter, it is worth mentioning some results on isolated cells from the anterior pituitary. Hormones are secreted from this endocrine gland on cell activation by neuropeptides released from the hypothalamus. Also, electrophysiological studies on isolated anterior pituitary cells have shown that they are excitable and have properties similar to neuroendocrine cells. In a mixed cell preparation (116) and in purified gonadotrophs (117), ω-conotoxin did not affect the potassium-induced rise in intracellular calcium concentration, although it was largely decreased by dihydropyridines. Surprisingly, ω-conotoxin inhibited by 33% the potassium-induced release of follicle-stimulating hormone (FSH) and luteinizing hormone (LH). Activation of the secretory process by gonadotropin-releasing hormone (GnRH) was differentially affected by ω-conotoxin, with FSH release being inhibited by only 56%, while LH secretion was decreased by 82%. Furthermore, in these cells the release of FSH and LH was inhibited 35 to 50% by nitrendipine. Thus, according to the classical definition of calcium channel subclasses, it would seem that gonadotrophs have two kinds of "L-type" channels, each with different sensitivities to ω-conotoxin.

Concluding Remarks

It seems evident that the actions of ω-conotoxin are less clear-cut than has been often assumed. There are puzzling differences in toxin effectiveness between species, especially so since the evolutionary strategy represented by the development of multiple peptide neurotoxins by the *Conus* snails arose presumably in large part in response to interspecies variability. Whether this reflects species-dependent differences in calcium channel molecular structure or simply in the distribution of certain subclasses of calcium channels that are toxin sensitive is in general difficult to know. This applies notably to functional studies where calcium currents are not directly measured. It thus appears premature to conclude that calcium-dependent transmitter release is driven by a given calcium channel subtype, based uniquely on the functional actions of ω-conotoxin and dihydropyridine derivatives. Furthermore, it should be noted that toxin effects on calcium currents in cell somata, in general, cannot be extrapolated to the calcium currents in nerve terminals that underlie neurosecretion. In any case, the electrophysiological data are also open to some debate as to the blocking effects of ω-conotoxin. While it was initially reported that both L- and N-type calcium channels were irreversibly inhibited in an essentially complete fashion, other studies now indicate that in certain cells, L-type calcium channels are only partially and reversibly blocked. As well, on the basis of ω-conotoxin block, it now is apparent that N-type calcium channels can be subdivided into sensitive and insensitive classes. It has been suggested by various authors that the use of ω-conotoxin, in conjunction with dihydropyridine derivatives, may well provide a more reliable means of defining neuronal high voltage-activated calcium channel subtypes, compared to a widely used scheme based on inactivation–activation kinetics and holding potential dependence. Last, the present lack of molecular biological definition of neuronal high voltage-activated calcium channels largely results from the absence of a specific, high-affinity ligand. It would not be surprising that perhaps the greatest contribution of ω-conotoxin to the calcium channel field will arise from its application as a ligand permitting purification of these neuronal calcium channel subclasses, eventually leading to sequencing and cloning of the presumably different channel protein structures.

Acknowledgments

We thank our colleagues, who kindly provided us with unpublished observations. Work in the authors' laboratories has been supported by the CNRS, INSERM, MRT, NIH, and the Université Louis Pasteur.

References

1. W. R. Gray, B. M. Olivera, and L. J. Cruz, *Annu. Rev. Biochem.* **57,** 665 (1988).
2. B. M. Olivera, W. R. Gray, R. Zeikus, J. M. McIntosh, J. Varga, J. Rivier, V. de Santos, and L. J. Cruz, *Science* **230,** 1338 (1985).
3. B. M. Olivera, J. Rivier, C. Clark, C. A. Ramilo, G. P. Corpuz, F. C. Abogadie, E. E. Mena, S. R. Woodward, D. R. Hillyard, and L. J. Cruz, *Science* **249,** 257 (1990).
4. D. Yoshikami, Z. Bagabaldo, and B. M. Olivera, *Ann. N.Y. Acad. Sci.* **560,** 230 (1989).
5. B. P. Bean, *Annu. Rev. Physiol.* **51,** 367 (1989).
6. P. Hess, *Annu. Rev. Neurosci.* **13,** 337 (1990).
7. R. J. Miller, *Science* **232,** 46 (1987).
8. D. Pelzer, S. Pelzer, and T. F. McDonald, *Rev. Physiol. Biochem. Pharmacol.* **114,** 107 (1990).
9. R. W. Tsien, *in* "Neuromodulation" (L. K. Kaczmarek and I. B. Levitan, eds.), pp. 206–242. Oxford Univ. Press, Oxford, England, 1987.
10. R. W. Tsien, P. Hess, E. W. McCleskey, and R. L. Rosenberg, *Annu. Rev. Biophys. Chem.* **16,** 265 (1987).
11. R. W. Tsien, D. Lipscombe, D. V. Madison, R. K. Bley, and A. P. Fox, *Trends Neurosci.* **11,** 431 (1988).
12. G. J. Augustine, M. P. Charlton, and S. J. Smith, *Annu. Rev. Neurosci.* **10,** 633 (1987).
13. J. R. Lemos, J. J. Nordmann, I. M. Cooke, and E. Stuenkel, *Nature (London)* **319,** 410 (1986).
14. J. J. Nordmann, G. Dayanithi, and J. R. Lemos, *Biosci. Rep.* **7,** 411 (1987).
15. E. F. Stanley, *Brain Res.* **505,** 341 (1989).
16. O. P. Hamill, A. Marty, E. Neher, B. Sakmann, and F. J. Sigworth, *Pfluegers Arch.* **391,** 85 (1981).
17. B. Sakmann and E. Neher (eds.), "Single-Channel Recording." Plenum, New York, 1983.
18. T. Godfraind, R. Miller, and M. Wibo, *Pharmacol. Rev.* **38,** 321 (1986).
19. M. M. Hosey and M. Lazdunski, *J. Membr. Biol.* **104,** 81 (1988).

20. D. J. Triggle and R. A. Janis, *Annu. Rev. Pharmacol. Toxicol.* **27,** 347 (1987).
21. D. N. Middlemiss and M. Spedding, *Nature (London)* **314,** 94 (1985).
22. L. M. Kerr and D. Yoshikami, *Nature (London)* **308,** 282 (1984).
23. M. Takemura, this volume [15].
24. C. M. Armstrong and D. R. Matteson, *Science* **227,** 65 (1985).
25. J.-L. Bossu, A. Feltz, and J. M. Thomann, *Pfluegers Arch.* **403,** 360 (1985).
26. E. Carbone and H. D. Lux, *Nature (London)* **310,** 501 (1984).
27. B. Nilius, P. Hess, and R. W. Tsien, *Nature (London)* **316,** 443 (1985).
28. M. C. Nowycky, A. P. Fox, and R. W. Tsien, *Nature (London)* **316,** 440 (1985).
29. W. Trautwein, M. Kameyama, J. Hescheler, and F. Hofmann, *Prog. Zool.* **33,** 163 (1986).
30. T. Aosaki and H. Kasai, *Pfluegers Arch.* **414,** 150 (1989).
31. E. Carbone, E. Sher, and F. Clementi, *Pfluegers Arch.* **416,** 170 (1990).
32. M. R. Plummer, D. E. Logothetis, and P. Hess, *Neuron* **2,** 1453 (1989).
33. B. P. Bean, *J. Gen. Physiol.* **86,** 1 (1985).
34. D. R. Matteson and C. M. Armstrong, *J. Gen. Physiol.* **87,** 161 (1986).
35. D. Swandulla and C. M. Armstrong, *J. Gen. Physiol.* **92,** 197 (1988).
36. R. Eckert and J. E. Chad, *Prog. Biophys. Mol. Biol.* **44,** 215 (1984).
37. C.-M. Tang, F. Presser, and M. Morad, *Science* **240,** 213 (1988).
38. M. C. Sanguinetti and R. S. Kass, *Circ. Res.* **55,** 336 (1984).
39. E. W. McCleskey, A. P. Fox, D. Feldman, L. J. Cruz, B. M. Olivera, and R. W. Tsien, *Proc. Natl. Acad. Sci. U.S.A.* **84,** 4327 (1987).
40. A. N. Savtchenko and A. N. Verkhratsky, *Gen. Physiol. Biophys.* **9,** 147 (1990).
41. D. H. Feldman, B. M. Olivera, and D. Yoshikami, *FEBS Lett.* **214,** 295 (1987).
42. A. P. Fox, M. C. Nowycky, and R. W. Tsien, *J. Physiol. (London)* **394,** 149 (1987).
43. R. H. Scott, J. F. Wootton, and A. C. Dolphin, *Neuroscience* **38,** 285 (1990).
44. E. Carbone and H. D. Lux, *Pfluegers Arch.* **413,** 14 (1988).
45. Y. Oyama, Y. Tsuda, S. Sakakibara, and N. Akaike, *Brain Res.* **424,** 58 (1987).
46. S. W. Jones and T. N. Marks, *J. Gen. Physiol.* **94,** 151 (1989).
47. H. Kasai, T. Aosaki, and J. Fukuda, *Neurosci. Res.* **4,** 228 (1987).
48. E. Carbone, A. Formenti, and A. Pollo, *Neurosci. Lett.* **111,** 315 (1990).
49. E. P. Seward and G. Henderson, *Pfluegers Arch.* **417,** 223 (1990).
50. L. M. Boland and R. Dingledine, *J. Physiol. (London)* **420,** 223 (1990).
51. K. Takahashi, M. Wakamori, and N. Akaike, *Neurosci. Lett.* **104,** 229 (1989).
52. P. Illes and J. T. Regenold, *Acta Physiol. Scand.* **137,** 459 (1989).
53. J. P. Leonard, J. Nargeot, T. P. Snutch, N. Davidson, and H. A. Lester, *J. Neurosci.* **7,** 875 (1987).
54. N. Dascal, T. P. Snutch, H. Lubbert, N. Davidson, and H. A. Lester, *Science* **231,** 1147 (1986).
55. A. J. Anderson and A. L. Harvey, *Neurosci. Lett.* **82,** 177 (1987).
56. C. A. Lindgren and J. W. Moore, *J. Physiol. (London)* **414,** 201 (1989).
57. R. Penner and F. Dreyer, *Pfluegers Arch.* **406,** 190 (1986).
58. H. Yawo, *J. Physiol. (London)* **428,** 199 (1990).
59. J. R. Lemos and M. C. Nowycky, *Neuron* **2,** 1419 (1989).

60. X. P. Sun, H. Takeuchi, Y. Okano, and Y. Nozawa, *Comp. Biochem. Physiol.* C **87C,** 363 (1987).

61. N. Suzuki, T. Kudo, H. Taragi, T. Yoshioka, A. Tanakadate, and M. Kano, *J. Cell. Physiol.* **144,** 62 (1990).

62. N. Suzuki and T. Yoshioka, *Neurosci. Lett.* **75,** 235 (1987).

63. M. Hans, P. Illes, and K. Takeda, *Neurosci. Lett.* **114,** 63 (1990).

64. C. R. Artalejo, M. A. Ariano, R. L. Perlman, and A. P. Fox, *Nature (London)* **348,** 239 (1990).

65. F. Edwards, A. Konnerth, B. Sakmann, and T. Takahashi, *Pfluegers Arch.* **414,** 600 (1989).

66. K. Enomoto, K. Sano, Y. Shibuya, and T. Maeno, *Proc. Jpn. Acad., Ser. B* **62,** 267 (1986).

67. K. Sano, K. Enomoto, and T. Maeno, *Eur. J. Pharmacol.* **141,** 235 (1987).

68. K. Koyano, T. Abe, Y. Nishiuchi, and S. Sakakibara, *Eur. J. Pharmacol.* **135,** 337 (1987).

69. I. Wessler, D. J. Dooley, H. Osswald, and F. Schlemmer, *Neurosci. Lett.* **108,** 173 (1990).

70. E. Ofiram-Uffenheimer, R. Rahamimoff, and R. Shapira, *J. Physiol. (London)* **409,** 49P (1988).

71. B. Clasbrummel, H. Osswald, and P. Illes, *Br. J. Pharmacol.* **96,** 101 (1989).

72. A. De Luca, C. G. Li, M. J. Rand, J. J. Reid, P. Thaina, and H. K. Wong, *Br. J. Pharmacol.* **101,** 437 (1990).

73. C. A. Maggi, R. Pattachini, P. Santicioli, I. T. Lippe, S. Giulliani, P. Geppetti, E. Del Bianco, S. Selleri, and A. Meli, *Naunyn-Schmiedeberg's Arch. Pharmacol.* **338,** 107 (1988).

74. D. Pruneau and J. A. Angus, *Eur. J. Pharmacol.* **184,** 127 (1990).

75. D. Pruneau and J. A. Angus, *Br. J. Pharmacol.* **100,** 180 (1990).

76. H. D. Allescher, S. Willis, V. Schusdziarra, and M. Clausen, *Neuropeptides* **13,** 253 (1989).

77. R. A. Keith, D. LaMonte, and A. I. Salama, *J. Autonom. Pharmacol.* **10,** 139 (1990).

78. K. Z. Shen and A. Surprenant, *J. Physiol. (London)* **431,** 609 (1990).

79. G. R. Seabrook and D. J. Adams, *Br. J. Pharmacol.* **97,** 1125 (1989).

80. J. A. Brock, T. C. Cunnane, R. J. Evans, and J. Ziogas, *Clin. Exp. Pharmacol. Physiol.* **16,** 333 (1989).

81. J. P. Pin and J. Bockaert, *Eur. J. Pharmacol.* **188,** 81 (1990).

82. I. J. Reynolds, J. A. Wagner, S. H. Snyder, S. A. Thayer, B. M. Olivera, and R. J. Miller, *Proc. Natl. Acad. Sci. U.S.A.* **83,** 8804 (1986).

83. L. D. Hirning, A. P. Fox, E. W. McCleskey, B. M. Olivera, S. A. Thayer, R. J. Miller, and R. W. Tsien, *Science* **239,** 57 (1988).

84. D. J. Dooley, A. Lupp, and G. Hertting, *Naunyn-Schmiedeberg's Arch. Pharmacol.* **336,** 467 (1987).

85. T. J. Feuerstein, D. J. Dooley, and W. Seeger, *J. Pharmacol. Exp. Ther.* **252,** 778 (1990).

86. R. A. Keith, T. J. Mangano, M. A. Pacheco, and A. I. Salama, *J. Autonom. Pharmacol.* **9,** 243 (1989).

87. M. Takemura, J. Kishino, A. Yamatodani, and H. Wada, *Brain Res.* **496,** 351 (1989).

88. H. Kamiya, S. Sawada, and C. Yamamoto, *Neurosci. Lett.* **91,** 84 (1988).

89. D. J. Dooley, A. Lupp, G. Hertting, and H. Osswald, *Eur. J. Pharmacol.* **148,** 261 (1988).

90. P. Dutar, O. Rascol, and Y. Lamour, *Eur. J. Pharmacol.* **174,** 261 (1989).

91. I. Rijnhout, D. R. Hill, and D. N. Middlemiss, *Neurosci. Lett.* **115,** 323 (1990).

92. H. Herdon and S. F. Nahorski, *Naunyn-Schmiedeberg's Arch. Pharmacol.* **340,** 36 (1987).

93. P. J. Owen, D. B. Marriott, and M. R. Boarder, *Br. J. Pharmacol.* **97,** 133 (1989).

94. A. Thate and K. Meyer, *Naunyn-Schmiedeberg's Arch. Pharmacol.* **339,** 359 (1989).

95. P. M. Lundy, K. Stauderman, J.-C. Goulet, and R. Frew, *Neurochem. Int.* **14,** 49 (1989).

96. J. Rivier, R. Galyean, W. R. Gray, A. Azimi-Zonooz, J. M. McIntosh, L. J. Cruz, and B. M. Olivera, *J. Biol. Chem.* **262,** 1194 (1987).

97. H. W. Sheer, *Can. J. Physiol. Pharmacol.* **68,** 1049 (1990).

98. J. B. Suszkiw, M. M. Murawsky, and R. C. Fortner, *Biochem. Biophys. Res. Commun.* **5,** 1283 (1987).

99. J. B. Suszkiw, M. M. Murawsky, and M. Shi, *J. Neurochem.* **52,** 1260 (1989).

100. J. J. Woodward, S. M. Rezazadeh, and S. W. Leslie, *Brain Res.* **475,** 141 (1988).

101. F. Hofmann and E. Habermann, *Naunyn-Schmiedeberg's Arch. Pharmacol.* **341,** 200 (1987).

102. H. N. Y. Pouillerel, K. K. Ussoor, M. C. P. Casimba, and K. T. Eyetis, *J. Con. Sci.* **69,** 123 (1948).

103. E. L. Stuenkel, *Brain Res.* **529,** 96 (1990).

104. G. Dayanithi, N. Martin-Moutot, S. Barlier, D. A. Colin, M. Kretz-Zaepfel, F. Couraud, and J. J. Nordmann, *Biochem. Biophys. Res. Commun.* **156,** 255 (1988).

104a. X. Wang, S. N. Treistman, and J. R. Lemos, *J. Physiol. (London),* in press.

105. S. Von Spreckelsen, K. Lollike, and M. Treiman, *Brain Res.* **514,** 68 (1990).

106. A. Raji and J. J. Nordmann, manuscript in preparation (1991).

107. A. L. Obaid, R. Flores, and B. M. Salzberg, *J. Gen. Physiol.* **93,** 715 (1989).

108. S. N. Ahmad and G. P. Miljanich, *Brain Res.* **453,** 247 (1988).

109. R. E. Yeager, D. Yoshikami, J. Rivier, L. J. Cruz, and G. P. Miljanich, *J. Neurosci.* **7,** 2390 (1987).

110. J. A. Umbach and C. B. Gundersen, *Proc. Natl. Acad. Sci. U.S.A.* **84,** 5464 (1987).

111. J. J. Ballesta, M. Palmero, M. J. Hidalgo, L. M. Gutierrez, J. A. Reig, S. Viniegra, and A. G. Garcia, *J. Neurochem.* **53,** 1050 (1989).

112. C.-R. Jan, M. Titeler, and A. S. Schneider, *J. Neurochem.* **54,** 355 (1990).

113. L. M. Rosario, B. Soria, G. Feuerstein, and H. B. Pollard, *Neuroscience* **29,** 735 (1989).

114. E. Sher, A. Pandiella, and F. Clementi, *FEBS Lett.* **235,** 178 (1988).

115. A. G. Garcia, F. Sala, J. A. Reig, S. Viniegra, J. Frias, R. I. Fronteriz, and L. Gandia, *Nature (London)* **308,** 69 (1984).

116. K. Meier, W. Knepel, and C. Schofl, *Endocrinology (Baltimore)* **122,** 2764 (1988).

117. M. Blotner, G. A. Shangold, E. Y. Lee, S. N. Murphy, and R. J. Miller, *Mol. Cell. Endocrinol.* **71,** 205 (1990).

[15] ω-Conotoxin GVIA and Its Receptors

Motohiko Takemura

Introduction

Voltage-sensitive calcium channels play crucial roles in neural functions, such as action potential spike formation, neurotransmitter release, and growth cone development. The discovery and synthesis of organic calcium channel antagonists (dihydropyridine derivatives, verapamil, diltiazem, etc.) have led to great progress in understanding the molecular mechanisms of voltage-sensitive calcium channels. These drugs have been used successfully as probes for the purification of the voltage-sensitive calcium channel from skeletal muscle and subsquent deduction of its primary structure from its cloned cDNA (1). Dihydropyridine receptors have also been found in the central nervous system; however, the stimulation-evoked release of neuro-transmitters, which depends entirely on extracellular calcium ion, is rather refractory to these organic calcium antagonists, therefore the mechanism of calcium entry into the axon terminal on electrical excitation is not yet completely understood.

ω-Conotoxin GVIA was first described as a toxin of *Conus geographus* that produces "persistent shaking" when administered intracranially to mice, but which does not interact with acetylcholine receptors or voltage-sensitive sodium channels (2). Electrophysiological studies showed that the toxin blocks a neuron-specific subtype [the N type described by Nowycky *et al.* (3)] of voltage-sensitive calcium channels (for reviews, see Refs. 4 and 5) that is insensitive to organic calcium channel antagonists such as 1,4-dihydropyri-dines, verapamil, and diltiazem. ω-Conotoxin has been successfully used as a pharmacological and neurochemical probe of neuronal voltage-sensitive calcium channels. The toxin effectively blocks transmitter release evoked by depolarization stimuli in neurons and so the subtype of voltage-sensitive calcium channels that is sensitive to this toxin seems to be responsible for excitation–secretion coupling in axon terminals. Synthetic ω-conotoxin has the same biological potencies as the natural toxin (6), and has greatly pro-moted studies on these toxin-sensitive channels. However, in such studies it must be remembered that (1) the toxin also affects L-type voltage-sensitive calcium channels, which are widely distributed in excitable cells and play crucial roles in the contraction of all types of muscle and excitation–secretion coupling of the endocrine cells, and (2) the calcium ion entry necessary for evoked release of some neurotransmitters, especially peptide neurotransmitters, occurs through L-type, or dihydropyridine-sensitive, calcium channels.

This chapter describes the methods used (1) to observe the inhibitory effects of the toxin on the evoked release of a putative neurotransmitter, histamine, (2) to evaluate the density of the toxin-binding sites in the membrane fractions of the brain using radioisotope-labeled toxin, and (3) to localize the toxin-binding sites in brain sections by *in vitro* autoradiography.

Neurochemical Studies on Inhibitory Effect of ω-Conotoxin GVIA Using *in Vitro* Slice Superfusion System

The sensitivity of the release of neurotransmitters in response to ω-conotoxin or dihydropyridines has been studied in the mammalian central nervous system (CNS), peripheral neurons, and in nonmammalian neuromuscular junctions and electric organs. The evoked release of acetylcholine, noradrenaline, dopamine, 5-hydroxytryptamine, and glutamate from mammalian neurons (7–10), and of vasopressin from the neural lobe of the pituitary gland (11), is reported to be sensitive to ω-conotoxin but not to dihydropyridine derivatives. In contrast, depolarization-evoked increase of the cytosolic free-calcium concentration in anterior pituitary cells (endocrine) (12) and release of noradrenaline from adrenal chromaffin cells (13) are sensitive to dihydropyridines but not to ω-conotoxin. The release of substance P from embryonic chick dorsal root ganglion neurons evoked by high K^+ stimulaltion is, however, sensitive to a rather high dose of dihydropyridine (14). The inhibitory effects of ω-conotoxin are restricted to central and peripheral neurons, and this toxin has no effects reported so far on the endocrine or exocrine cells. Therefore, the sensitivity to ω-conotoxin for the evoked release of a substance subserves as an additional criterion to define that substance as a neurotransmitter. The release of histamine, a possible neurotransmitter or neuromodulator, in response to ω-conotoxin and dihydropyridine was examined using brain slices and an *in vitro* superfusion technique (15). The method used in brain slice superfusion experiments has been described in several reviews (e.g., Refs. 16 and 17). Experimental conditions for studying the release of neuroactive substances other than histamine have also been described for the *in vitro* superfusion technique (18–23; see also references cited in Ref. 24).

The hypothalamus was excised from rat brains perfused with 60 ml of ice-cold modified Krebs–Henseleit solution, containing (mM): NaCl, 124; KCl, 4.8; KH_2PO_4, 1.2; $MgSO_4$, 1.3; $CaCl_2$, 1.2; glucose, 5.5; and $NaHCO_3$, 25; the solution is saturated with 95% O_2/5% CO_2. In order to optimize histamine release, the glucose concentration was lowered to 5.5 mM, otherwise 10.0

mM glucose should be used. Perfusion was carried out through the ascending aorta under pentobarbital anesthesia. The excised hypothalamus was chilled in ice-cold solution for 5 min and then sliced by hand with a razor in ice-cold Krebs–Henseliet solution. All the slices from one hypothalamus were put into a 200-μl plastic chamber filled with the same solution at 37°C. The chamber was incubated at 37°C and the tissue was superfused with the same solution at a flow rate of 50 μl/min. Later it was found that a flow rate of 250 μl/min resulted in greater release over the basal level after depolarization (25). After perfusion for 60 min to allow the tissue to reach a new steady state, the superfusate was collected every 5 min in a plasic tube containing 60% (w/v) perchloric acid to give a final concentration of 2% (w/v). The samples were centrifuged at 10,000 g and 4°C for 20 min and histamine concentration in the supernatant was determined by an automated high-performance liquid chromatography (HPLC)–fluorometric method (26). Depolarization stimulation was applied by superfusion with high K$^+$ solution (solution containing 40 mM KCl substituted isosmotically for NaCl). Electrical stimulation through a platinum electrode installed in the superfusion chamber was also effective (25, 27). Depolarization stimulations were applied to the tissue for a 10-min period with 40-min intervals. Synthetic ω-conotoxin GVIA (purchased from the Peptide Institute, Mino-o, Japan; identical samples can be obtained from Peninsula, Belmont, CA) or nilvadipine (kindly supplied by Fujisawa Pharmaceutical Co., Osaka, Japan) was administered for 40 min after the effect of first depolarization stimulation had been observed. Then the second depolarization stimulation was applied in the presence of these agents. As the dihydropyridines are ultraviolet sensitive, the superfusion chamber, solution reservoir, and connecting tubes should be shielded from the light. We used nilvadipine because this substance is a relatively light-resistant dihydropyridine derivative. The effects of the agents on the basal release were estimated by comparing the fractional release rates preceding the first and second (with the agent) stimulations. The effects of the agents on the stimulation-evoked release were estimated by comparing the fractional release rates during the second stimulation in their presence and absence. The reversibilities of the effects were evaluated by comparing the release rate during the third stimulation, which was applied after a 40-min washout of the agents. To determine the significance of the differences, we divided the amount of the fractional release by the mean basal release by each slice, pooled the data for slices treated in the same way, and calculated the mean values and standard errors. The differences in the means were examined by Student's t test.

In our experiment neither ω-conotoxin nor nilvadipine at up to 1.0×10^{-6} M had any effect on the basal release of histamine. Nilvadipine at up to $1.0 \times 10^{-6} M$ had no effect on the depolarization-evoked release, but ω-conotoxin at

1.0×10^{-9} to 1.0×10^{-6} M inhibited this depolarization-evoked release dose dependently with an IC_{50} value of 2.7×10^{-9} M. The effective concentrations of ω-conotoxin for inhibiting stimulation-evoked transmitter release, Ca^{2+} uptake by neurons, and the calcium current, determined in other experiments, ranged from 1 pM (8) to 40 μM (28), with IC_{50} values being estimated as between 4 nM (7) and 1 μM (11, 22). The difference in the reported values may be due to the fact that the effect of the toxin is time dependent (29). Therefore, initially, the effect of about 1 μM ω-conotoxin should be examined after preincubation for 30–60 min. If an inhibitory effect is observed, it is recommended that the dose dependency or time dependency of the effect then be examined by the same experimental protocol.

Biochemical Assay of ^{125}I-labeled ω-Conotoxin GVIA Binding Sites

ω-Conotoxin binding sites were studied using ^{125}I-labeled or [^{3}H]propionyl-labeled toxin. The toxin was iodinated with Iodogen (Pierce, Rockford, IL) and purified by gel-permeation and reversed-phase chromatographies (30). Iodination was also performed by the chloramine-T method with subsquent purification by gel-permeation and ion-exchange chromatographies (31). Iodinated ω-conotoxin is now also available commercially [New England Nuclear (Boston, MA) or Amersham (Arlington Heights, IL)]. The mono[^{3}H]-propionyl derivative of the toxin was also prepared and used successfully for identification of toxin binding sites (32). The labeled toxin could be stored at 4°C for 1 month without loss of binding activity, but the nonspecific binding increased after longer storage.

The binding sites were observed in avian and mammalian synaptosomes, synaptic plasma membranes, and crude membrane fractions of brain (24, 30–42), crude homogenates of neuronal cell lines (43), membrane fractions of small intestine (44) (the presence of toxin binding sites in the small intestine may reflect neuronal components of this organ), and the electric organ of the electric ray (45). As the toxin binding sites in rat brain subcellular fractions are concentrated in synaptosomes or synaptic plasma membranes (31, 33), these fractions are good material for studies on toxin binding activity. Crude membrane fractions and crude homogenates may also be used, but freeze–thawing these fractions destroys their toxin binding sites (36), probably by activating lysosomal enzymes.

The association time constant (k_{-1}) of the toxin was calculated to be 1.3–2.6×10^{10} min^{-1} M^{-1} (36, 38) or 2.52×10^{9} min^{-1} M^{-1} (35) at 25°C, 4.1×10^{8} at 37°C (37), and 7.1×10^{9} at 4°C (36). The dissociation time constant (k_{1}) was calculated to be 0.0006–0.006 min^{-1} (36–38) at 25 or 37°C, and much lower (38) or about the same (41) at 4°C. Thus, the dissociation rate of the toxin is very low, and an equilibrium binding assay is practically impossible. The saturation binding assays at 4, 25, or 37°C were arbitrarily stopped after incubation for 60–240 min. Chick, rat, and bovine brains contain binding sites for the toxin with "apparent" dissociation constants (K_D) of 0.7–60 pM, although these are not true equilibrium values because of the very slow rate of the dissociation of the toxin described above. The binding capacity (B_{max}) of this site was calculated to be 0.3–3 pmol/mg membrane protein (24, 30, 32, 35–38, 40–43). When incubations were conducted at 4°C for 90 min, an additional binding site with a K_D of 0.5–4 nM and B_{max} of 2–4 pmol/mg protein was observed in rat and bovine brains (24, 32, 41, 42). The first report of identification of the ω-conotoxin binding site in the chick brain demonstrated that half-maximal binding occurs at a subnanomolar concentration of the toxin (30). Thus, it is not clear whether or not chick brain also contains this low-affinity binding site for the toxin. In later studies demonstrating the existence of only one class of binding sites, the toxin concentrations used were too low to investigate the low-affinity site (35–38, 40, 43). Different incubation times, incubation media, or incubation temperatures may also give different results. The toxin binding to either of the two sites was not affected by incubation with organic calcium channel antagonists (30, 31, 35, 36, 41, 43), indicating that the binding sites for these two ligands have no cooperativity. The concentration of the toxin used in electrophysiological experiments on calcium current inhibition and neurochemical experiments on neurotransmitter release inhibition (discussed in the previous section) was similar to the dissociation constant of the low-affinity site. Toxin binding was reported to be inhibited by metal ions and inorganic cations, toxins that are closely related to ω-conotoxin (30–32, 35, 36, 38, 40, 41, 43, 46) and venom of the spider *Plectreurys tristes* (38). The affinity of ω-conotoxin for the binding sites was increased by dynorphin A and related peptides, probably through a nonopiate mechanism (38). The binding of the toxin to the high-affinity site of bovine brain synaptic membranes was inhibited stereospecifically by diltiazem, but not by other organic calcium channel antagonists, and so the inhibition may be unrelated to L-type calcium channels (32).

For the saturation binding assay, 1–100 μg of the membrane preparation was incubated in 0.5 ml of 5 mM HEPES–Tris buffer, pH 7.4 [note a high concentration of Tris may inhibit the toxin binding (35)], containing 0.32 M sucrose, 1 mg/ml bovine serum albumin, 0.01 mg/ml lysozyme, 0.1 mM phenylmethylsulfonyl fluoride, 1 mg/ml bacitracin, and various concentration of labeled toxin. Nonspecific binding of the toxin was measured by addition of the 1 μM cold toxin. Incubation was conducted for 90 min at 4°C and then the mixture was diluted with 1.0 ml of ice-cold 5 mM HEPES-Tris buffer (pH 7.4) containing 160 mM choline chloride, 1.5 mM CaCl$_2$, and 1 mg/ml bovine serum albumin and rapidly filtered through glass fiber filters (GF/C; Whatman, Clifton, NJ) under vacuum. The filters were washed three times with 2-ml volumes of the same solution as that used for dilution (25, 30, 33, 42). Incubation in 20 mM Tris-HCl (pH 7.5) containing 1 mg/ml bovine serum albumin and washing with 5 ml of 20 mM Tris-HCl (pH 7.5) containing 0.15 M NaCl and 1 mg/ml bovine serum albumin seemed to give similar results (31, 32, 41). The density of ω-conotoxin-binding sites in the lower brain regions is reported to change with age in rats (39). The high-affinity binding site was solubilized satisfactorily from bovine brain. In these experiments binding was measured after rapid filtration through polyethyleneimine-treated glass fiber filters or after rapid gel filtration through a Sephadex G-75 column (32).

The target molecule of ω-conotoxin in synaptosomal membranes was identified by cross-linking of the labeled toxin (31, 34, 35). With disuccinimidyl suberate (DSS) as a cross-linking reagent, chick brain gave a specifically labeled band of 210K (34) or 170K in nonreducing conditions and of 140K in reducing conditions (35) in sodium dodecyl sulfate–polyacrylamide gel electrophoresis. When DSS was used for cross-linking, rat brain did not show specific labeling (35). However, photoaffinity labeling of the toxin derivative with N-(5-azido-2-nitrobenzoyloxy)succinimide, components of 310K, 240K, and 34K (31) or 220K and 33K (35) were visualized in rat brain, as was a 220K component in chick brain (35). Thus there may be some differences in the assemblies of toxin-binding molecules in different species. It is speculated that the toxin binding sites are composed of molecules of 220K, 140K, and 30K and that the 140K and 30K molecules are linked by disulfide bonds. No apparent differences in the labeling pattern of rat brain were seen using different concentrations of toxin to label high- or low-affinity sites, suggesting that the two sites are on the same polypeptide molecule (31). More experimental data are, however, needed for further understanding of the molecular nature of the toxin-binding molecule, that is, the putative neuron-specific subtype of the voltage-sensitive calcium channel.

Anatomical Study of ^{125}I-Labeled ω-Conotoxin GVIA Binding Sites

The distribution of ω-conotoxin binding sites in the brain was studied by binding assays on membrane preparations from discrete regions of the brain (35, 36, 39). More detailed information on the distribution of these sites in discrete regions of the brain of rats (25, 42, 47) and mice (48) was obtained using ^{125}I-labeled ω-conotoxin and *in vitro* autoradiographic techniques. For detection of ω-conotoxin binding sites, sections of rat or mouse brain of 10- to 20-μm thickness were cut in a cryostat at about $-10°C$ and placed on glass slides coated with chrome–alum/gelatin. In our study, rats under sodium pentobarbital anesthesia [50 mg/kg, intraperitoneal (ip)] were perfused intra-cardially with 200 ml of 0.5% (w/v) paraformaldehyde in 0.1 M sodium phosphate buffer (pH 7.4) before removal of the brain to improve the integrity of the sections during incubation and washing procedures. This prefixation did not influence the distribution of the binding sites (25, 42). Others have reported the distribution of toxin binding sites in freshly frozen sections (47, 48). After drying the sections on slides for 1–2 hr at 4°C, they were preincubated with 0.32 M sucrose and 0.01 mg/ml lysozyme in 5 mM HEPES-Tris (pH 7.4) (47) or this solution supplemented with bovine serum albumin at 1 mg/ml, 0.1 mM phenylmethylsulfonyl fluoride, and bacitracin at 1 mg/ml (25, 42) for 10 or 30 min. The inclusion of bovine serum albumin reduced nonspecific binding and the inclusions of phenylmethylsulfonyl fluoride and bacitracin reduced degradation, if any, of the toxin and its receptors during experimental procedures. The sections were then incubated in the same solution containing 0.5 nM ^{125}I-labeled ω-conotoxin for 90 min at 4°C (25, 42) with or without 1 μM competitor or for 30 min at 20°C (47). At lower temperature binding sites are better preserved. The sections incubated at 4°C were then washed six times (10 min each) with 200 ml of buffer containing 160 mM choline chloride, 1.5 mM CaCl$_2$, and bovine serum albumin at 1 mg/ml in 5 mM HEPES-Tris (pH 7.4). Six washings were optimal to obtain a clear difference between specific bindings and the nonspecific binding. The sections incubated at 20°C were washed at 4°C with a solution of 160 mM NaCl, 1.5 mM CaCl$_2$, and bovine serum albumin at 1 mg/ml in 5 mM HEPES (pH 7.4) (47). In this experiment, 0.25 μM competitor was added to determine nonspecific binding. The sections were dried at 4°C and exposed to Ultrofilm [3]H (LKB-Produkter AB, Bromma, Sweden) at −20°C for 7–10 days. The duration of exposure necessary differs with the concentration and the specific radioactivity of the toxin used, but 7–10 days was suitable when 2.96–3.33 MBq/nmol (80–90 μCi/nmol) radioligand was used. The sections of freshly frozen mouse brains were stored at −40°C for 15 hr after drying and incubated in a solution containing 0.5 nM labeled toxin, bovine serum albumin at 1 mg/ml, 150 mM choline chloride, and 10 mM HEPES-Tris (pH 7.4), with or without competitor (1 μM) for 30 min at room temperature without preincubation. Then the sections on slides were washed four times with phosphate-buffered saline and fixed in 2% (w/v) paraformaldehyde/0.2% (v/v) glutaraldehyde/phosphate-buffered saline for 10 min. Then they were washed three times with phosphate-buffered saline and once with distilled water, dried, and exposed to photographic emulsion. The specific radioactivity of the labeled toxin used in this experiment was 1000 Ci/mmol and the exposure time was 5 days at 4°C (48).

In the experiments described above, low affinity binding sites (if there are two classes) were detected. These binding sites were distributed unevenly throughout the brain. Details of the relative densities of binding sites have been reported (24). It is noteworthy that there were clear differences between the distributions of ω-conotoxin binding sites and sites for organic calcium antagonists reported previously. The difference was especially clear in the hypophysis. These differences indicate that the ω-conotoxin binding sites observed under these conditions are not the L-type voltage-sensitive calcium channel/organic calcium antagonist receptors. The density of toxin binding sites was higher in areas with complex synaptic connections, and no binding sites were detected in white matter tracts (24, 42, 47, 48).

Maeda *et al.* (48) reported an interesting correlation between the density of toxin binding sites and the density of parallel fibers of the granule cells in the molecular layer of the cerebellum in Purkinje cell degeneration mutant (*pcd*) and *weaver* mutant mice. In the cerebellum of rats and mice, the molecular layer has the highest density of ω-conotoxin binding sites. However, when compared to other brain regions, the density of ω-conotoxin binding sites in the molecular layer of the cerebellum is "moderate" (24, 48). In *pcd* mice almost all the Purkinje cells are lost but granule cells are only moderately affected. The densities of toxin binding sites in the molecular layers of *pcd* mice and normal mice were comparable. On the other hand, *weaver* (*wv*) mutant mice are characterized by degeneration of granule cells without change in interneurons and Purkinje cells, except for poor and disoriented dendritic arborization of the Purkinje cells. Autoradiograms of the cerebellum showed no ω-conotoxin binding in this type of mutant. This result indicates that the toxin binding sites in the molecular layer of the cerebellum are present on the parallel fibers of the granular cells, not on the Purkinje cell soma, dendrites, or interneurons (48).

Tetramethylrhodamine and biotin derivatives of ω-conotoxin were used for microscopic detection of binding sites in cultured hippocampal neurons (49). Both derivatizations increase the dissociation constant of the toxin for its binding site 15- to 30-fold, which means that its affinity decreases substantially. The derivatized toxins retained activity to inhibit the calcium current in hippocampal cells, as shown by the patch-clamp technique (49). The localization of toxin binding sites in hippocampal cultured cells was observed using these toxin derivatives. The staining of toxin binding sites in the cell populations was heterogeneous, and about 10% of the cells were not stained with these toxin derivatives. In the cells to which the toxin derivatives were bound, the staining was observed on cell bodies and processes. The toxin binding sites on cell processes were colocalized with MAP-2, a dendritic marker protein (49).

These results clearly show the presence of toxin binding sites on the cell soma and dendrites. So there may be some differences in the localizations of the toxin binding sites on neurons in the hippocampus and the cerebellum, or this may be the case only for cultured neurons. The characteristics of toxin binding sites may also differ at different stages of cell differentiation and maturation. More investigations are needed on the localization of toxin binding sites on neuronal cells.

Conclusions

ω-Conotoxin was reported to block both N- and L-type voltage-sensitive calcium channels in nerve preparations. Recent electrophysiological reports, however, have shown that the toxin blocks only N-type channels and does not affect L-type channels in neurons (20, 43, 50). The reason for these discrepant reports may be because L-type channel action could not be separated sufficiently in previous studies, or because the sensitivities of L-type channels to ω-conotoxin differ in different cells. There are differences in the primary structures of dihydropyridine receptors in skeletal and cardiac muscles (51). Therefore, it would not be surprising to find that the toxin blocks the L-type channels of nonneuronal tissue but does not block those in neuronal cells.

The low-affinity binding site of ω-conotoxin in rat brain may not be that of L-type voltage-sensitive calcium channels or dihydropyridine binding sites, because the distributions of the two clearly differ in brain regions.

A new subtype of voltage-sensitive calcium channels, P-channel, has been found in the cerebellar Purkinje cells and the terminal of squid giant axons (52). This subtype of calcium channel is inhibited by a funnel web spider venom fraction, but not by dihydropyridines or ω-conotoxin (52). The toxin used in this experiment was a low-molecular-weight compound, probably a derivative of polyamines (53). There is also a report of a proteinaceous toxin from the same spider venom that inhibits calcium channels; three structurally related proteins with calcium antagonistic activity were purified from the venom and one of them was found to inhibit ω-conotoxin binding, whereas the other two did not (52). Voltage-sensitive calcium channels in the nervous tissues can be classified into three subclasses; ω-conotoxin sensitive, dihydropyridine sensitive, and both ω-conotoxin and dihydropyridine insensitive. The third subclass may be further classified using these new, potent tools for recognizing voltage-sensitive calcium channels.

The action of ω-conotoxin was first demonstrated in electrophysiological studies (54). This toxin has also been used to distinguish the subtypes of voltage-sensitive calcium channels (e.g., Ref. 20). These studies are not described in detail in this chapter. Readers interested in electrophysiological studies on the effect of this toxin should refer to other papers describing appropriate techniques.

Acknowledgments

The neurochemical studies using brain slices described here were conducted in collaboration with Mr. J. Kishino, Dr. J. Ono, and Dr. A. Yamatodani, the biochemical binding study with Dr. H. Fukui, Department of Pharmacology II, and the anatomical studies with Dr. H. Kiyama of the Department of Neuroanatomy, and Dr. M. Tohyama, Department of Anatomy II. The author thanks all those involved in these experimental projects, and also Prof. H. Wada for supervision throughout and Dr. F. Gusovsky for reading the manuscript. He also thanks Fujisawa Pharmaceuticals Company for a generous gift of nilvadipine. This work was supported by grants from the Ministry of Education, Science, and Culture of Japan.

References

1. T. Tanabe, H. Takeshima, A. Mikami, V. Flockerzi, H. Takahashi, K. Kangawa, M. Kojima, H. Matsuo, T. Hirose, and S. Numa, *Nature (London)* **328,** 313 (1987).
2. B. M. Olivera, J. M. McIntosh, L. J. Cruz, F. A. Luque, and W. R. Gray, *Biochemistry* **23,** 5087 (1984).
3. M. C. Nowycky, A. P. Fox, and R. W. Tsien, *Nature (London)* **316,** 440 (1985).
4. R. J. Miller, *Science* **235,** 46 (1987).
5. S. Watson and A. Abbott, *Trends Pharmacol. Sci., Suppl.* **29,** 29 (1990).
6. Y. Nishiuchi, K. Kumagaye, Y. Noda, T. X. Watanabe, and S. Sakakibara, *Biopolymers* **25,** S61 (1986).
7. D. J. Dooley, A. Lupp, and G. Hertting, *Naunyn-Schmiedeberg's Arch. Pharmacol.* **336,** 467 (1987).
8. L. D. Hirrning, A. P. Fox, E. W. McCleskey, B. M. Olivera, S. A. Thayer, R. J. Miller, and R. W. Tsien, *Science* **239,** 57 (1988).
9. H. Kamiya, S. Sawada, and C. Yamamoto, *Neurosci. Lett.* **91,** 84 (1988).
10. I. J.Reynolds, J. A. Wagner, S. H. Snyder, S. A. Thayer, B. M. Olivera, and R. J. Miller, *Proc. Natl. Acad. Sci. U.S.A.* **83,** 8804 (1986).
11. G. Dayanithi, N. Martin-Moutot, S. Barlier, D. A. Colin, M. Kretz-Zaepfel, F. Couraud, and J. J. Nordmann, *Biochem. Biophys. Res. Commun.* **156,** 255 (1988).
12. K. Meier, W. Knepel, and C.Schöfl, *Endocrinology (Baltimore)* **122,** 2764 (1988).
13. P. J. Owen, D. B. Marriott, and M. R. Boarder, *Br. J. Pharmacol.* **97,** 133 (1989).
14. S. G. Rane, G. G. Holz IV, and K. Dunlap, *Pfluegers Arch.* **409,** 361 (1987).
15. M. Takemura, J. Kishino, A. Yamatodani, and H. Wada, *Brain Res.* **496,** 351 (1989).

16. F. Orrego, *Neuroscience* **4,** 1037 (1979).

17. E. R. Korpi and S. S. Oja, *J. Neurochem.* **43,** 236 (1984).

18. S. Mochida and H. Kobayashi, *Neurosci. Lett.* **72,** 205 (1986).

19. E.Carbone and H. D. Lux, *Pfluegers Arch.* **413,** 14 (1988).

20. M. R. Plummer, D. E. Logothetis, and P. Hess, *Neuron* **2,** 1453 (1988).

21. J. Rivier, R. Galyean, W. R. Gray, A. Azimi-Zonooz, J. M.McIntosh, L. J. Cruz, and B. M. Olivera, *J. Biol. Chem.* **262,** 1194 (1987).

22. P. M. Lundy and R. Frew, *Eur. J. Pharmacol.* **156,** 325 (1988).

23. J. J. Woodward, S. M. Rezazadeh, and S. W. Leslie, *Brain Res.* **475,** 141 (1988).

24. M. Takemura, H.Kiyama, H. Fukui, M. Tohyama, and H. Wada, *Neuroscience* **32,** 405 (1989).

25. J. Ono, A. Yamatodani, J. Kishino, M. Takemura, T. Mikami, S. Okada, and H. Wada, *Neurosci. Res.* **11,** (suppl.), S123 (1990).

26. A. Yamatodani, H. Fukuda, H. Wada, T. Iwaeda, and T. Watanabe, *J. Chromatogr.* **344,** 115 (1985).

27. J. F. Van der Werf, A. Bast, G. J. Bijloo, A. Van der Vliet, and H. Timmerman, *Eur. J. Pharmacol.* **138,** 199 (1987).

28. R. E. Yeager, D. Yoshikami, J. Rivier, L. J. Cruz, and G. P. Miljanich, *J. Neurosci.* **7,** 2390 (1987).

29. Y. Oyama, Y. Tsuda, S. Sakakibara, and N. Akaike, *Brain Res.* **424,** 58 (1987).

30. L. J. Cruz and B. M. Olivera, *J. Biol. Chem.* **261,** 6230 (1986).

31. T. Abe and H. Saisu, *J. Biol. Chem.* **262,** 9877 (1987).

32. T. Yamaguchi, H. Saisu, H. Mitsui, and T. Abe, *J. Biol. Chem.* **263,** 9491 (1988).

33. M. Takemura, H. Fukui, and H. Wada, *Biochem. Biophys. Res.Commun.* **149,** 982 (1987).

34. L. J.Cruz, D. S. Johnson, and B. M. Olivera, *Biochemistry* **26,** 820 (1987).

35. J. Barhanin, A. Schmid, and M. Lazdunski, *Biochem. Biophys. Res. Commun.* **150,** 1051 (1988).

36. J. A. Wagner, A. M. Snowman, A. Biswas, B. M. Olivera, and S. H. Snyder, *J. Neurosci.* **8,** 3354 (1988).

37. B. Marqueze, N. Martin-Moutot, C. Levêque, and F. Couraud, *Mol. Pharmacol.* **34,** 87 (1988).

38. P. Feigenbaum, M. L. Garcia, and G. J. Kaczorowski, *Biochem. Biophys. Res. Commun.* **154,** 298 (1988).

39. D. J. Dooley, M. Lickert, A. Lupp, and H. Osswald, *Neurosci. Lett.* **93,** 318 (1988).

40. H.-G. Knaus, J. Striessnig, A. Koza, and H. Glossmann, *Naunyn-Schmiedeberg's Arch. Pharmacol.* **336,** 583 (1987).

41. T. Abe, K. Koyano, H. Saisu, Y. Nishiuchi, and S. Sakakibara, *Neurosci. Lett.* **71,** 203 (1986).

42. M. Takemura, H. Kiyama, H. Fukui, M. Tohyama, and H. Wada, *Brain Res.* **451,** 386 (1988).

43. E. Sher, A. Pandiella, and F. Clementi, *FEBS. Lett.* **235,** 178 (1988).

44. S. Ahmad, J. Rausa, E. Jang, and E. E. Daniel, *Biochem. Biophys. Res. Commun.* **159,** 119 (1989).

45. S. N. Ahmad and G. P. Miljanich, *Brain Res.* **453,** 247 (1988).

46. B. M. Olivera, L. J. Cruz, V. de Santos, G. W. LeCheminant, D. Griffin, R. Zeikus, J. M. McIntosh, R. Galyean, J. Varga, W. R. Gray, and J. Rivier, *Biochemistry* **26,** 2086 (1987).

47. L. M. Kerr, F. Filloux, B. M. Olivera, H. Jackson, and J. K. Wamsley, *Eur. J. Pharmacol.* **146,** 181 (1988).

48. N. Maeda, K. Wada, M. Yuzaki, and K. Mikoshiba, *Brain Res.* **489,** 21 (1989).

49. O. T. Jones, D. L. Kunze, and K. J. Angelides, *Science* **244,** 1189 (1989).

50. H. Kasai and T. Aosaki, *Pfluegers Arch.* **411,** 695 (1988).

51. A. Mikami, K. Imoto, T. Tanabe, T. Niidome, Y. Mori, H. Takeshima, S. Narumiya, and S. Numa, *Nature (London)* **340,** 230 (1989).

52. R. Llinás, M. Sugimori, J.-W. Lin, and B. Cherksey, *Proc. Natl. Acad. Sci. U.S.A.* **86,** 1689 (1989).

53. M. E. Adams, V. P. Bindokas, L. Hasegawa, and V. J. Venema, *J. Biol. Chem.* **265,** 861 (1990).

54. L. M. Kerr and D. Yoshikami, *Nature (London)* **308,** 282 (1984).

[16] Dendrotoxin Acceptor Sites: Identification and Labeling of Brain Potassium Channels

Roger G. Sorensen and Mordecai P. Blaustein

Progress in the structural characterization of ion channels has been greatly aided by the identification of toxins and venom components that bind with high affinities to these proteins. For example, α-bungarotoxin, from the venom of the krait, *Bungarus multicinctus,* has been identified as a selective blocker of the nicotinic acetylcholine receptor cation channel, and tetrodotoxin, from puffer fish of the suborder Gymnodontes, has been identified as a selective blocker of Na^+ channels. These toxins have been employed as selective ligands for the purification and subsequent structural characterization of these two ion channel proteins (1, 2).

Various venoms have been found to contain toxins that affect K^+ channel activity (3, 4). Several such toxins are the dendrotoxins, a homologous family of low-molecular-weight (ca. 7000) polypeptides found in the venoms of mamba (*Dendroaspis*) snakes (5, 6), that have sequence homologies similar to the Kunitz type of proteinase inhibitors (7). The dendrotoxins block several types of Ca^{2+}-independent, voltage-gated K^+ channels (8–11), and have been used for the characterization and purification of these ion channels (12–17). Here we describe the isolation and use of the dendrotoxins for the study of voltage-gated K^+ channels.

Purification of Dendrotoxin Homologs from *Dendroaspis angusticeps* Venom

Five polypeptide neurotoxins that block K^+ channels can be isolated from the venom of the Eastern green mamba snake, *Dendroaspis angusticeps*. Their purification is achieved by a two-step chromatographic procedure (5). The first step involves separation of the venom components by gel-filtration chromatography. Lyophilized venom (Sigma Chemical Co., St. Louis, Mo; or Latoxan, Rosans, France), 1 g in 5 ml of 0.1 M ammonium acetate, pH 6.8, is applied to a Sephadex G-50 column (2.6 × 90 cm). The column is resolved (flow rate of 0.5 ml/min) with the ammonium acetate buffer, and peptide fractions are monitored at 280 nm. Five A_{280} absorbing peaks are obtained (Fig. 1). The third peak (fraction III, polypeptides of average M_r 5000) contains K^+ channel-blocking activity. Fraction III is lyophilized to concentrate the polypeptides, and redissolved in 5 ml of 0.05 M ammonium acetate, pH 6.8.

The second step involves the separation of the components of fraction III by cation-exchange high-performance liquid chromatography (HPLC). Approximately 10 mg of fraction III protein (in 1 ml) is applied to a 4.6 × 220 mm Aquapore CX-300 cation-exchange column (Applied Biosystems, Foster City, CA) that has been equilibrated in 0.05 M ammonium acetate, pH 6.8. Adsorbed peptides are eluted (flow rate of 1 ml/min) with a linear ascending gradient from 0.05 to 0.8 M ammonium acetate, pH 6.8. The dendrotoxins elute at ammonium acetate concentrations greater than 0.5 M (Fig. 2). The dendrotoxins are lyophilized and stored at $-20°C$. The dendrotoxins are readily dissolved in H_2O or aqueous buffers (stock solutions are made at 1 mg protein/ml), and remain stable in solution for several months when stored at 4°C.

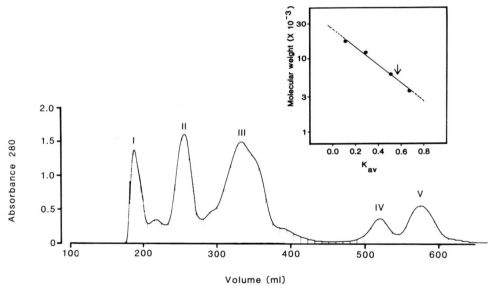

FIG. 1   Sephadex G-50 gel-filtration chromatography of *D. angusticeps* venom. The five primary protein fractions obtained (fractions I through V) are indicated. *Inset:* calibration of the column using myoglobin, cytochrome *c*, aprotinin, and the β chain of insulin (decreasing order by molecular weight). K_{average} $(K_{\text{av}}) = V_e - V_0/V_t - V_0$. V_e, elution volume; V_0, void volume; V_t, total volume. The arrow indicates the position of fraction III. (From Ref. 5 with permission.)

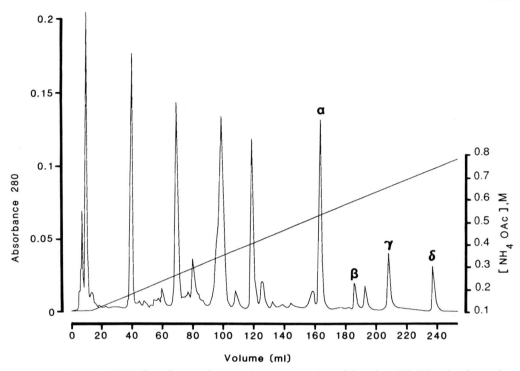

Fɪɢ. 2   HPLC cation-exchange chromatography of fraction III. The dendrotoxins that block synaptosome K^+ channels are indicated by α (α-DaTX), β (β-DaTX), γ (γ-DaTX), and δ (δ-DaTX). Recently, β-DaTX has been further resolved into two components, β_1-DaTX and β_2-DaTX, by similar chromatographic methods (unpublished observations). (From Ref. 5 with permission.) .

   Five dendrotoxins that possess K^+ channel-blocking activity are separated by this procedure; they are designated α-DaTX, β_1-DaTX, β_2-DaTX, γ-DaTX, and δ-DaTX, the order in which they are eluted from the cation-exchange column. The K^+ channel-blocking activity of the toxins is conveniently determined in an *in vitro* assay by measuring rubidium efflux (18, 19) from tracer (^{86}Rb)-preloaded rat brain synaptosomes (pinched off and re-sealed presynaptic nerve terminals). With this assay, it has been shown [(5), and unpublished observations] that α-DaTX, β_2-DaTX, and δ-DaTX preferentially block rapidly inactivating (A-type) K^+ channels, whereas β_1-DaTX and γ-DaTX preferentially block noninactivating (or slowly inactivating) (delayed rectifier-type) K^+ channels. The polypeptide, α-DaTX, is the most prevalent K^+ channel-blocking peptide in the venom, and is the same peptide that has been commonly referred to as dendrotoxin (5).

Separation of fraction III polypeptides has also been attempted by cation-exchange chromatography on Mono S (Pharmacia LKB Biotechnology, Piscataway, NJ) fast-protein liquid chromatography (FPLC) columns, and by conventional chromatography on its sister support, S-Sepharose Fast Flow (Pharmacia LKB), using linear ammonium acetate gradients similar to those described above. These supports can be used to resolve α-DaTX, γ-DaTX, and δ-DaTX, but not the β-dendrotoxins (unpublished observations).

The venom of the black mamba, *Dendroaspis polylepis polylepis*, also contains dendrotoxin homologs. The isolation of these polypeptides has been achieved by chromatographic procedures similar to those described above, including a gel-filtration chromatography step for the initial fractionation of the venom, followed by various ion-exchange and reversed-phase chromatography separations (20, 21). We have used the same methods as are described above, i.e., Sephadex G-50 and HPLC cation-exchange chromatography, to isolate the dendrotoxin homologs present in *D. polylepis polylepis* venom. Those venom components include DTX-I, a homolog with high affinity for the dendrotoxin receptor, which has been used successfully for the purification of the dendrotoxin-sensitive K^+ channel (16, 17).

Radioiodination of Dendrotoxins

The dendrotoxins are radiolabeled for use in ligand (receptor)-binding assays. This is conveniently done by direct methods in the presence of chloramine-T (12) or Iodogen (Iodobeads, Pierce Chemical Co., Rockford, IL) (13). Conjugation methods using Denny–Jaffe reagent (New England Nuclear, Boston, MA), or Bolton–Hunter reagent (Amersham Corp., Arlington Heights, IL) have met with little success.

The labeling procedure is as follows: Typically, 5–10 μg dendrotoxin (10 μl total volume), 10 μl 0.5 M NaH_2PO_4, pH 7.0, and 10 μl (1 mCi) $Na^{125}I$ (Amersham or New England Nuclear) are added to a 1.5-ml microcentrifuge tube. Black *et al.* (12) also include 0.02% Triton X-100 in the reaction mixture, but we have found little difference in the specific activities of the radiolabeled toxins obtained in the absence or presence of this detergent.

The reaction is started by the addition of 5 μl of 0.25 mg/ml chloramine-T in 0.1 M NaH_2PO_4, pH 7.0 (prepared just before use), added twice at 30-sec intervals. The reaction is quenched by the addition of 500 μl of 0.1 M NaH_2PO_4, pH 7.09, containing 0.05 mg/ml tyrosine and 2 mg/ml NaI.

Radioiodinated toxin is recovered by gel-filtration chromatography on Sephadex G-25 (10-ml disposable column; Bio-Rad, Richmond, CA) equilibrated in 0.1 M NaH$_2$PO$_4$, pH 7.0. The toxin is eluted from the column with the phosphate buffer.

For labeling with Iodogen, the labeling reaction is initiated by the addition of 10 μl (10 μg) dendrotoxin to the reaction mixture, which contains 10 μl 0.5 M NaH$_2$PO$_4$, pH 7.0, 10 μl (1 mCi) Na^{125}I, 10 μl H$_2$O rather than chloramine-T, and one or two Iodobeads. The reaction is allowed to proceed for 2–5 min at ambient temperature. The reaction is terminated by dilution with 0.5 ml of 0.1 M NaH$_2$PO$_4$, pH 7.0, containing 2 mg/ml NaI (the addition of tyrosine is not necessary). The reaction vessel is rinsed with an additional 0.5 ml of phosphate buffer. This is added to the diluted reaction mixture, which is permitted to stand for an additional 5 min to allow the Iodogen to inactivate. The mixture is then applied to the Sephadex gel-filtration column to recover the radioiodinated toxin.

Alternatively, the reaction is stopped by the addition of 500 μl 20 mM NaH$_2$PO$_4$, pH 7.0, containing 200 mM NaCl and 2 mg/ml NaI. The reaction mixture is applied to 2- to 5-ml columns containing CM-Sepharose CL-6B anion-exchange resin (12), or SP-Sephadex C-25 anion-exchange resin (13) equilibrated in the above solution without NaI. The column is washed with 20 mM NaH$_2$PO$_4$, pH 7.0, containing 200 mM NaCl to remove unincorporated ^{125}I. The radiolabeled toxin is then eluted from the support by increasing the NaCl concentration in the phosphate buffer to 700 mM.

The molar absorption coefficient (ε) for α-DaTX has been reported as 10,500 M^{-1} cm^{-1} [278 nm, neutral pH (6)], 9009 [280 nm, unbuffered H$_2$O (unpublished observations, 1990)] and 3950 [280 nm, 50 mM HEPES, pH 7.0 (unpublished observations, 1990)], and 10,060 [280 nm, no conditions given (14)]. Because of the small amounts of toxin used for radiolabeling (5–10 μg, M_r 7000), the spectrophotometric measurement of the amount of dendrotoxin recovered after radioiodination approaches the limit of detection by this method. Furthermore, the molar absorption coefficients for the other dendrotoxins have not been determined. Therefore, specific activity is usually determined by trichloroacetic acid (TCA) precipitation (12). Aliquots (10 μl) of the diluted reaction mixtures prior to column chromatography are precipitated with ice-cold 10% (w/v) TCA in the presence of 1% (w/v) bovine serum albumin in 1.5-ml microcentrifuge tubes. The mixtures are allowed to stand on ice for 10 min and the precipitated materials are collected by microcentrifugation for 10–15 min. The pellets are counted for γ radiation. The specific activities obtained typically range from 150 to 300 Ci/mmol for α-DaTX, and from 75 to 150 Ci/mmol for β_1-DaTX (assuming 100% of the toxin is recovered after TCA precipitation).

Labeling of Membrane-Bound Acceptor Sites

Membrane Preparation

Dendrotoxin binding to several rat forebrain membrane preparations has been routinely measured. A common procedure for synaptic membrane preparation begins with the isolation of synaptosomes (5). The synaptosomes (P_2 pellet) are subsequently lysed by incubation in hypotonic solution (5 mM Tris, pH 8.1) on ice for 30 min, and centrifuged (30,000 g for 30 min at 4°C) to collect the membrane pellet.

This preparation can be further enriched for synaptic plasma membrane (SPM) content by layering the resuspended membranes onto a discontinuous sucrose density gradient as described by Salvaterra and Matthews (22). The resulting synaptic membrane preparation (collected at the 28.5–34% sucrose interface after centrifugation) contains less than 10% contamination each by myelin and mitochondria. The density of dendrotoxin-binding sites per (milligram of membrane protein is increased up to fivefold in this SPM preparation, relative to that of the lysed synaptosome preparation.

Binding Assay

The assay of toxin binding to brain membrane preparations is readily accomplished by a rapid centrifugation technique. The brain membrane preparation (1 mg protein/ml) is incubated at 37°C in solution A (145 mM NaCl, 5 mM KCl, 1.4 mM MgCl$_2$, and 20 mM HEPES, pH 7.0), usually containing 1 mM radioiodinated toxin and various amounts of the nonradiolabeled toxins or other test compounds. After a 30-min incubation to achieve binding equilibrium, 0.2 ml of the binding mixture is layered on top of 0.2 ml dinonyl phthalate/silicone oil (65 : 35) in 1.5-ml microcentrifuge tubes. The membrane-bound acceptor–toxin complex is collected by microcentrifugation (at least 8700 g) through the oil mixture for 4 min at ambient temperature. The membrane pellets are washed once with solution A and counted for γ radiation. The dinonyl phthalate/silicone oil mixture can be omitted and the membranes pelleted directly by microcentrifugation with little change in background or nonspecific binding. A typical experiment is shown for α-DaTX binding (Fig. 3). Scatchard analysis reveals a single saturable binding site, with a K_D of 0.69 ± 0.09 nM (15), after subtraction of nonspecific binding by computer-assisted data analysis, LIGAND (Elsevier-BIOSOFT, Milltown, NJ).

Toxin binding to brain membranes is affected by a variety of factors (15). For example, binding is dependent on the ionic strength of the binding

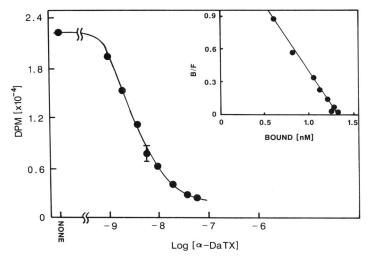

Fig. 3 α-DaTX binding to synaptic membranes. The main graph shows the competitive displacement of bound radioiodinated α-DaTX by increasing amounts of the unlabeled toxin. The corresponding Scatchard plot is presented in the inset. (From Ref. 15 with permission.)

mixture. Toxin binding is promoted in solutions containing high salt concentrations (e.g., 150 mM NaCl, or 145 mM NaCl plus 5 mM KCl), and is reduced to less than 5% of these levels under reduced salt conditions (e.g., 20 mM Tris/HEPES, pH 7.0, or 20 mM sodium phosphate, pH 7.4).

Toxin binding is also dependent on the sepcies of monovalent cation present in the binding mixture. Binding is optimal (defined as 100%) in the presence of 150 mM NaCl (the highest concentration tested), and decreases as Na$^+$ is replaced isosmotically (150 mM ion concentration) by other alkali metal ions: K$^+$ (76%) > Li$^+$ (65%) > Rb$^+$ (46%) > Cs$^+$ (0%). Indeed, Cs$^+$ (IC$_{50}$ 5–6 mM) is a potent inhibitor of toxin binding in the presence of 150 mM Na$^+$.

pH also affects toxin binding: optimal binding occurs at pH 6–7, and decreases with increasing pH. This decrease in specific binding of the toxin to its acceptor site with increasing pH results from both a decrease in total binding of the toxin to the membrane preparation, and an increase in the level of nonspecific binding (as measured in the presence of excess unlabeled toxin).

Several investigators (12–14) routinely include the divalent cations, Ca^{2+} or Sr^{2+}, in their binding mixtures. However, under the conditions described above, we found that Ba^{2+} (IC_{50} 5 mM) and Ca^{2+} (IC_{50} 10 mM) are potent inhibitors of dendrotoxin binding (15).

The composition of the binding mixture may also affect the discrimination of dendrotoxin–binding site interactions. For example, Breeze and Dolly (14) observed that β-bungarotoxin (β-BuTX) is a very weak ($IC_{50} > 1$ μM) inhibitor of ^{125}I-labeled DaTX binding to rat brain membranes when assayed in Krebs/phosphate solution containing 0.74 mM $SrCl_2$ or $CaCl_2$. When measured in imidazole buffer (50 mM imidazole/HCl, pH 7.4, 90 mM Nacl, 5 mM KCl, 1.5 mM $SrCl_2$ or $CaCl_2$), β-BuTX becomes a much more potent (IC_{50} 60 nM) inhibitor of dendrotoxin binding.

Dendrotoxin Binding to Solubilized Receptor

Receptor Solubilization

Dendrotoxin acceptor sites are solubilized from brain membranes by detergent extraction [1% (v/v) Triton X-100 or 0.8% (v/v) zwittergent 3–12; Calbiochem Corp., San Diego, CA] in the presence of K^+. Typically, the brain membrane preparation (4 mg protein/ml final concentration) is incubated in the detergent-containing solubilization buffer [150 mM KCl, 2 mM $MgCl_2$, 10 mM HEPES, pH 7.0, 10% (v/v) glycerol, 0.8% (v/v) zwittergent 3-12 or 1% (v/v) Triton X-100, 0.25% (w/v) soybean lecithin, as adapted from Ref. 16] containing a proteinase inhibitor cocktail (23). This cocktail may contain, for example, 0.5 mM phenylmethylsulfonyl fluoride (PMSF) or 0.25 mM benzamidine to inhibit serine proteinases, 1 mM iodoacetamide to inhibit thiol proteinases, 1 mM 1,10-phenanthroline or 1 mM EDTA to inhibit metalloproteinases, and 1 μM pepstatin A carboxylproteinases. The cocktail is prepared as a 100-fold concentrated stock solution in ethanol.

The mixture is incubated on ice for 15–60 min, and the solubilized membrane proteins are recovered in the supernatant after centrifugation (100,000 g for 1 hr at 4°). Triton X-100 solubilizes 60–70% of the DaTX receptor, and 50–60% of the membrane protein (Ref. 16 and unpublished observations, 1990). Alternatively, zwittergent 3–12 solubilizes 50–60% of the dendrotoxin receptor, and 60–70% of the membrane protein (15). Other detergents, such as deoxycholate, cholate, octylglucoside, and 3-[(3-cholamidopropyl)dimethylammonio]-1-propane sulfonate (CHAPS), at 0.1–1% (v/v) concentration, are much less effective in solubilizing the receptor from brain membranes (15).

The presence of 0.25% (w/v) soybean lecithin in the solubilization buffer stabilizes the solubilized receptor (15, 16). There does not appear to be a requirement for any specific phospholipid, as comparable results are obtained with phosphatidylcholine (lecithin), phosphatidylserine, or phosphatidylethanolamine, each at 0.25% (15).

The species of monovalent cation used in the extraction buffer affects the recovery of solubilized toxin receptor-binding activity (15). This cation requirement is different from that required for toxin binding to the membrane-bound receptor. The dendrotoxin receptor should be solubilized in the presence of 150 mM KCl, rather than 150 mM NaCl, which is used for the assay of the membrane-bound receptor. We found that the highest levels of dendrotoxin binding were obtained when the receptor was detergent extracted in the presence of K^+ (15). Dendrotoxin binding increased with increasing osmolarity and ionic strength up to a maximum level measured in the presence of 200 mM K^+ (unpublished observations, 1990). Dendrotoxin binding remained unchanged as the KCl concentration was further increased to 700 mM. Other alkali metal ions can substitute for K^+, but the retention of toxin-binding activity is reduced. The effectiveness of these cations (at 150 mM) relative to that obtained with K^+ is (percentage binding): K^+ (100%) > Rb^+ (55%) > Cs^+ (44%) > Li^+ (37%) > Na^+ (25%). As in the case of the membrane-bound receptor, Ba^{2+} and Ca^{2+} inhibit dendrotoxin binding to the solubilized receptor with IC_{50} values of 8–10 mM.

Binding Assay

Toxin binding to the soluble receptor can be measured by a rapid gel-filtration method. Solubilized brain proteins (4–5 mg protein/ml) are incubated in the detergent extraction solution containing radiolabeled toxin (usually 1 nM) for 30 min at 37°C. During this incubation, Sephadex G-50 spun columns are prepared. Sephadex G-50 is swollen in buffered K-solution (150 mM KCl, 1.4 mM MgCl$_2$, 20 mM HEPES, pH 7.0). Columns (1.5-ml bed volume) are prepared in 2-ml disposable chromatography columns (Bio-Rad or Pierce Chemical Co.) by gravity packing. The columns are placed in 15 × 100 mm polystyrene tubes and centrifuged at 800 g (2200 rpm) for exactly 90 sec in a table-top centrifuge (IEC HN-SII; Damen, Needham Heights, MA) without brake. K-solution (0.2 ml) is applied to the columns, and the columns are recentrifuged for exactly 90 sec without brake. This is repeated several times until 0.2-ml samples are consistently collected in the eluate. The spun columns are now ready for sample application. Do not let the columns dry while waiting for application of the binding mixtures. To prevent drying, the prepared columns may be stored at 4°C prior to use. Additionally, the columns can be rehydrated by applying 0.2-ml aliquots of K-solution and centrifuging as decribed above just before applying the binding mixture.

Aliquots (0.2 ml) of the binding mixture are applied to the columns, and the columns are centrifuged for exactly 90 sec without brake. Free toxin is retained by the column packing. The eluate, containing the toxin–receptor complex, is counted for γ radiation. We found that 95% of unbound toxin is retained by the column, and that more than 98% of the toxin–receptor complex is collected in the eluate. Plastic test tubes (15 $\times$ 100 mm) are used as holders to collect the eluates because these tubes fit conveniently into the racks of a Packard (Sterling, VA) Minaxi γ counter.

Figure 4 shows the results from a typical experiment in which we measured α-DaTX binding to zwittergent 3–12-solubilized brain membrane protein. Receptor solubilization decreased the affinity of α-DaTX for its receptor by about a factor of 10 (K_D = 7.0 $\pm$ 1.1 nM, vs K_D = 0.7 nM for the membrane-bound receptor), with a 30% recovery of the original membrane receptor sites (B_{max} = 0.56 $\pm$ 0.11 pmol toxin bound/mg protein) (15).

Others (16, 17) have used a filtration method to separate bound from free toxin. After equilibrium binding, aliquots (0.2 ml) of the binding mixtures are applied to glass fiber filters [e.g., Whatman (Clifton, NJ GF/C or Schleicher & Schuell (Keene, NH) No. 24] that have been pretreated with 0.2 to 0.5% (w/v) polyethyleneimine (24). The filters are washed several times with

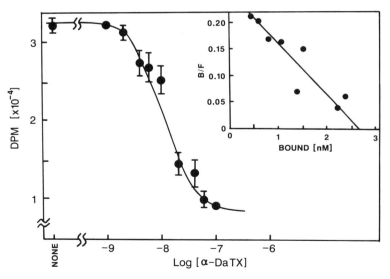

FIG. 4 α-DaTX binding to soluble synaptic membrane receptors. The main graph shows the competitive displacement of bound radioiodinated α-DaTX by increasing amounts of the unlabeled toxin. The corresponding Scatchard plot is presented in the inset. (From Ref. 15 with permission.)

K-solution and counted for γ radiation. Although inherently easier than the spun column method, we found that large amounts of radiolabeled toxin bind to these filters. This causes high background counts that are associated with low signal-to-noise ratios.

Dendrotoxin Receptor Purification

The logical extension of the methods described above is to use the dendrotoxins to monitor the purification of their receptors, the voltage-gated K^+ channels. Receptor purification using the dendrotoxins, α-DaTX or δ-DaTX isolated from *D. angusticeps* venom, has proven to be difficult for as yet unknown reasons. On the other hand, the dendrotoxin homolog, DTX-I, isolated from *D. polylepis polylepis* venom, has been used successfully to purify a dendrotoxin-sensitive K^+ channel (16, 17, 25, 26). These purification schemes use detergent solubilization procedures similar to the one described above (i.e., solubilization in solutions containing high K^+ concentrations and employing Triton X-100 as the detergent), and rely on affinity chromatography on DTX-I affinity supports to isolate the dendrotoxin receptor from the other solubilized brain membrane proteins.

Summary

The methods presented here describe the isolation of several dendrotoxins from *D. angusticeps* and *D. polylepis polylepis* venoms. These toxins have been used as ligands for the identification and characterization of their acceptor sites, which are located on dendrotoxin-sensitive, voltage-gated K^+ channels. Furthermore, several investigators (16, 17) have employed a DTX-I affinity chromatography support as an integral part of the protocol for the purification of a dendrotoxin receptor protein, a voltage-gated K^+ channel. Several of the other dendrotoxins should also become important tools for future work on the purification and characterization of various voltage-gated K^+ channels.

References

1. R. M. Stroud, M. P. McCarthy, and M. Shuster, *Biochemistry* **29,** 11009 (1990).
2. J. S. Trimmer and W. S. Agnew, *Annu. Rev. Physiol.* **51,** 401 (1989).
3. E. Moczydlowski, K. Lucchesi, and A. Ravindran, *J. Membr. Biol.* **105,** 95 (1988).

4. N. A. Castle, D. G. Haylett, and D. H. Jenkinson, *Trends NeuroSci.* **12,** 59 (1989).
5. C. G. Benishin, R. G. Sorensen, W. E. Brown, B. K. Krueger, and M. P. Blaustein, *Mol. Pharmacol.* **34,** 152 (1988).
6. A. L. Harvey and E. Karlsson, *Naunyn-Schmiedeberg's Arch. Pharmacol.* **312,** 1 (1980).
7. M. J. Dufton, *Eur. J. Biochem.* **153,** 647 (1985).
8. J. V. Halliwell, I. B. Othman, A. Pelchen-Matthews, and J. O. Dolly, *Proc. Natl. Acad. Sci. U.S.A.* **83,** 493 (1986).
9. R. Penner, M. Petersen, F.-K. Pierau, and F. Dreyer, *Pfluegers Arch.* **407,** 365 (1986).
10. E. Benoit and J.-M. Dubois, *Brain Res.* **377,** 374 (1986).
11. C. E. Stansfeld and A. Feltz, *Neurosci. Lett.* **93,** 49 (1988).
12. A. R. Black, A. L. Breeze, I. B. Othman, and J. O. Dolly, *Biochem. J.* **237,** 397 (1986).
13. H. Rehm, J.-N. Bidard, H. Schweitz, and M. Lazdunski, *Biochemistry* **27,** 1827 (1988).
14. A. L. Breeze and J. O. Dolly, *Eur. J. Biochem.* **178,** 771 (1989).
15. R. G. Sorensen and M. P. Blaustein, *Mol. Pharmacol.* **36,** 689 (1989).
16. H. Rehm and M. Lazdunski, *Proc. Natl. Acad. Sci. U.S.A.* **85,** 4919 (1988).
17. D. N. Parcej and J. O. Dolly, *Biochem. J.* **257,** 899 (1989).
18. D. K. Bartschat and M. P. Blaustein, *J. Physiol.* (*London*) **361,** 419 (1985).
19. D. K. Bartschat and M. P. Blaustein, *J. Physiol.* (*London*) **361,** 441 (1985).
20. D. J. Strydom, *Eur. J. Biochem.* **69,** 169 (1976).
21. H. Schweitz, J.-N. Bidard, and M. Lazdunski, *Toxicon* **28,** 847 (1990).
22. P. M. Salvaterra and D. A. Matthews, *Neurochem. Res.* **5,** 181 (1980).
23. A. J. Barrett (ed.), *Res. Monogr. Cell Tissue Physiol.* **2** (1977).
24. R. F. Bruns, K. Lawson-Wendling, and T. Pugsbey, *Anal. Biochem.* **32,** 74 (1983).
25. H. Rehm, S. Pelzer, C. Cochet, E. Chambaz, B. L. Tempel, W. Trautwein, D. Pelzer, and M. Lazdunski, *Biochemistry* **28,** 6455 (1989).
26. V. E. S. Scott, D. N. Parcej, J. N. Keen, J. B. C. Findlay, and J. O. Dolly, *J. Biol. Chem.* **265,** 20094 (1990).

[17] Endothelins and Sarafotoxin in Neural Tissues

Christian Frelin and Jean-Philippe Breittmayer

Endothelins and sarafotoxins belong to the same family of closely related, 21-amino acid residue peptides. They have powerful vasoconstricting and cardiotonic properties (1). Sarafotoxins have been purified from the venom of the snake *Atractaspis engaddensis* (2). Among the four different toxins that have been isolated, sarafotoxin S6b (SRTX) is the most potent (3). Endothelin-1 (Et-1) is produced by vascular endothelial cells and may act as a paracrine factor that regulates the vascular tone. Mammalian genomes code, in fact, for two additional forms of endothelins: endothelin-2 (Et-2) and endothelin-3 (Et-3) (4). While Et-1 and Et-2 are very similar in structure and properties, Et-3 is distinct. Immunoreactive Et-1- and Et-3-like materials have been identified in brain extracts (5) and at least two molecularly defined receptor subtypes for endothelins are expressed in the brain (6, 7), suggesting that endothelins have important functions in neural tissues in addition to their cardiovascular actions (8). In this chapter, we describe some of the methods used to analyze the action of peptides of the endothelin family in brain cells.

Endothelin Receptors

Radiolabeled endothelin peptides with specific radioactivities of about 2000 Ci/mmol and unlabeled peptides are all commercially available from a diversity of sources. Binding experiments are performed using tissue or cell homogenates or intact cells using conventional methods (9, 10). Nonspecific binding obtained in the presence of a large excess of unlabeled ligand is usually less than 10% of the total binding. At the concentration of labeled ligand (0.1 nM) and temperature (25–37°C) used in most experiments, stable binding is achieved only after 1–2 hr of incubation. It should be kept in mind that, during such long times of association, degradation of endothelins, for instance by neutral endopeptidase (11), or internalization of endothelin–receptor complexes by intact cells (12), may occur and influence the conclusions drawn. Dissociation of the endothelin–receptor complexes is a very slow process. For instance, in cerebellar homogenates, less than 10% of bound ^{125}I-labeled Et-1 dissociates during a 14-hr incubation in the presence of a large excess of unlabeled ligand (9). The irreversible character of the binding of endothelins to their receptors is an important parameter that should be considered when the physiological role(s) of these peptides is evaluated.

Binding sites for endothelins are widely distributed in the brain. Yet some heterogeneity exists. Highest densities are found in the cerebellum, thalamus, and hypothalamus. Lowest densities are in caudate and cerebral cortex (13–15). In cerebellar homogenates (9), Et-1 recognizes a single class of saturable binding sites (K_d = 0.3 nM, B_{max} = 0.3 pmol/mg of protein) that poorly discriminates between the different endothelin peptides [K_d (Et-2) = 1 nM, K_d (Et-3) = 0.2 nM, K_d (SRTX) = 0.2 nM]. The properties of this "nonselective" receptor site are similar to those of the ET_B receptor subtype that has recently been cloned from rat lung (7). Brain tissues express high levels of mRNA coding for the ET_B receptor (7). Endothelin receptors with a pharmacological profile similar to that of ET_B receptors are found in neuronal cells [e.g., cerebellar granule cells (16, 17)], in astrocytes (17, 18), and in endothelial cells from brain microvessels (19).

A second receptor subtype for endothelins is present in endothelial cells from brain microvessels (10). It has a high affinity for Et-1 (K_d = 0.8 nM, B_{max} = 0.4 pmol/mg of protein) and for Et-2 (K_d = 0.7 nM), a low affinity for Et-3 (K_d = 450 nM), and an intermediate affinity for SRTX (K_d = 27 nM). These properties are similar to those of the receptor found in vascular smooth muscle cells and in cardiac cells. It may correspond to the ET_A receptor subtype cloned from bovine lung (6). High levels of expression of the mRNA coding for the ET_A receptor are also observed in the brain (6).

Affinity-labeling experiments have been performed using ^{125}I-labeled Et-1 and Et-3 and bifunctional cross-linking reagents. In rat brain membranes, two membrane proteins with molecular weights of 53,000 (Et-1 and Et-3) and 38,000 (Et-3) have been labeled (20).

Identification of Receptor Subtypes Using Binding Experiments

Receptor heterogeneity is a complicating factor when labeled Et-1 is used to titrate binding sites in membrane or cell preparations. Because Et-1 recognizes the different receptor subtypes with nearly identical affinities, Scatchard plots for the specific ^{125}I-labeled Et-1 binding (using unlabeled Et-1 to define nonspecific binding) may be linear even when more than one class of receptor sites are present. Receptor subtypes are best characterized in binding assays using two types of experiments. ET_B receptors (defined by their high affinity for both Et-1 and Et-3) are titrated using ^{125}I-labeled Et-3, nonspecific binding being determined using a large excess of either Et-1 or Et-3. ET_A receptors (defined by their high affinity for Et-1 and low affinity for Et-3) are best titrated by ^{125}I-labeled Et-1 using unlabeled Et-1 to define nonspecific binding. When ^{125}I-labeled Et-1 is used as a labeled probe, it is advisable, however, to perform all experiments in the presence of 10–30 nM unlabeled Et-3. Under these conditions, ET_B receptor subtypes that could eventually be present in the preparation are saturated with Et-3 and do not contribute to the specific ^{125}I-labeled Et-1-binding component. Heterogeneity of endothelin receptors in a preparation may also be detected using SRTX as a competitor for ^{125}I-labeled Et-1 binding. Provided that ET_A and ET_B receptors are present in similar amounts (see, e.g., Ref. 21), the Hill coefficient for SRTX inhibition of Et-1 binding is markedly less than 1. When ET_A receptors greatly outnumber ET_B receptors (see, e.g., Ref. 19), ^{125}I-labeled Et-1 and Et-3 can be used as specific probes for ET_A and ET_B receptors, respectively.

Activation of Phospholipase C by Endothelins

The two types of endothelin receptor that have been cloned so far belong to the G protein-coupled receptor superfamily (6, 7). A general action of endothelins in brain slices (22), granule cerebellar cells (16), endothelial cells from brain microvessels (10), and astrocytes (18) is to stimulate phosphoinositide hydrolysis, usually via a pertussis toxin-insensitive mechanism. A pertussis toxin-sensitive inhibition by Et-1 of adenylate cyclase was reported in mouse striatal astrocytes (23).

Preparation of Suspended, Indo-1-loaded Cells

Activation of phospholipase C by endothelins and SRTX leads to the production of inositol 1,4,5-trisphosphate, which triggers the release of Ca^{2+} from intracellular stores. Endothelins are the most potent agonist found so far to increase $[Ca^{2+}]_i$ in astrocytes (18). Changes in $[Ca^{2+}]_i$ in response to endothelins may be observed in cells loaded with a Ca^{2+}-sensitive fluorescent probe using classical spectrofluorimetric techniques (see, e.g., Ref. 24). They may also be monitored by flow cytometry. The technique was first used to follow changes in $[Ca^{2+}]_i$ in activated lymphocytes (25). It was then adapted to cells freshly dissociated from their culture plates and more recently to cells dispersed from intact organs. A single emission wavelength being allowed, Indo-1 rather than Fura-2 is used as a probe for Ca^{2+}. Cortical astrocytes (1-month-old primary cultures) or endothelial cells from brain microvessels in 75-cm^2 Falcon (Los Angeles, CA) flasks are incubated for 2 hr at 37°C in serum-supplemented culture medium containing 5 μM Indo-1/AM (Sigma, St. Louis, MO, or Boehringer, Mannheim, Germany). The culture medium is then removed and cells rinsed twice with serum-free culture medium. Cells are then dissociated from their dishes using a balanced salt solution supplemented with 5 mM EDTA and 0.05% (v/v) trypsin at room temperature. It is essential that the exposure to the trypsin solution does not exceed 5 min, in order to keep large responses to the peptides. The cell suspension is then diluted into complete culture medium containing 10% (v/v) serum and centrifuged at 1000 g. Cells are resuspended into an Earle's salt solution (140 mM NaCl, 5 mM KCl, 1.8 mM CaCl$_2$, 0.8 mM MgSO$_4$, 5 mM glucose buffered at pH 7.4 using 25 mM HEPES–Tris) and kept in the dark at room temperature for at least 1 hr until analysis. This delay allows unhydrolyzed Indo-1/AM to leak out of the cells and cells to recover from the dissociation procedure.

Flow Cytometric Analysis of [Ca^{2+}]$_i$ Distribution in Brain Cells

An ATC 3000 cell sorter (Odam-Bruker, Wissembourg, France) is well suited for analyzing intracellular Ca^{2+} levels and their variations in suspended cells. Ultraviolet excitation is from an argon laser (Coherent, Innova, 90, Auburn, CA) tuned at 351–364 nm. By using selected interference filters and long-pass filters (Fig. 1), blue (490–500 nm) and violet (400–410 nm) fluorescence emissions are measured. The blue fluorescence corresponds to the fluorescence emission of free Indo-1. The violet fluorescence corresponds to an isobestic point of the Indo-1 fluorescence emission spectrum and is used to correct for the cell-to-cell variations in Indo-1 load. The ratio of the violet to blue fluorescences is a measure of the intracellular Ca^{2+} concentration. The two fluorescence emissions, the ratio of the violet to blue fluorescences, the electric volume, and the wide-angle light scatter (side scatter) are measured cell by cell and collected in real time using an Aspect computer.

Figure 2 presents typical distributions of the electric volume (A), side scatter (B), and violet (C) and blue (D) fluorescences for a preparation of Indo-1-loaded brain capillary endothelial cells. It indicates a wide range of Indo-1 load in individual cells (C). This fact is often overlooked and justifies the use of a fluorescence ratio to correct for cell-to-cell variability in the intracellular concentration of the probe. Figure 2 also illustrates the gating procedure used to exclude from the analysis dead cells and debris. By selecting "healthy" cells, it narrows the distribution of the Indo-1 fluorescence ratio, increases the signal-to-noise ratio, and provides an increased sensitivity of the measures. Figure 3 shows the distribution of the violet-to-blue fluorescence ratio in a population of brain capillary endothelial cells using the gates defined in Fig. 2. It indicates a narrow and symmetrical distribution of the Indo-1 fluorescence ratio (i.e., of [Ca^{2+}]$_i$). Usually the mean and the mode

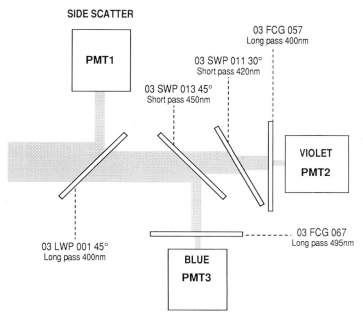

FIG. 1 Optical path and filters used to measure Indo-1 fluorescence ratio by flow cytometry. Side scatter and violet and blue fluorescences are detected by the three photomultiplier tubes (PMT). Violet fluorescence (400–410 nm) is detected by PMT2. Blue (490–500 nm) is detected by PMT3. Filters were from Melles-Griot (Irvine, CA).

of the distribution of the Indo-1 fluorescence ratio do not differ by more than 3 units. They may differ by more than 30 units in ungated cell populations.

Calibration

Calibration of the fluorescence signals using conventional methods (26) cannot be used in flow cytometry for only the fluorescence of intracellularly trapped Indo-1 is measured. Attempts to calibrate the Indo-1 fluorescence ratio to $[Ca^{2+}]$ as described by Chused et al. (27) for lymphocytes were unsuccessful using excitable cells in general. One reason could be that excitable cells do not tolerate very high intracellular Ca^{2+} levels. Loading cells with large amounts of Ca^{2+} rapidly leads to cell death, as evidenced by an increase in the side scatter and a leakage of Indo-1 out of the cells.

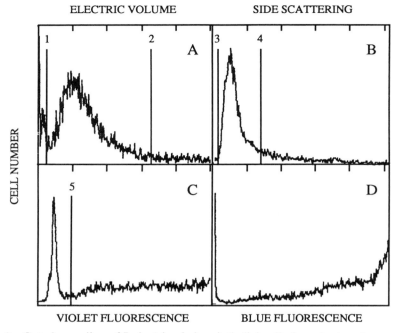

FIG. 2   Gated sampling of Indo-1-loaded endothelial cells from brain microvessels. The different panels show the distributions of the electric volume (A), of the wide-angle scatter (B), of the violet fluorescence (C), and of the blue fluorescence (D) obtained by flow cytometry. In (A) and (B) a linear abscissa is used. In (C) and (D), a log scale is used. As a consequence, cells with a background level of violet fluorescence are clustered and appear as a peak on the left side of (C). Only cells with an electric volume between cursors 1 and 2 (A), with a side scatter between cursors 3 and 4 (B), and a violet fluorescence > cursor 5 (C) are selected for analysis. Gating on the electric volume excludes debris (i.e., events with a volume < cursor 1) and cell aggregates (i.e., events with a volume > cursor 2) from the analysis. Gating on side scatter mainly excludes damaged cells (cells with a side scatter > cursor 4). Finally, gating on the violet fluorescence excludes leaky cells that are weakly loaded with Indo-1 (violet fluorescence < cursor 5). In some instances, the distribution of Indo-1 loads (violet fluorescence) is markedly bimodal. In that case, gates may be narrowed to select a smaller fraction of the cell population. In typical experiments, 50–80% of total recorded events are gated and analyzed. The number of gated cell analyzed in this experiment is 5000. In experiments in which changes in $[Ca^{2+}]_i$ are analyzed, the different distributions are displayed on a screen and superposed to the traces recorded before the addition of an agonist. By such means, it is possible to control the integrity of the cells analyzed during each experiment. Changes in the cell volume, side scatter, or in the violet fluorescence indicate that some cellular damage or a leakage of the probe has occurred during the experiment and caution should be exercised about the validity of the results. Only experiments in which cellular integrity is maintained are considered.

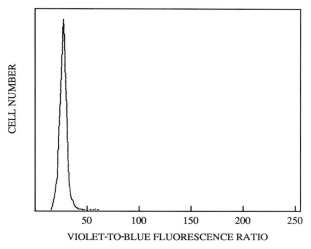

FIG. 3   Distribution of the Indo-1 fluorescence ratio in a gated population of brain capillary endothelial cells. Data presented correspond to the experiment shown in Fig. 2. Indo-1 fluorescence ratio is not based on absolute values. The scale on the abscissa is subdivided into 256 units. The position of the peak ratio on the abscissa depends on the setting (voltage and gain) of the photomultiplier tubes. These settings are adjusted for each batch of cells to obtain a mean apparent ratio of about 30. All settings are then kept constant. An increase in $[Ca^{2+}]_i$ results in a rightward shift in the distribution of the fluorescence ratio. In most cases, the distribution remains unimodal, indicating that all cells behave similarly. In some instances [see, for example, C. Frelin, P. Vigne, and J.-P. Breittmayer, *Mol. Pharmacol.* **38,** 904 (1990)], a unimodal distribution transforms into a bimodal distribution under the influence of an agonist, indicating a heterogeneity of the cell responses. Unimodal distribution of $[Ca^{2+}]_i$ levels is observed in endothelin-treated brain capillary endothelial cells and astrocytes. This is an indication that endothelin receptors are present in most (if not all) cells of the populations analyzed.

Analysis of Transient Changes in $[Ca^{2+}]_i$ in Response to Endothelins

By adjusting the cell density in the sample tube and the differential hydrostatic pressure between sample and sheath, typical flow rates of 500–1000 cells/ sec can be obtained. Under these conditions, a mean Indo-1 fluorescence ratio, computed on 3000–5000 gated events, can be sampled every 5–10 sec, thus allowing one to monitor the changes in $[Ca^{2+}]_i$ that occur in response to application of endothelins.

Suspended cells are diluted into 1 ml of Earle's salt solution at a density of 2–4 $\times$ 10^5 cells/ml and the resting Indo-1 fluorescence ratio measured.

An aliquot of an endothelin solution [prepared in 0.1% (v/v) bovine serum albumin] is then added to the cells. After gentle vortexing, the mean Indo-1 fluorescence ratio (computed over 3000–5000 gated events) is continuously monitored over a 2- to 8-min period. The first measure is usually obtained 8 to 10 sec after the addition of the agonist. This delay, which is due to the time required to handle tubes and for the cells to reach the laser beam, could not be reduced further. Experiments are usually carried out at room temperature. Very similar results have been obtained at 37°C using a thermostatted tube holder (Odam-Bruker) and prewarmed incubation solutions.

The flow cytometry technique has been successfully used to study the action of endothelin peptides on $[Ca^{2+}]_i$ in rat brain astrocytes, C6 and NN glioma cells (18), cultured aortic smooth muscle cells (28), and cardiac cells freshly dissociated from newborn rat hearts (29). Typical traces of the changes in the Indo-1 fluorescence ratio in brain capillary endothelial cells following an exposure to 100 nM Et-1 are shown in Fig. 4. Et-1 induces a rapid rise in $[Ca^{2+}]_i$ which peaks at about 10 seconds and then declines to a secondary and sustained plateau phase. The transient peak is mainly due to the release of intracellular Ca^{2+} stores for it is almost unaffected when $[Ca^{2+}]_o$ is decreased from 1.8 mM to 50 nM. Conversely, the plateau phase of $[Ca^{2+}]_i$ elevation is mainly due to Ca^{2+} entry as evidenced by the experiment shown in the lower panel of Fig. 4.

Single-cell measurements of Indo-1 fluorescence usually show a high cell-to-cell variability of the responses to agonists. This may be a great problem when a quantitative analysis of the data is attempted. Such variability is not observed with flow cytometry, for each mean Indo-1 fluorescence ratio is computed on a large number of cells (usually 3000–5000). Accordingly, very reproducible mean values of the fluorescence ratio are obtained for the same batch of cells and may be used for a quantitative analysis of the responses. For instance, a careful analysis of the dose–response curves for the action of endothelins on $[Ca^{2+}]_i$ in brain capillary endothelial cells allowed us to conclude that only one of the two endothelin receptor subtypes that are expressed by the cells is coupled to phospholipase C and to an intracellular mobilization of Ca^{2+} (19). The sensitivity of the technique is also well suited to study the plateau phase of $[Ca^{2+}]_i$ elevation in response to endothelins and to analyze the pharmacological properties of the Ca^{2+} permeation pathways involved.

A diversity of actions of endothelins in the brain is expected, for neurons, astrocytes, and capillary endothelial cells express functional endothelin receptors. Endothelins are produced by neurons (30) and possibly by brain vascular endothelial cells (31; see, however, Ref. 10). Endothelins may act as neuropeptides in the spinal cord (32, 33), in the posterior pituitary system (34), and in cerebellar granule cells (35). Endothelins are powerful Ca^{2+}-mobilizing peptides (18, 24) and mitogens for astrocytes (17, 24) and have

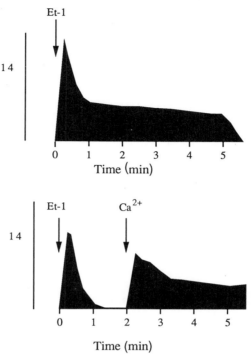

Fig. 4   Intracellular Ca^{2+} transients induced by Et-1 in endothelial cells from brain microvessels. Changes in the mean Indo-1 fluorescence ratio are monitored by flow cytometry following the addition of 100 nM Et-1 to Indo-1-loaded, suspended brain capillary endothelial cells. In the upper panel, $[Ca^{2+}]_0$ is 1.8 mM. In the lower panel, cells were incubated in a 50 mM Ca^{2+} solution (containing 1.2 mM EGTA and 0.5 mM CaCl$_2$). After 2 min $[Ca^{2+}]_o$ was raised to 3 mM by the addition of concentrated CaCl$_2$ to the incubation solution. The vertical scale represents a 14-unit increase in the mean Indo-1 fluorescence ratio. Precision is usually <0.3 units.

been proposed to be mediators of the sequelae of cerebral infarction (36). Finally, it is of interest that both ET_A- and ET_B-like receptors are present in astrocytes and in endothelial cells from brain microvessels that closely associate *in vivo* to form the blood–brain barrier.

Acknowledgments

This work was supported by the CNRS and the Association pour la Recherche sur le Cancer. We are grateful to Dr. P. Vigne for helpful discussions.

References

1. M. Yanagisawa, H. Kurihara, S. Kimura, Y. Tomobe, M. Kobayashi, Y. Mitsui, K. Goto, and T. Masaki, *Nature (London)* **332,** 441 (1988).
2. C. Takasaki, N. Tamiya, A. Bdolah, Z. Wollberg, and E. Kochva, *Toxicon* **26,** 543 (1989).
3. A. Bdolah, Z. Wollberg, G. Fleminger, and E. Kochva, *FEBS Lett.* **256,** 1 (1989).
4. A. Inoue, M. Yanagisawa, S. Kimura, Y. Kasaya, T. Miyauchi, K. Goto, and T. Masaki, *Proc. Natl. Acad. Sci. U.S.A.* **86,** 2863 (1989).
5. H. Matsumoto, N. Suzuki, H. Onda, and M. Fujino, *Biochem. Biophys. Res. Commun.* **164,** 74 (1989).
6. S. Arai, S. Hori, I. Aramori, H. Ohkubo, and S. Nakanishi, *Nature (London)* **348,** 730 (1990).
7. T. Sakurai, M. Yanagisawa, Y. Takuwa, H. Miyazaki, S. Kimura, K. Goto, and T. Masaki, *Nature (London)* **348,** 732 (1990).
8. T. Masaki and M. Yanagisawa, *Cardiovasc. Drug Rev.* **8,** 373 (1990).
9. C. R. Hiley, C. R. Jones, J. T. Pelton, and R. Miller, *Br. J. Pharmacol.* **101,** 319 (1990).
10. P. Vigne, R. Marsault, J.-P. Breittmayer, and C. Frelin, *Biochem. J.* **266,** 415 (1990).
11. M. Sokolovski, R. Galron, Y. Kloog, A. Bdolah, F. E. Indig, S. Blumberg, and G. Fleminger, *Proc. Natl. Acad. Sci. U.S.A.* **87,** 4702 (1990).
12. T. J. Resink, T. Scott-Burden, C. Boulanger, E. Weber, and F. R. Buhler, *Mol. Pharmacol.* **38,** 244 (1990).
13. I. Ambar, Y. Kloog, E. Kochva, Z. Wollberg, A. Bdolah, U. Oron, and M. Sokolovski, *Biochem. Biophys. Res. Commun.* **157,** 1104 (1988).
14. C. R. Jones, C. R. Hiley, J. T. Pelton, and M. Mohr, *Neurosci. Lett.* **97,** 276 (1989).
15. C. Koseki, M. Imai, Y. Hirata, M. Yanagisawa, and T. Masaki, *Am. J. Physiol.* **256,** R858 (1989).
16. W. W. Lin, C. Y. Lee, and D. M. Chuang, *Eur. J. Pharmacol.* **166,** 581 (1989).
17. M. W. MacCumber, C. A. Ross, and S. H. Snyder, *Proc. Natl. Acad. Sci. U.S.A.* **87,** 2359 (1990).
18. R. Marsault, P.Vigne, J.-P. Breittmayer, and C. Frelin, *J. Neurochem.* **54,** 2142 (1990).
19. P. Vigne, A. Ladoux, and C. Frelin, *J. Biol. Chem.* **266,** 5925 (1991).
20. I. Ambar, Y. Kloog, and M. Sokolovski, *Biochemistry* **29,** 6415 (1990).
21. R. Takayanagi, K. Ohnaka, C. Takasaki, M. Ohashi, and H. Nawata, *Regul. Pept.* **32,** 23 (1991).
22. Y. Kloog, I. Ambar, E. Kochva, Z. Wollberg, A. Bdolah, and M. Sokolovski, *FEBS Lett.* **242,** 387 (1989).
23. P. Marin, J. C. Delumeau, O. Durieu-Trautmann, D. LeNguyen, J. Prémont, A. D. Strosberg, and P. O. Couraud, *J. Neurochem.* **56,** 1270 (1991).
24. S. Supattapone, A. W. M. Simpson, and C. C. Ashley, *Biochem. Biophys. Res. Commun.* **165,** 1115 (1989).

25. J. A. Ledbetter, C. H. June, L. S. Grosmaire, and P. Rabinovitch, *Proc. Natl. Acad. Sci. U.S.A.* **84,** 1384 (1987).
26. G. Grynkiewicz, M. Poenie, and R. Y. Tsien, *J. Biol. Chem.* **260,** 3440 (1985).
27. T. M. Chused, H. A. Wilson, D. Greenblatt, Y. Ishida, L. J. Edison, R. Y. Tsien, and F. D. Finkelman, *Cytometry* **8,** 396 (1987).
28. C. Van Renterghem, P. Vigne, J. Barhanin, A. Schmid-Alliana, C. Frelin, and M. Lazdunski, *Biochem. Biophys. Res. Commun.* **157,** 977 (1988).
29. P. Vigne, J.-P. Breittmayer, R. Marsault, and C. Frelin, *J. Biol. Chem.* **265,** 6782 (1990).
30. A. Giaid, S. J. Gibson, N. B. N. Ibrahim, S. Legon, S. R. Bloom, M. Yanagisawa, T. Masaki, I. M. Varndell, and J. M. Polak, *Proc. Natl. Acad. Sci. U.S.A.* **86,** 7634 (1989).
31. S. Yoshimoto, Y. Ishizaki, H. Hurihara, T. Sasaki, M. Yoshizumi, M. Yanagisawa, Y. Yazaki, T. Masaki, K. Takakura, and S. Murota, *Brain Res.* **508,** 283 (1990).
32. T. Yoshizawa, S. Kimura, I. Kanazawa, Y. Uchiyama, M. Yanagisawa, and T. Masaki, *Neurosci. Lett.* **102,** 179 (1989).
33. O. Shimni, S. Kimura, T. Yoshizawa, T. Sawamura, T. Uchiyama, Y. Sugita, I. Kanazawa, M. Yanagisawa, and T. Masaki, *Biochem. Biophys. Res. Commun.* **162,** 340 (1989).
34. T. Yoshizawa, O. Shinmi, A. Giaid, M. Yanagisawa, S. J. Gibson, S. Kimura, Y. Uchiyama, J. M. Polak, T. Masaki, and I. Kanazawa, *Science* **247,** 462 (1990).
35. W. W. Lin, C. Y. Lee, and D. M. Chuang, *Biochem. Biophys. Res. Commun.* **167,** 593 (1990).
36. T. Asano, I. Ikegaki, Y. Suzuki, S. Satoh, and H. Shihuya, *Biochem. Biophys. Res. Commun.* **159,** 1345 (1989).

[18] Fasciculin: Neuropharmacology of a Potent Anticholinesterase Polypeptide

Federico Dajas, Rodolfo Silveira, and Carlos Cerveñansky

Introduction

Neurotoxins from snake venoms have proven to be valuable tools for the understanding of synaptic transmission mechanisms (1–3). In addition to postsynaptic neurotoxins, some snakes from the Elapidae family have presynaptic toxins that act on the storage and release of neurotransmitters (4–7). Some time ago, it was realized that the venom from a snake of this family, *Dendroaspis angusticeps* (green mamba), contained a polypeptide that when injected into mice provoked long-lasting and generalized muscle fasciculations and gland secretion (8). This syndrome has been described after acute intoxication with anticholinesterase (AChE) agents (9), supporting the idea that one or more venom substances might inactivate cholinesterases.

The first biochemical and histochemical evidence for the existence of an independent peptide with anticholinesterase activity in the venom of *D. angusticeps* was provided by Dajas and co-workers in Montevideo in 1983 (8). Two toxins with this activity were isolated. These toxins caused severe, generalized muscle fasciculations for 5–7 hr after intraperitoneal injection (0.5–3 μg/g) into mice, followed by a gradual recovery. Due to the symptoms that they produced, these two toxins were called fasciculin 1 and 2 (8).

Four peptides with activities similar to those of fasciculin 2 from the green mamba *D. angusticeps* have since been isolated from *Dendroaspis* venoms (10). By far, most of the biochemical and neurobiological work has been done mainly with fasciculin 2, and it will be referred hereinafter as fasciculin (FAS).

Biochemical Properties of Fasciculin

Fasciculin is a 61-amino acid residue peptide with 4 disulfide bridges (M_r 6735, from amino acid sequence, Fig. 1), structurally homologous to the short-chain neurotoxins present in elapid snake venoms (7). The amino acid sequence was known (11) before basic aspects of its biological activity became clear (8, 12–14).

Methods in Neurosciences, Volume 8

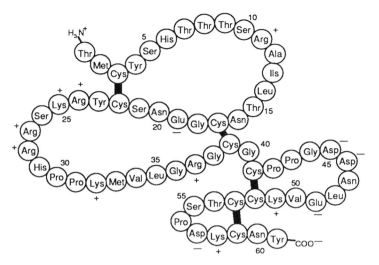

Fɪɢ. 1   Amino acid sequence of fasciculin 2, an anticholinesterase peptide isolated from *D. angusticeps* snake venom.

The anticholinesterase activity of FAS displays an interesting pattern, so far not elucidated in detail, against AChEs from different sources (see Table I). For example, rat brain soluble and membrane-bound enzymes purified by affinity chromatography from striatum show a K_1 of about $5 \times 10^{-11} M$, while chicken brain and insect head enzymes are insensitive to concentrations up

TABLE I   Some Cholinesterases Inhibited by Fasciculin[a]

Enzyme source	$K_i (M)$[b]
Acetylcholinesterase	
Human erythrocytes	2.2×10^{-10}
Human cerebrospinal fluid	2×10^{-10}
Rat brain	0.45×10^{-10}
Guinea pig brain	1.0×10^{-10}
Butyrylcholinesterase	
Human plasma G_4 form	0.5×10^{-6}
Horse plasma	$0.02{-}3.0 \times 10^{-6}$ [c]

[a] Adapted from Ref. 14.
[b] pH 7.4, ionic strength 0.16 M, at 37°C.
[c] pH 7.4, ionic strength 2 mM.

to 8 μM. On the other hand, FAS is able to discriminate between AChE activity (i.e., human red blood cells, human cerebrospinal fluid, rat brain) and butyrylcholinesterase (BuChE) activity (i.e., human plasma, rat brain) by a factor of up to 10,000.

Among the AChE activities tested, no differences in inhibition could be related directly to differences in molecular forms or solubility properties of the enzyme molecule (13).

Acetylcholinesterase inhibition by FAS follows noncompetitive kinetics, and binding to a peripheral anionic site on the enzyme molecule has been postulated according to displacement studies with the fluorescent probe propidium and Ca^{2+} (12). It has been also postulated that FAS may show antiproteolytic activity against some trypsin-like enzymes, but with a relative low affinity (14).

Isolation and Purification Procedures

Details regarding each separation step are given in Figs. 2–5.

Freeze-dried or desiccated venom from *D. angusticeps** is first submitted to gel filtration on Sephadex G-50 with 0.1 M ammonium acetate, pH 6.8. The fraction containing peptides in the M_r 5K–8K range (peak III, Fig. 2) is freeze dried. The next step is cation-exchange chromatography on Bio-Rex 70 (Bio-Rad, Richmond, CA). This high-capacity resin must be preequilibrated with 0.2 M ammonium acetate and the pH adjusted with 2.5 M solutions of either acetic acid or ammonium hydroxide until pH 7.30 is reached. Once the column is packed and the resin properly equilibrated, the elution starts with about 100 ml of 30 mM ammonium acetate. Then the sample is dissolved in the same buffer, applied, and eluted until a baseline recording is achieved before the gradient elution is started, as described in the caption to Fig. 3. Peak 5 from this run is FAS 2, and after pooling as indicated it is dialyzed against 10 mM ammonium acetate (or diluted to one-half with water) prior to freeze drying.

In following this protocol usually about 20 mg of FAS 2 could be obtained per gram of dried venom in a fairly pure state, with FAS 1 being the major impurity (see Fig. 4A). If additional purification is required, then a second run in Bio-Rex 70 under the same conditions removes most contaminating peaks (see Fig. 4B). Depending on the quantities needed, an high-performance liquid chromatography (HPLC) ion-exchange or reversed-phase step can be carried out with material pooled from the Bio-Rex 70 run, as shown in Fig. 3 (see also Figs. 4A and 5). In both cases peaks with the desired activity can be freeze dried directly with retention of full activity.

* Some venom suppliers are Sigma Chemical Company (St. Louis MO), Jabria BV (Hierden, Holland), and Laxotan (Rosans, France).

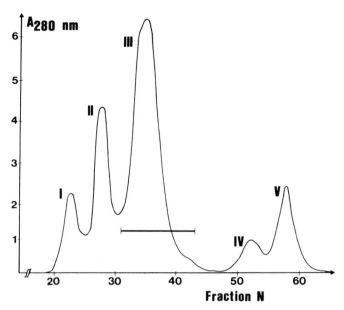

FIG. 2   Gel filtration on Sephadex G-50 (1.6 × 120 cm) of 0.3 g of *D. angusticeps* venom dissolved in 9 ml of the running buffer, 0.1 *M* ammonium acetate, pH 6.8. Flow rate, 11.0 ml/hr; fraction size, 3.68 ml. Fraction III containing FAS was pooled as indicated and freeze dried.

Fasciculin concentration can be calculated from spectrophotometric measurements at 276 nm (molar absorptivity at this maximum is 4900) (15). A solution containing 1 mg/ml of FAS would have an absorbance of 0.73 at 276 nm (10).

The tendency of FAS to stick to plastic and glass containers is very noticeable in dilute solutions, thus the addition of bovine serum albumin (BSA) or horse immunoglobulin G (IgG) (about 0.1 mg/ml) is advised. Under these conditions solutions frozen at −20°C preserve their activity for many months.

Pharmacological Effects of Fasciculin on Peripheral Nervous System

From a pharmacological point of view it is interesting to note that FAS (at concentrations of 0.15 μg/ml) augments twitch responses to indirect stimulation in mouse phrenic nerve–hemidiaphragm preparations, although it is not active on the chick biventer cervicis nerve–muscle preparation (16). In electrophysiological experiments, FAS (1.5 nM–0.15 μM) produces a 50–100% in-

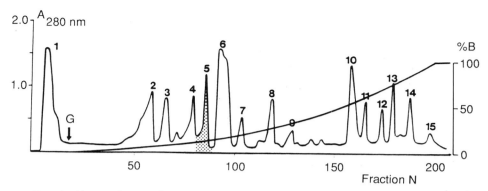

FIG. 3   Ion-exchange chromatography on Bio-Rex 70 (1.9 × 30.5 cm) equilibrated with 0.20 M ammonium acetate, pH 7.30. Sample: fraction III (Fig. 1) from 0.85 g of starting venom dissolved in 25 ml of 30 mM ammonium acetate, pH 7.30. The elution with a concave gradient (started as indicated) of 30 mM vs 1.25 M ammonium acetate, pH 7.30, was performed with an Ultrograd gradient mixer (LKB, Uppsala, Sweden). (Similar results are obtained with two cylinders with diameters 9 cm (30 mM ammonium acetate) and 6 cm [1.25 ammonium acetate, 2.0-liter gradient volume (see Ref. 10)]. Fraction size, 8.91 ml; flow rate, 35.7 ml/hr. Peak 5 (pooled as indicated) corresponds to fasciculin 2.

crease in the amplitude of end-plate potentials and miniature end-plate potentials and a twofold increase in their time course. The onset of FAS action is seen in 2–5 min, and the maximum effect is generally found between 10 and 30 min. The action of FAS is well sustained throughout a 3-hr exposure period, and it is not reversed by a 30-min washing with normal physiological saline solution (17).

Similar fractions from *D. angusticeps* venom potentiate the actions of acetylcholine (ACh) on rabbit intestine and frog rectus abdominis preparations and enhance the responses of guinea pig ileum to nerve stimulation (18).

The pharmacological effects of FAS are consistent with an anticholinesterase action. Fasciculin represents the first anticholinesterase polypeptide from natural sources that is active under physiological conditions.

Pharmacology of Fasciculin in Central Nervous System

General Properties of Acetylcholinesterases

Even though AChE is one of the most studied enzymes, most of its functions in different parts of the organism are largely unknown. The enzyme is widely distributed physiogenetically and in individuals, e.g., in mammals it can be found in blood cells, muscle, and brain (13).

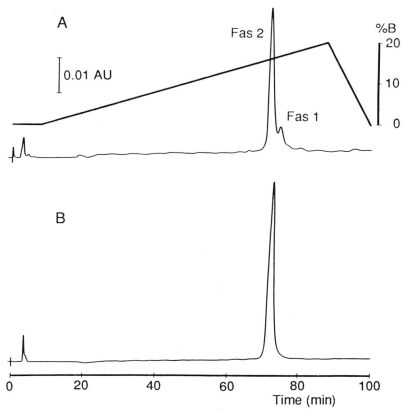

Fig. 4   HPLC-ion exchange of fasciculin 2. Column, TSK SP-SPW (7.5 × 70 mm); flow rate, 0.70 ml/min. Eluents: (A) water, (B) 1 M ammonium acetate, pH 6.8. Gradient: 0 to 8 min, $\%B = 0$; 8 to 88 min, linear gradient up to $\%B = 20$; 88 to 100 min, down to $\%B = 0$. Detection: UV recording at $A_{276\ nm}$. Samples: (A) about 100 μg of fasciculin from Bio-Rex 70 peak 5 pooled as indicated in Fig. 3; (B) 125 μg of fasciculin purified by a second run in Bio-Rex 70 under similar conditions as stated in Fig. 3. AU, absorbance unit.

The wide distribution of AChEs as well as their molecular variety suggest that different functions would be attributable to different forms in diverse localizations.

The breakdown of ACh was long considered the only function attributed to AChE in the central nervous system (CNS). Nevertheless, some authors have started to postulate that AChE may have functions different from the cholinergic ones (19).

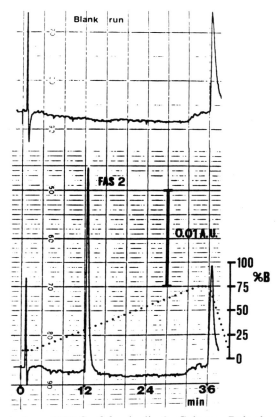

FIG. 5   Reversed-phase HPLC of fasciculin 2. Column, Bakerbond (J. T. Baker, Phillipsburg, NJ) WP-butyl (4.6 × 50 mm); flow rate, 0.8 ml/min. Eluents: (A) 0.1 M ammonium acetate, pH 6.9; (B) 0.1 M ammonium acetate, pH 6.9 in 40% 2-propanol. Gradient: 10% B for 2 min; 10 to 75% B in 30 min; 75% B for 3 min; reequilibration in 10% B. Detection: UV recording at $A_{276 \text{ mn}}$. Sample: 58 μg of fasciculin as in Fig. 4B.

The distribution of AChE in tissues having little or no ACh and choline acetyltransferase has long proved to be a puzzle to the biochemist. In the brain, large quantities of AChE, but relatively little of the cholinergic marker, choline acetyltransferase, are found in diverse areas that include the hypothalamus, globus pallidus, raphe nucleus, red nucleus, cerebellum, and the substantia nigra (20).

Some years ago, evidence was presented that soluble AChE was secreted in the CNS in a physiological manner (21), a result that was confirmed afterward (22). On the other hand, a peptidase role has been attributed to AChE in the brain (23, 24).

In this context, because FAS inhibits both the cholinolytic and proteolytic functions of AChE, it has become an useful tool for studying the diverse functions of AChE in the CNS.

Biochemical Effects of Fasciculin Injection into the Striatum

To study the effects of FAS in the CNS, the striatum (caudate putamen nuclei of the basal ganglia) was chosen as a characteristic structure where AChE shows mainly a cholinolytic function.

Acetylcholine is one of the most important striatal neurotransmitters and the intrinsic nature of cholinergic neurons in the striatum is now well determined (25, 26).

Furthermore, some well-known interactions, such as dopamine–ACh, ACh—γ-aminobutyric acid (GABA), and glutamate–ACh (27–29), provide these cholinergic neurons with a decisive regulatory role of striatal functioning.

Stereotaxic injection of FAS into the rat caudate putamen was carried out at doses of 5–250 ng/rat. Fifteen minutes after injection an AChE inhibition of up to 90% was shown and the inhibition persisted in the range of 50% for 15–21 days after injection (30). Similar experiments performed with the well-known anticholinesterase physostigmine showed 25% inhibition for only 1 hr after injection.

Regarding the persistence of AChE inhibition induced by FAS, it is likely that FAS provokes an irreversible inhibition of the enzyme and *de novo* synthesis is needed to replenish the enzymatic activity. However, the turnover rate of AChE has been estimated to be about 3 days in the CNS (31). Thus, the reasons for this long-term inhibition remain unclear at present.

The potent and long-lasting inhibition of striatal AChE is accompanied by a selective decrease of cholinergic muscarinic receptors 7 days after FAS without affecting benzodiazepine or dopamine (DA) receptors (32). In spite of the fact that direct assessments of ACh levels after FAS have not yet been performed, it is very likely that FAS-induced AChE inhibition provokes an increase of cholinergic activity which in turn would lead to the cholinergic receptor down regulation.

To study the effects of FAS on striatal metabolism further, the levels of monoamines and metabolites were assessed using HPLC with electrochemical detection. Rats sacrificed 24 hr and 7 days after FAS injection showed no changes in monoamine levels or monoamine turnover (32).

The lack of effects on the monoaminergic neurotransmission is in agreement with the reported unchanged levels of DA, serotonin (5-HT), or their metabolites after intrastriatal or systemic diisopropyl fluorophosphate (DFP) administration (33–35).

Fasciculin and Control of Motor Behavior in Basal Ganglia

The nigrostriatal, striatonigral, and nigrothalamic pathways are important connections of the basal ganglia and their relevance is mainly shown by the control they exert on motor behavior, as is dramatically shown in Parkinson's disease after degeneration of the dopaminergic nigrostriatal pathway.

The motor effects of lesions or pharmacological challenges of nigrostriatal pathways have been taken as a test model for different drugs such as neuroleptics. The circling behavior demonstrated as turning after unilateral lesion or different drug treatments of the nigrostriatal pathway (36, 37) and the cataleptic behavior expressed as a motionless picture after bilateral actions on the same structures are good examples of behavioral effects of pharmacological actions on the basal ganglia.

Unilateral injection of 0.5 µg of FAS in the striatum provokes, 24 hr after treatment, ipsilateral turning after apomorphine (APO) challenge. This effect is blocked by atropine and is not seen 7 days after FAS (32). When bilaterally injected in both striata, FAS provokes catalepsy, a motor syndrome clearly shown 24 hr after FAS, that is also reversed by atropine and disappears spontaneously after 7 days (M. Castelló, B. Bolioi, and F. Dajas; unpublished observations, 1991).

Taking into account the basic basal ganglia circuitry, which includes a dopaminergic nigrostriatal pathway that forms a feedback loop with a striatonigral GABA-ergic connection having a striatal cholinergic interneuron, it is likely that hyperactivity of the cholinergic core of this loop provoked by unilateral FAS could lead to a massive activation of the GABA-ergic output, which induces an ipsilateral motor inhibition, contralateral dominance, and therefore ipsilateral circling. Bilateral FAS administration produces a general activation of GABA-ergic output expressed as a cataleptic syndrome.

The inhibition by atropine of both ipsilateral turning or catalepsy induced by FAS and the disappearance of both syndromes 7 days after FAS (when muscarinic down regulation is installed) show the prominent role of the striatal cholinergic component of the basal ganglia circuitry for the control of motor behavior.

These results also demonstrate that the cholinolytic function of striatal AChE is functionally the most significant, in spite of the fact that effects in some other neurotransmitter connections like the peptidergic striatonigral pathways have not yet been assessed.

To study the role of AChE in the control of motor behavior in the basal ganglia, FAS was injected into the substantia nigra (SN) (0.5-µg total dose).

Rats turn contralaterally after FAS injection, a behavior that is potentiated by APO and only partially blocked by atropine (Fig. 6). Although AChE is reduced by about 90% in the treated SN, analyses of catecholamines and metabolites do not show significant changes.

The classical DA hypothesis of circling behavior as mainly a DA-driven effect (38, 39) is not directly applicable in this case, given the absence of biochemical changes in DA levels and DA metabolites in the SN and in the striatum after FAS. It is likely that in DA agonism provoked by APO, the transitory down regulation of DA metabolism would allow that actions on

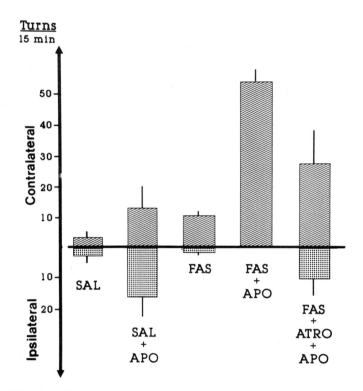

FIG. 6   Effects of different treatments on the rotational behavior produced by intranigral FAS injection. Twenty-four hours after FAS (0.5 μg in 0.3 μl) or saline (0.3 μl) injection into the right substantia nigra, the rats were tested in a rotometer for 15 min. After that, the animals received apomorphine (1 mg/kg, sc) and were tested again during 15 min. A group of FAS-injected animals was treated with atropine (20 mg/kg, ip) 20 min before apomorphine and the rotational behavior was also recorded for 15 min. (n = 12–15 in each group.) SAL, saline; APO, apomorphine; ATRO, atropine.

other neurotransmitter systems (such as those provoked by FAS in the cholinergic one) could be expressed, thereby provoking a disbalance that finally ends in circling.

A further demonstration that FAS effects on the SN are independent from the dopaminergic nigrostriatal pathway is given by the injection of 6-hydroxydopamine (6-OHDA) into the SN. Eighty percent of rats lesioned in the SN with 6-OHDA turn ipsilaterally spontaneously, a trend that is changed to 100% turning to the side of the lesion after APO administration (5 mg/kg, ip, 5 days after FAS). This turning is reverted in 70% of rats when FAS is injected in the SN previously lesioned with 6-OHDA.

In both intact and 6-OHDA-lesioned animals, intraperitoneal administration of atropine to rats previously treated with FAS shows only a partial blockade of the turning, indicating that, in contrast with striatal effects, cholinergic hyperactivity provoked by FAS in the SN is only partially responsible for turning behavior and that unknown functions of AChE could also be affected by FAS.

Locus Coeruleus Acetylcholinesterase and Fasciculin

The locus coeruleus (LC) is the nucleus of the hindbrain that gives rise to a massive noradrenaline (NA)-containing projection throughout the neuroaxis (40). Although no cholinergic afferents have been described, muscarinic and nicotinic ACh receptors, as well as a high AChE activity, have been found in LC neurons (41, 42). The LC is now recognized as the core of stress-adaptive mechanisms, anxiety, and depression.

Stereotaxic injection of FAS into the LC provokes a significant increase of NA levels that are insensitive to atropine treatment (43). When an AChE inhibitor with no intracellular effects (like BW 284C51) is applied stereotaxically, it also provokes an increase in NA levels that is sensitive to atropine treatment (43).

It would therefore appear that in the LC extracellular AChE would demonstrate mainly a cholinolytic action and the intracellular enzyme a noncholinolytic one, probably related to tyrosine monooxygenase activation.

Concluding Remarks

From all of the above-described results it appears that FAS is an extremely useful tool for studying the different functions of AChE in different brain structures *in vivo*. First of all, it clearly differentiates BuChE from AChE activities, and AChEs from different sources. Furthermore, FAS has allowed us to further demonstrate the key significance of the striatal AChE in the cholinergic mechanisms involved in the control of motor behavior.

According to FAS effects, the AChE present in catecholaminergic nuclei in the CNS would have different modulatory functions, being independent of DA metabolism in the SN and being involved in NA regulation in the LC.

Acknowledgments

The work on fasciculins has been supported by IPICS (International Program in the Chemical Sciences, Uppsala University, Sweden), IFS (International Foundation for Science), and PEDECIBA (Programa de Desarrollo de las Ciencias Básicas, Montevideo, Uruguay). The continuous support and advise of Professor E. Karlsson is greatly appreciated. The authors wish to express their gratitude to Professor R. Liminga, of Uppsala University, and people working at the Neurochemistry Division, Instituto de Investigaciones Biologicas Clemente Estable. The secretarial help of A. García is greatly appreciated.

References

1. C. Chang and C. Lee, *Arch. Int. Pharmacodyn.* **144,** 241 (1963).
2. H. Fertuck and M. Salpeter, *J. Cell Biol.* **69,** 144 (1976).
3. A. Speth, F. Chen, J. Lindstrom, R. Kobayashi, and H. Yamamura, *Brain Res.* **131,** 350 (1967).
4. C. Y. Lee, *Annu. Rev. Pharmacol.* **12,** 265 (1972).
5. R. B. Kelly and F. R. Brown, *J. Neurobiol.* **5,** 135 (1974).
6. T. Abe, S. Alema, and R. Miledi, *Eur. J. Biochem.* **80,** 1 (1967).
7. E. Karlsson, *Handb. Exp. Pharmacol.* **52,** 159 (1979).
8. D. Rodríguez-Ithurralde, R. Silveira, L. Barbeito, and F. Dajas, *Neurochem. Int.* **5,** 267 (1983).
9. D. Grob, *Handb. Exp. Pharmacol., Suppl.* **15,** 989 (1963).
10. E. Karlsson, P. Mbugua, and D. Rodríguez-Ithurralde, *Pharmacol. Ther.* **30,** 259 (1985).
11. C. C. Viljoen and D. P. Botes, *J. Biol. Chem.* **248,** 4915 (1973).
12. E. Karlsson, P.Mbugua, and D. Rodríguez-Ithurralde, *J. Physiol. (Paris)***79,** 232 (1984).
13. F. Dajas, C. Cerveñansky, R. Silveira, and L. Barbeito, *in* "Neurotoxins in Neurochemistry" (J. O. Dolly, ed.), pp. 241–251. Ellis Horwood, London, 1988.
14. C. Cerveñansky, F. Dajas, A. Harvey, and E. Karlsson, *Int. Encycl. Pharmacol. Ther.* (in press).
15. K. B. Augustinsson, H. Eriksson,and Y. Faijersson, *Clin. Chim. Acta* **89,** 239 (1978).
16. A. L. Harvey, A. J. Anderson, P. M. Mbugua, and E. Karlsson, *J. Toxicol. Toxin. Rev.* **3,** 91 (1984).

17. A. J. Anderson, A. L. Harvey, and P. M. Mbugua, *Neurosci. Lett.* **54,** 123 (1985).
18. J. Wangai, K. Thairu, B. S. Bharaj, and B. V. Telang, *Acta Physiol. Acad. Sci. Hung.* **60,** 75 (1982).
19. S. A. Greenfield, *in* "Cholinesterases" (M. Brain, E. A. Barnwood, and D. Sket, eds.), pp. 289–337. de Gruyter, Berlin, 1984.
20. R. M. Kobayashi, M. Brownstein, J. M. Saavedra, and M. Palkovits, *J. Neurochem.* **24,** 637 (1975).
21. S. Greenfield and A. D. Smith, *Brain Res.* **177,** 445 (1979).
22. S. A. Greenfield, A. Cheramy, V. Leviel, and J. Glowinsky, *Nature (London)* **284,** 355 (1980).
23. D. Small, *Neurosci. Lett.* **95,** 307 (1988).
24. D. Small and I. W. Chubb, *J. Neurochem.* **51,** 69 (1988).
25. J. Bolam, B. Wainer, and A. Smith, *Neuroscience* **12,** 711 (1984).
26. J. Lehmann and S. Langer, *Neuroscience* **10,** 1105 (1983).
27. G. Bartholini, H. Stadler, M. Gadea Ciria, and K. Lloyd, *Adv. Biochem. Psychopharmacol.* **16,** 391 (1977).
28. G. Bartholini, B. Scatton, P. Worms, B. Zivkovic, and K. Lloyd, *in* "GABA and the Basal Ganglia" (G. di Chiara and G. L. Gessa, eds.), pp. 119–127. Raven, New York, (1981).
29. B. Scatton and G. Bartholini, *Brain Res.* **200,** 174 (1980).
30. F. Dajas, B. Bolioli, M. Castelló, and R. Silveira, *Neurosci. Lett.* **77,** 87 (1987).
31. R. J. Wenthold, H. R. Mahler, and W. J. Moore, *J. Neurochem.* **22,** 941 (1974).
32. B. Bolioli, M. E. Castelló, D. Jerusalinsky, M. Rubinstein, J. Medina, and F. Dajas, *Brain Res.* **504,** 1 (1989).
33. S. Robinson, A. Rice, and K. Hambrecht, *J. Neurochem.* **46,** 1632 (1986).
34. P. Potter, M. Hadjiconstantinou, J. Rubinstein, and N. Neff, *Eur. J. Pharmacol.* **106,** 607 (1985).
35. J. Fernando, B. Hoskins, and I. Ho, *Pharmacol. Biochem. Behav.* **20,** 951 (1984).
36. M. Herrera-Marschitz and U. Ungerstedt, *Eur. J. Pharmacol.* **98,** 165 (1984).
37. M. Herrera-Marschitz and U. Ungerstedt, *Eur. J. Pharmacol.* **109,** 349 (1985).
38. N. E. Andén, *in* "Advances in Parkinsonism" (W. Birkmayer and O. Hornykiewicz, eds.), pp. 169–177. Editiones Roche, Basel, Switzerland, 1976.
39. U. Ungerstedt and G. W. Arbuthnott, *Brain Res.* **24,** 485 (1970).
40. S. Loughlin and J. Fallon, *in* "The Rat Nervous System" (G. Paxions, ed.), Vol. 2, pp. 79–93. Academic Press, Orlando, Florida, 1985.
41. A. Albanese and L. L. Butcher, *Brain Res.* **5,** 127 (1980).
42. P. R. Lewis and F. E. Schon, *J. Anat.* **120,** 373 (1975).
43. V. Abó, L. Viera, R. Silveira, and F. Dajas, *Neurosci. Lett.* **98,** 253 (1988).

[19] Geographutoxins

Hideshi Nakamura, Kazuki Sato, and Yasushi Ohizumi

The piscivorous cone snail *Conus geographus* belongs to the large genus *Conus* of gastropod mollusks involving about 300 species. Most species are found in tropical areas and have a well-developed venom apparatus to catch their prey, e.g., fishes. A survey of toxic components of the marine snail revealed that of the *Conus* species examined, *C. geographus* is most dangerous to vertebrate organisms and the toxicity is due to several types of peptide toxins (1). Collection of *Conus geographus,* therefore, must be carried out with special care.

Geographutoxin I (GTX I) and II (GTX II) have been isolated as the muscle sodium channel toxins from *C. geographus* and the amino acid sequences (2) of GTX I and II and the disulfide pairings (3) of GTX I have been determined. Geographutoxin I and II discriminate neuronal and muscle sodium channels (4) and are classified as μ-conotoxins, GIIIA and GIIIB, respectively. Geographutoxins are now available by solid-phase synthesis (5, 6), as well as from natural sources. Geographutoxin II (μ-conotoxin GIIIB) is also commercially available.

GTX I:
$$\underset{15}{}$$

GTX I: Arg-Asp-Cys-Cys-Thr-Hyp-Hyp-Lys-Lys-Cys-Lys-Asp-
(positions 5 and 10 marked)

Arg-Gln-Cys-Lys-Hyp-Gln-Arg-Cys-Cys-Ala-NH$_2$
(positions 15 and 20 marked)

GTX II: Arg-Asp-Cys-Cys-Thr-Hyp-Hyp-Arg-Lys-Cys-Lys-Asp-
(positions 5 and 10 marked)

Arg-Arg-Cys-Lys-Hyp-Met-Lys-Cys-Cys-Ala-NH$_2$
(positions 15 and 20 marked)

Assay Method

Pharmacological Experiments

Male mice (ddy, 25–30 g) and bullfrogs (100–200 g) are used. The mouse hemidiaphragms are excised and suspended in a Krebs–Ringer bicarbonate solution of the following composition (mM): NaCl, 120; KCl, 4.8; CaCl$_2$, 1.2; MgSO$_4$,

1.3; KH_2PO_4, 1.2; $NaHCO_3$, 25.2; and glucose, 5.8 at pH 7.4 and are aerated with 95% O_2–5% CO_2. Sartorius preparations are isolated from both legs of the bullfrogs, cut into pieces longtudinally, and mounted in organ baths. The baths are filled with 20 ml of frog Ringer's solution containing (mM) NaCl, 115; KCl, 2.5; $CaCl_2$, 1.8; and N-2-hydroxyethylpiperidine-N'-2-ethylsulfonic acid (HEPES), pH 7.4, which is gassed with 100% O_2. All experiments on the sartorius muscle are done at room temperature (21–23°C). A resting tension of 1 g is applied to hemidiaphragm and sartorius preparations and contractions are recorded isometrically on a pen recorder through the force–displacement transducer. The hemidiaphragm and sartorius preparations are stimulated directly with 5-msec pulses (submaximal voltage) at a frequency of 0.1 Hz and with 3-msec pulses at a frequency of 0.1 Hz, respectively.

Electrophysiological Experiments

Action Potential

The isolated bullfrog sartorius is set in a chamber containing 5 ml of the frog Ringer's solution, which is gassed with 100% O_2. The muscle is fixed at both ends by tweezers and stretched to decrease the displacement by contractions. The middle point of the muscle is lifted 5 mm by a bent glass bar to make a node on contractions. A muscle fiber in the lifted portion is penetrated by glass microelectrodes (5–10 MΩ, filled with 3 M KCl solution) under direct view in a dissecting microscope. One of the microelectrodes is used for recording the membrane potential and the other for injecting either direct or pulse current. The muscle fibers within each sartorius have nearly the same value for the resting potential (-80 to -87 mV), depending on the preparation. In order to maximize the maximum rate of rise of the action potential, the membrane potential is maintained at -90 mV by injecting a direct current continuously. The fiber is stimulated with a 10-msec pulse (200–500 nA) to evoke an action potential.

Voltage-Clamp Experiments

Male C57 black mice 0 days of age (day of birth, P_0; body weight, 1.2 ± 0.1 g) to 20 days postnatal (P_{20}; 8.8 ± 0.4 g) are used. Mice are killed by rapid decapitation under ether anesthesia. Single fibers are isolated from flexor digitorum brevis muscles of the right and left hind limbs by collagenase digestion followed by gentle trituration through a Pasteur pipette as described previously (7). The muscle fibers and the fragments range between 32 and 370 μm in length and 8 and 15 μm in diameter.

A plastic dish containing isolated muscle fibers in 300 μl of the recording medium is mounted on the stage of an inverted phase-contrast microscope. The recording medium consists of 5 mM NaCl, 145 mM tetraethylammonium (TEA) chloride, 5 mM KCl, 1.5 mM CaCl$_2$, 1 mM MgCl$_2$, 5 mM glucose, and 5 mM 3-(N-morpholino)propanesulfonic acid (MOPS; adjusted to pH 7.4 by TEA hydroxide). The medium contains a lower concentration of Na$^+$ than ordinary mammalian salines to minimize series resistance artifacts. In half of the experiments on muscle fibers from mice younger than P$_4$, recordings are also performed in a medium containing 15 mM Na$^+$ (135 mM TEA chloride, the other ion composition remaining unchanged). Geographutoxin II is dissolved in the recording medium at a concentration of 4 μM, and 100 μl of this solution is added to the dish to obtain a final concentration of 1 μM. Recordings are performed at room temperature (20 ± 2°C). A List EPC-7 patch-clamp system (List Electronic, Germany) is used for whole-cell voltage-clamp recordings as described by Hamill *et al.* (8). Patch pipettes are pulled in two steps and fire polished. The pipettes are filled with 130 mM CsF, 18 mM CsCl, 2 mM NaCl, and 10 mM MOPS solution (adjusted to pH 7.2 with CsOH). The tip resistances of the pipettes range between 0.5 and 0.9 MΩ in the recording medium. Ag|AgCl electrodes are immersed directly in the recording solutions.

Binding Experiments

Muscle homogenates of male rat diaphragm (9) and T-tubular membranes of rabbit skeletal muscle (10) are prepared as described previously. Binding of [³H]saxitoxin to skeletal muscle homogenates and T-tubular membranes is measured by a rapid filtration procedure. The homogenates and the membranes are incubated with [³H]saxitoxin in standard binding medium consisting of 130 mM choline, 5 mM HEPES (adjusted to pH 7.4 with Tris base), 5.5 mM glucose, 6.8 mM MgSO$_4$, and 5.4 mM KCl in the presence or absence of 1.8 mM CaCl$_2$ at 36°C.

Preparative Method

Isolation of Geographutoxins I and II from the Marine Snail *Conus geographus*

Collection and Extraction

The specimens of *C. geographus* (Fig. 1) are collected from coral reefs in waters around Onna village, Kunigami-gun, Okinawa and the gastropods are frozen, shipped via air to Tokyo, and stored at −20°C. The body is

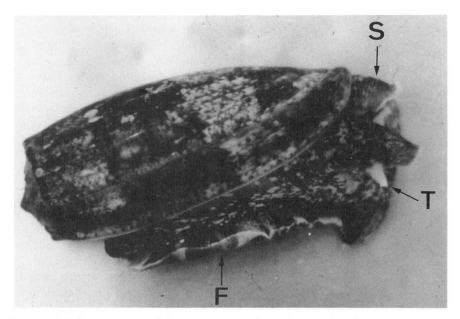

FIG. 1   A living specimen of *C. geographus* collected at coral reefs in waters around Onna village, Kunigami-gun, Okinawa (ca. 10 cm long, 4 cm wide). F, foot; S, siphon; T, tentacle.

removed from the outer shell after thawing and the venom ducts are dissected (Fig. 2) on a stainless-steel plate cooled by ice. The venom ducts (8.24 g) obtained from 30 specimens (average 8.5 cm long) are cut into small pieces, homogenized in 80 ml of 0.2 *M* acetic acid using a Polytron homogenizer and centrifuged at 3000 rpm at 0°C. The surpernatant is collected and the extraction is repeated twice. The extracts are lyophilized to give a pale yellow residue (1.6 g) that is further extracted with 0.2 *M* acetic acid (30, 20, and 20 ml) to yield crude toxins (1.24 g) after lyophilization. The material is purified by the following chromatography procedures at 5°C, except that the high-performance liquid chromatography (HPLC) is done at room temperature (around 20°C). Purification is done by monitoring inhibitory effects on twitch response of the mouse hemidiaphragm to direct stimulation. Aliquots of extracts in water or fractions of each purification steps are added to the organ bath containing 10 ml Krebs–Ringer bicarbonate solution; inhibitory effects are judged after 30 min.

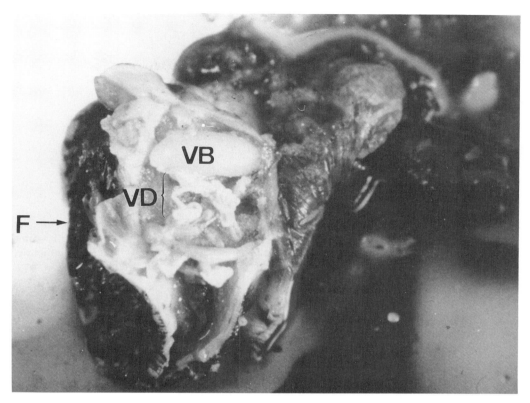

Fig. 2   Photograph of *C. geographus*. Venom apparatus is exposed. VD, venom duct; VB, venom bulb; F, foot.

Purification Procedure

Step 1: Sephadex G-50 Gel Filtration

The crude material is dissolved in 0.03 M sodium phosphate buffer containing 0.15 M NaCl, pH 5.6, and applied to a Sephadex G-50 column (Pharmacia, Piscataway, NJ) (2.6 × 55 cm), previously equilibrated with the same buffer, and eluted under the same conditions. Five-milliliter fractions are collected and the absorbance at 254 nm and the inhibitory effects are measured (Fig. 3). The active fractions (28 to 44) are pooled.

Step 2: CM-Sephadex Chromatography

The pooled solution from step 1 is directly applied to a CM-Sephadex C-25 column (2.6 × 50 cm), previously equilibrated with 0.03 M sodium phosphate

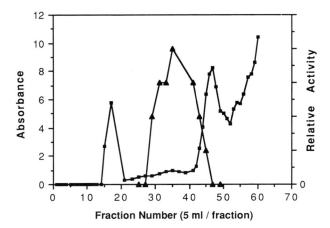

FIG. 3   Chromatography of crude *C. geographus* venom on a Sephadex G-50 column eluted with 0.2 *M* acetic acid. Absorbance at 254 nm (■) and the relative inhibitory effects on mouse hemidiaphragm (▲) were measured and fractions 28 to 44 were pooled as the active fractions.

buffer containing 0.15 *M* sodium chloride, pH 5.6 and eluted first with the same buffer and then with a linear gradient made with 1000 ml of 0.03 *M* sodium phosphate buffer containing 0.15 *M* sodium chloride, pH 5.6 in the mixing chamber and 1000 ml of the same buffer containing 1 *M* sodium chloride in the reservoir. Twenty-milliliter fractions are collected and the activity of each fraction is measured. The active fractions (93 to 107 and 108 to 122) are separately concentrated in a filtering chamber with a membrane filter (UM05; Amicon, Danver, MA) and lyophilized to give crude GTX I (188 mg) and GTX II (190 mg), respectively (see Fig. 4).

Step 3: HPLC Purification

The crude GTX I is dissolved in water (5 ml) and purified on an HPLC column (MCI gel CQP-10, 7.6 × 600 mm; Mitsubishi Chemical Industries, Tokyo, Japan) using 0.15 *M* ammonium formate in water as the mobile phase (Fig. 5). Solution is injected to give a peak at a retention time (t_R) of 7.4 min (flow rate, 3 ml) corresponding to GTX I. The fractions containing GTX I obtained from about 14 injections are pooled.

Step 4: Sephadex G-25 Chromatography

The combined fractions from step 3 are lyophilized and chromatographed on a Sephadex G-25 column (Pharmacia, 1.7 × 52 cm) using 0.2 *M* acetic acid eluent to yield 12.2 mg of colorless powdered GTX I after lyophilization.

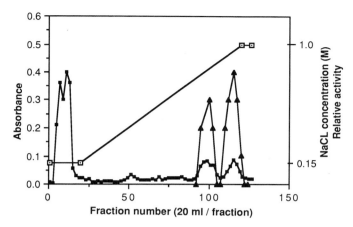

FIG. 4   Chromatography of the Sephadex G-50 purified venom on a CM-Sephadex column. Peptides were eluted with a linear gradient of NaCl from 0.15 to 1 M in 0.03 M sodium phosphate buffer, pH 5.6 (□). Absorbance at 254 nm (■) and the relative activity (▲) were measured.

The crude GTX II is also purified by the same procedure as in steps 3 (t_R 8.6 min) and 4, to afford 12.9 mg of GTX II as a colorless powder.

Preparation of Geographutoxins I and II by Solid-Phase Synthesis

Materials

Derivatized L-amino acids used in the synthesis are purchased from Peptide Institute, Inc. (Minoh, Japan). The α-amino functionality is protected with a *tert*-butyloxycarbonyl (Boc) group and side-chain functional groups are protected as follows: benzyl for threonine, hydroxyproline, and aspartic acid; 4-methylbenzyl for cysteine; *p*-toluenesulfonyl for arginine; 2-chlorobenzyloxycarbonyl for lysine. *p*-Methylbenzhydrylamine (MBHA) resin (Peptide Institute, Inc.) contains 0.64 mmol amino group/g. 1,2-Ethanedithiol (EDT), 1-hydroxybenzotriazole (HOBt), 1,3-diisopropylcarbodiimide (DIPCDI), and 1-acetylimidazole (peptide synthesis grade) are obtained from Watanabe Chemical Industries (Hiroshima, Japan). Diisopropylethylamine (DIPEA) redistilled for solid-phase synthesis is obtained from MilliGen/Biosearch (division of Millipore, Bedford, MA). Anisole and ethyl methyl sulfide are obtained from Aldrich Chemical Company, Inc. (Milwaukee, WI), Trifluoroacetic acid (TFA), dichloromethane (CH_2Cl_2), and N,N-dimethylformamide (DMF) are peptide synthesis grade and acetonitrile is HPLC grade.

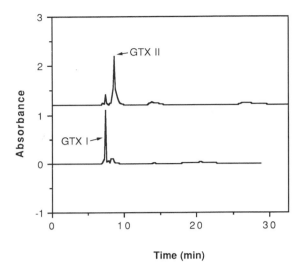

FIG. 5 Chromatographic purification of geographutoxin I (GTX I) (lower trace) and II (GTX II) (upper trace) on an MCI gel CPQ-10 column. Peptides were eluted with 0.15 M ammonium formate in water and absorbance at 230 nm was monitored.

Solid-Phase Synthesis

A linear protected GTX I is synthesized on MBHA resin (0.94 g) using a Biosearch model 9500 peptide synthesizer with a standard protocol for Boc chemistry: deblocking step (20 min) with 45% TFA in CH_2Cl_2 containing 2.5% anisole and 2% EDT (v/v); neutralization with 10% DIPEA in CH_2Cl_2 (v/v); coupling in 50% DMF in CH_2Cl_2 (v/v) using 0.4 M DIPCDI for 120 min. A fivefold excess of each protected amino acid is used based on the original substitution of MBHA resin. Unreacted amino groups on the peptide resin are acetylated by treatment with 0.3 M 1-acetylimidazole in CH_2Cl_2 for 20 min. After 22 coupling cycles, the N-terminal Boc-protecting group is removed to give a side chain-protected peptide resin (3.76 g).

Cleavage from the Resin and Formation of Disulfide Bridges

The peptide resin (3.76 g) is treated with a mixture of 38 ml liquid HF, 5.7 ml anisole, 0.95 ml ethanedithiol, and 0.95 ml ethyl methyl sulfide at 0°C for 60 min. After removal of HF under vaccum, the residue is triturated with ethyl acetate and filtered. The mixture is further washed with ethyl acetate (150 ml) and the peptide is extracted from the mixture with 2 M aqueous acetic acid (100 ml) and diluted to 750 ml with distilled water. The pH of the solution is adjusted to 7.8 with ammonium hydroxide. The solution stirred slowly in an open beaker at room temperature for 48 hr. The cyclization reaction is monitored by HPLC with a column (4.6 × 250 mm) provided by a Shim-pack Prep-ODS (H) kit (Shimazu Co., Kyoto, Japan). Elution is performed with a linear gradient from 5 to 35% (v/v) CH_3CN in 0.1% (v/v) TFA for 30 min at the flow rate of 1 ml/min. A major component in crude linear peptides elutes at 12.8 min and, after being stored for 48 hr, a major cyclized peptide peak appears at 10.8 Min. After being acidified (pH 4–5) with acetic acid, the solution is lyophilized to give 1.26 g of crude product.

Purification Procedure

Step 1: Sephadex G-50F Chromatography

The crude product dissolved in 30% (v/v) acetic acetic (20 ml) is applied on a Sephadex G-50 F column (5 × 100 cm) and eluted with the same solvent. Eluate is monitored by absorbance at 280 nm and the flow rate is 19 ml/10 min for each fraction. The fractions containing monomers (79 to 92) are collected and lyophilized.

Step 2: Carboxymethylcellulose Chromatography

The partially purified peptide (753 mg) is further purified on a carboxymethyl-cellulose column (CM-52, Whatman, Clifton, NJ) (1.8 × 20 cm) developed with a linear gradient generated by adding 500 ml of 0.6 M ammonium acetate at pH 6.5 to 500 ml of 0.01 M ammonium acetate at pH 4.5. Eluate is monitored by absorbance at 280 nm and the flow rate is 11 ml/10 min for each fraction. Peak fractions are analyzed by HPLC with the analytical column mentioned above, using an isocratic elution with 6% CH_3CN in 0.1% TFA. Fractions 38 to 42 are collected and lyophilized.

Step 3: HPLC Purification

The product (232 mg) is dissolved in 9 ml of distilled water and each 0.5-ml portion is purified by HPLC with a preparative column (2 × 25 cm) provided by a Shimpack Prep-ODS (H) kit. Elution is performed with a linear gradient from 2 to 17% CH_3CN in 0.1% TFA in 30 min at a flow rate of 15 ml/min. Peak fractions eluted at the retention time of 17.8 min are pooled and lyophilized. The trifluoroacetate of GTX I obtained was passed through a Sephadex G-25F column (1.8 × 100 cm) using 2 M acetic acid as eluent to be converted to acetate (69 mg). The overall yield of this highly purified peptide is 4%, starting from MBHA resin.

Geographutoxin II is synthesized (3% yield, starting from MBHA resin) by the same procedure described for GTX I, with the following modifications: a linear gradient to 0.8 M ammonium acetate for ion-exchange chromatography is used, and the retention time on the analytical HPLC column under the linear gradient condition is 12.8 min.

Properties

Purity

Geographutoxins I and II isolated from *C. geographus* showed almost a single peak on HPLC analysis and gave satisfactory amino acid analysis. These materials were used for amino acid sequencing and pharmacological studies at a concentration determined by amino acid analysis. Both synthetic GTX I and II showed a single peak on HPLC and were identical with the natural products in all respects, including biological activities, amino acid analysis, HPLC retention time, fast atom bombardment (FAB) mass spectrum, circular dichroism (CD) spectrum, and ^{1}H NMR spectrum.

Pharmacological Properties

Geographutoxin II was three times more potent than GTX I. The 50% lethal toxicity (LD_{50}) of GTX I and II to mice was 340 and 110 μg/kg, respectively. Geographutoxin II (3×10^{-9} to $10^{-7} M$) inhibited the twitch response of the mouse hemidiaphragm to direct stimulation in a concentration-dependent manner. In bullfrog sartorius muscles, GTX II caused a similar inhibitory effect on the twitch response, but at a higher concentration (6×10^{-7} to $3 \times 10^{-6} M$) (Fig. 6).

Electrophysiological Properties

Geographutoxin II ($10^{-6} M$) inhibited or abolished the action potential evoked in sartorius muscle and distinguished two different types of voltage-sensitive Na^+ currents. Geographutoxin II-sensitive and insensitive currents correspond to currents with high and low tetrodotoxin sensitivity, respectively.

Binding Properties

Geographutoxin II inhibited [^{3}H]saxitoxin binding to receptor sites associated with voltage-sensitive Na^+ channels in skeletal muscle homogenates and T-tubular membranes with $K_{0.5}$ values of 60 nM for homogenates and 35 nM for T-tubular membranes.

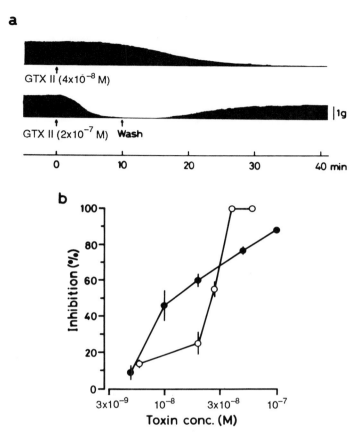

FIG. 6 Inhibition of the contractile response of the hemidiaphragm to direct electrical stimulation (0.1 Hz, 5 msec, supermaximal voltage) by geographutoxin II (GTX II). (a) Typical inhibition patterns of twitch responses by GTX II. (b) Dose-inhibitory response curve for GTX II (○) or TTX (●). The tensions of twitch responses were measured 60 min after exposure to the toxins. Each point and bar represent the mean ± SEM (n = 3–5). Conc, concentration. (From Ref. 11.)

References

1. B. M. Olivera, J. R. Rivier, C. Clark, C. A. Rakilo, G. P. Corpuz, F. C. Abogadie, E. E. Mena, S. R. Woodward, D. R. Hillyard, and L. J. Cruz, *Science* **246,** 257 (1990); J. Kobayashi, H. Nakamura, Y. Hirata, and Y. Ohizumi, *Toxicon* **20,** 823 (1982).
2. S. Sato, H. Nakamura, Y. Ohizumi, J. Kobayashi, and Y. Hirata, *FEBS Lett.*

155, 277 (1983); L. J. Cruz, W. R. Gray, B. M. Olivera, R. D. Zeikus, L. Kerr, D. Yoshikami, and E. Moczydlowski, *J. Biol.Chem.* **260,** 9280 (1985).

3. Y. Hidaka, K. Sato, H. Nakamura, J. Kobayashi, Y. Ohizumi, and Y. Shimonishi, *FEBS Lett.* **264,** 29 (1990).

4. Y. Ohizumi, H. Nakamura, J. Kobayashi, and W. A. Catterall, *J. Biol. Chem.* **261,** 6249 (1986).

5. K. Sato, H. Nakamura, J. Kobayashi, R. Kato, A. Muroyama, and Y. Ohizumi, *in* "Peptide Chemistry 1989: Proceedings of the 27th Symposium on Peptide Chemistry" (N. Yanaihara, ed.), pp. 97–102. Protein Res. Found., Osaka, Japan, 1990.

6. L. J. Cruz, G. Kupryszewski, G. W. LeCheminant, W. R. Gray, B. M. Olivera, and J. Revier, *Biochemistry* **28,** 3437 (1989).

7. A. Bekoff and W. J. Betz, *J. Physiol.* (*London*) **271,** 25 (1977).

8. O. P. Hamill, A. Marty, E. Neher, B. Sakmann, and F. J. Sigworth, *Pfluegers Arch.* **391,** 85 (1981).

9. S. J. Sherman and W. A. Catterall, *J. Gen. Physiol.* **80,** 753 (1982).

10. S. D. Kraner, J. C. Tanaka, and R. L. Barchi, *J. Biol. Chem.* **260,** 6341 (1985).

11. Y. Ohizumi, S. Minoshima, M. Takahashi, A. Kajiwara, H. Nakamura, and J. Kobayashi, *J. Pharmacol. Exp. Ther.* **239,** 243 (1986).

[20] Presynaptic Activity of α-Latrotoxin: Purification and Properties

Ya. T. Terletskaya, N. H. Himmelreich, and
Yu. V. Sokolov

Introduction

The venom of black widow spider *Latrodectus mactans tredecimguttatus* contains, as its major protein component, the toxin called α-latrotoxin (LTX) (1). It has been shown by electrophysiological techniques that the main effect of LTX consists of a massive stimulation of transmitter release from the neuromuscular junctions of vertebrates, which eventually leads to blocking of the synaptic transmission (2, 3).

α-Latrotoxin is an acidic protein (isoelectric point ranges from pH 5.2 to 5.5), with a molecular weight of about 130,000. It consists of only a single polypeptide chain, and is devoid of any proteolytic and lipolytic activity (2).

Numerous studies have been undertaken to determine the nature (the molecular mechanism) of the neurotoxic activity of LTX. The characteristics of the neurotoxin can be summarized as follows:

1. α-Latrotoxin binds to the high-affinity receptor on presynaptic plasma membranes and pheochromocytoma cells PC-12.
2. α-Latrotoxin has the ability to promote an influx of divalent cations through selective channels in presynaptic membranes.
3. α-Latrotoxin can penetrate, in a specific way, into liquid bilayers.
4. α-Latrotoxin has the ability to induce the fusion of artificial phospholipid structures.

These properties of LTX make a significant contribution to the understanding of the molecular mechanism of toxin-induced synaptic action, but the actual mechanism of the neurotoxin action of LTX is still unknown.

This chapter describes the methodological approaches for the isolation and assays of LTX properties.

Methods in Neurosciences, Volume 8

Purification of α-Latrotoxin

α-Latrotoxin is purified from glands of female black widow spiders. The spiders are collected in August and September in Middle Asia. Chelicera, containing the venom glands, are removed to prepare LTX. It is necessary to emphasize that chelicera can be used freshly dissected with or without homogenization, can be stored at −80°C for prolonged periods of time (2–3 months), or lyophilized. The experimental studies presented here have been performed using extracts of the freshly dissected or frozen glands of adult females, because extracts from lyophilized material are much less active and often give inconsistent results.

All procedures are performed at 4°C unless otherwise specified. The freshly dissected glands of approximately 1000 spiders are immersed into 50–60 ml 20 mM Tris-HCl buffer, pH 8.0, and extracted for 2–3 hr. The extract is centrifuged at 105,000 g for 30 min at 4°C and supernatant is stored in aliquots of 1 mg protein/ml buffer at −80°C until use. About 150 mg (wet weight) of the frozen glands is used for isolation of LTX, and if lyophilized glands are used, 50 mg is mixed with 10 ml of 20 mM Tris-HCl buffer, pH 8.0, and incubated at 4°C for 12–15 hr. The extract is centrifuged at 10,000 g for 30 min at 4°C and supernatant is used immediately for isolation of LTX.

α-Latrotoxin is usually purified from the extracts by anion-exchange chromatography (4, 5) or affinity chromatography (6). These techniques provide fast separation and high resolution of LTX, with its structural integrity and biological activities intact.

In this chapter we describe the separation achieved using an FPLC (fast protein liquid chromatography) system for preparative scale chromatography with a strong anion-exchange Mono Q prepacked HR 5/5 column (5). All solvents, salts, and buffers used are of analytical grade, and chromatographic gradients are controlled by the gradient programmer GF 250, according to the manufacturer's instructions concerning flow rate, recorder chart speed, activation and deactivation of the fraction collector, motor valve position, changes in the slope of the elution gradient, etc. The gradients are also programmed in terms of time. Separation of LTX is optimized and the conditions for maximum resolution are as follow: practical sample loadings for proper resolution usually range from 5 to 10 mg of protein/run; buffer A consists of 20 mM Tris-HCl, pH 8.0, and buffer B consists of 1 M NaCl in buffer A; a linear gradient of 0–40% buffer B is run in 18 min, followed by a gradient of 40–100% buffer B in 2 min; the flow rate is maintained at 1 ml/min; detection is made at 280 nm. α-Latrotoxin is clearly seen as a major peak at a concentration of 0.33 M NaCl. This fraction is collected and pooled from several identical runs. Reproducibility is excellent, with a 5% variance coefficient. The time of separation is about 20 min, therefore up to three samples can be processed per hour. The purity of the LTX fraction is checked by sodium dodecyl sulfate-polyacrylamide gel electrophoresis (SDS-PAGE). The protein concentration is routinely measured by UV spectroscopy, assuming an extinction coefficient ε_{280} of $1.36 \times 10^5 M^{-1}$ cm^{-1} for LTX (7). The final yield of LTX approaches 4–6% of the original venom protein content. The purified neurotoxin is stored in aliquots of 50 μg of protein/200 μl and retaines its structural integrity and biological activities for about 6 months at $-70°$C. It should be stressed that LTX tends to degrade when stored. The toxicity of LTX in mice is 18 μg/kg weight (LD$_{50}$).

This FPLC method is a promising one because of its speed, simplicity, and reproducibility.

Measurement of α-Latrotoxin Effect on γ-Aminobutyric Acid Release from Synaptosomes

Electrophysiological studies of the effects of black widow spider venom on single neuromuscular junctions, using the methods of intracellular and extracellular recording, have shown that after adding black widow spider venom the miniature end-plate potential (MEPP) frequency rose from control values of 0.5–1.5 sec^{-1} to peak values of 300–1000 sec^{-1} (8). After reaching a peak, MEPP frequency declines. Interpretation of the marked increase in MEPP frequency implies that the venom reacts with the nerve terminal membrane, thereby inducing the release of transmitter. This proceeds until the total store of transmitter has been exhausted.

It has been shown that LTX accounts entirely for the effects of venom at vertebrate synapses. It affects all nerve endings regardless of the involved transmitter. In most studies, the release of acetylcholine, norepinephrine, or γ-aminobutyrate (GABA) is investigated.

In this chapter, biochemical approaches to studying LTX synaptosomes interactions are described in detail, particularly the uptake and release procedures for GABA.

For uptake studies, a synaptosomal suspension prepared as described by Cotman (9) (2 mg of protein/ml) is added to normal salt solution (126 mM NaCl, 5 mM KCl, 1.4 mM MgCl$_2$, 1.0 mM CaCl$_2$, 1.0 mM NaH$_2$PO$_4$, 10 mM glucose, and 20 mM HEPES, pH 7.4) or sodium-free medium that has the same composition as normal salt medium except that NaCl is replaced by sucrose (252 mM). In normal salt medium, the total uptake of [^{14}C]GABA is measured; in sodium-free medium, the sodium-independent portion is measured. Sodium-dependent uptake is calculated by subtracting the uptake values found in samples containing sodium-free medium from the values of total uptake. High-affinity uptake occurred almost exclusively in the sodium-dependent portion of uptake.

Routine assays of high-affinity GABA uptake are performed as follows: aliquots of synaptosomal suspension are incubated at 30°C in sodium or sodium-free media in the presence of 10 μM aminooxyacetate for 10 min. The uptake is started by addition of 5×10^{-7} [^{14}C]GABA (232 mCi/mmol). The uptake is stopped after 7 min by fivefold dilution of samples in ice-cold media of appropriate composition without [^{14}C]GABA and transferral of samples to an ice bath. The synaptosomes are then precipitated by centrifugation at 5000 g (4°C) for 5 min, resuspended in cold media at concentrations of 0.5 mg protein/ml, and used for efflux studies. (All solutions used for [^{14}C]GABA efflux experiments contain 10^{-5} M aminooxyacetate.)

The suspension preloaded with [^{14}C]GABA right before efflux experiments is incubated for 5 min at 30°C and then the initial level of [^{14}C]GABA is measured. At definite time intervals ranging from 0.5 to 15 min, 0.5-ml aliquots are removed and filtered through Whatman (Clifton, NJ) GF/C filters (prewashed by a solution of 126 mM NaCl, 5 mM KCl, 20 mM HEPES, pH 7.4). The filters are washed two times with 4 ml of ice-cold washing solution and pellets on the filter papers are solubilized in 1% (w/v) SDS. The radioactivity is determined using a liquid scintillation counter. The protein recovery of synaptosomal suspension in the filtration procedure is 93 ± 6%.

It has been shown that [^{14}C]GABA efflux from synaptosomes loaded with [^{14}C]GABA in both sodium and sodium-free media is a very slow process. Only 10% of the [^{14}C]GABA within the synaptosomes is released after 15 min.

On addition of LTX to synaptosomes loaded with [^{14}C]GABA in a sodium-dependent process, the rate of neurotransmitter release substantially increases. No influence of toxin is observed when synaptosomes are loaded with [^{14}C]GABA in a sodium-independent process.

Based on these observations, the hypothesis that LTX induces the process of exocytosis was suggested. This suggestion is supported by morphological data about the toxin-induced decrease of vesicle numerical density in synaptosomes (10).

Channel-Forming Activity Assays of α-Latrotoxin

Most studies on the mode of action of LTX have revealed the ionophore-like activity of this toxin. α-Latrotoxin was found to function by forming channels through the synaptic plasma membrane, which becomes highly permeable to cations, particularly to Ca^{2+}. The idea of LTX forming the transmembrane cation channels was supported by the data on correlation between the processes of LTX incorporation into synaptosomes and formation of ionic channels (11).

In order to examine the ionophoric activity of LTX it was necessary to determine how LTX affects (1) Ca^{2+} influx into synaptosomes, (2) Ca^{2+} efflux from synaptosomes, and (3) the level of cytosolic free Ca^{2+} concentration. This problem can be solved using a combination of $^{45}Ca^{2+}$ exchange technique and cytosolic free calcium concentration measurements. The dynamics of calcium movement in intact synaptosomes have been studied using $^{45}Ca^{2+}$. The level of cytosolic Ca^{2+} was measured with the fluorescent Ca^{2+} indicator quin 2.

Calcium Ion Influx

All steps are normally carried out at room temperature immediately after obtaining synaptosomal preparations. The synaptosomes are resuspended at 4 mg of protein/ml in a medium at pH 7.4, containing 126 mM NaCl, 5 mM KCl, 1.4 mM MgCl$_2$, 1.0 mM CaCl$_2$, 1.0 mM NaH$_2$PO$_4$, 10 mM glucose, and 20 mM HEPES. Calcium-45 (0.5 nCi/ml) is added after preincubation for 15 min to ensure a return to steady state conditions. Aliquots (100 μl) are taken and layered onto a Sephadex G-50 column (1-ml bed volume) preequilibrated with 50 mM Tris-HCl, 2 mM CaCl$_2$, pH 7.4. The elution buffer contains 100 mM NaCl, 10 mM Tris-HCl, pH 7.4, and no added Ca^{2+}. Synaptosomes are eluted with 0.8 ml of this buffer. After elution synaptosomes are solubilized in SDS (final concentration 1%) and then synaptosomal $^{45}Ca^{2+}$ is quantitated by scintillation counting, using an aqueous cocktail.

This method permits removing $^{45}Ca^{2+}$ not taken up by synaptosomes and bound to the synaptosomal surface.

α-Latrotoxin is added to the synaptosomal suspension simultaneously with $^{45}Ca^{2+}$. After a certain lag period, it induces the marked rise in $^{45}Ca^{2+}$ influx. The duration of the lag period and the rate of $^{45}Ca^{2+}$ influx depends on LTX concentrations.

If the synaptosomes are pretreated with LTX in a Ca^{2+} medium for more than 5 min, $^{45}Ca^{2+}$ influx induced by toxin substantially decreases.

Calcium Ion Efflux

In the studies of Ca^{2+} efflux the synaptosomes are loaded with $^{45}Ca^{2+}$ under different conditions: (1) in the medium with normal value of external Ca^{2+} and (2) in the medium with Ca^{2+} six times higher than the normal value.

In the first experiments, suspensions of synaptosomes at 12–16 mg of protein/ml are incubated in the presence of 1 mM CaCl$_2$ and 1 μCi/ml ^{45}Ca^{2+} for 30 min. Thirty minutes is sufficient for loading the tracer. It is followed by the synaptosomal suspension diluted 10-fold with the same buffer, but with no added ^{45}Ca^{2+}, and 0.1-ml aliquots are removed at definite time intervals. Calcium-45 within synaptosomes is determined as described above.

The second technique is carried out as follows. The synaptosomal suspension (12–16 mg protein/ml) is incubated in the presence of sixfold elevated CaCl$_2$ (6 mM) and ^{45}Ca^{2+} (1 μCi/ml) for 30 min. Then ^{45}Ca^{2+}-loaded synaptosomes are diluted with 5 vol of Ca^{2+}-free medium to lower the concentration of external calcium to the normal value. Exposure of synaptosomes to high-Ca^{2+} medium causes them to take up the excessive Ca^{2+}. This helps to observe the net Ca^{2+} efflux from synaptosomes (12). It has been shown that ^{45}Ca^{2+} efflux from synaptosomes loaded with ^{45}Ca^{2+} by either method does not change in the presence of LTX at concentrations of 1–20 nM.

Measurement of Intrasynaptosomal Free Calcium Ion

Incorporation of Quin 2 into Synaptosomes

Quin 2 does not readily cross the plasma membrane: therefore free Ca^{2+} in the cell is determined by using the lipid-soluble parent molecule, quin 2A/M, in which carboxylic acid groups are blocked with acetoxymethyl groups (13). Quin 2A/M can be loaded easily into synaptosomes.

The technique for loading quin 2 into synaptosomes was described by Ashley *et al.* (14) and consists of the following: the synaptosomes are diluted in the medium containing 126 mM NaCl, 5 mM KCl, 1.4 mM MgCl$_2$, 1.0 mM CaCl$_2$, 1.0 mM NaH$_2$PO$_4$, 10 mM glucose, and 20 mM HEPES, pH 7.4, at a concentration of 1.5–2.0 mg protein/ml. Quin 2A/M, stored as a 6 mM solution in dimethyl sulfoxide (DMSO) at $-20°$C, is added to a synaptosomal suspension to a final concentration of 50 μM [final concentration of DMSO is initially 1% (v/v)]. The suspension is incubated at 37°C for 20 min. Then the suspension is diluted 10-fold in warm (37°C) medium and incubated for 40 min to allow completion of intracellular hydrolysis of the blocking groups, yielding free quin 2. The synaptosomes are then precipitated by centrifugation at 5000 g for 5 min, resuspended in cold medium at a concentration of 0.15–0.3 mg protein/ml, and kept on ice until fluorescent measurements are made (for no more than 2 hr). One-milliliter aliquots are incubated for 5 min at 37°C just before fluorescence measurements.

Measurements of Quin 2 Signals

Fluorescent signals from quin 2-loaded synaptosomes are recorded by a spectrofluorometer with thermostatting and stirring capabilities. Experiments are conducted at 37°C with constant stirring. An excitation wavelength of 339 nm and emission wavelength of 490 nm are used. Prior to the experiments, quin 2A/M conversion to free acid is measured by observing a shift in the emission from a peak at 430 nm for the ester to a peak of 490 nm for the acid.

When working with synaptosomes attention must be paid to autofluorescence. The excitation wavelength of 339 nm lies in the ultraviolet band and is capable of stimulating the fluorescence of several cellular constituents providing measurable signals within the visible spectrum (490 nm). All studies must be accompanied by investigations of the same amount of non-quin 2-loaded synaptosomes.

The technique for calibration of quin 2 signals is similar to that described by Tsien et al. (15). The following parameters must be determined by the fluorescence measurements:

F: the magnitude of Ca^{2+}-dependent fluorescence of synaptosomes at resting $[Ca^{2+}]_i$.

F^*: the magnitude of the peak fluorescence achieved after stimulation of the suspension of the quin 2-loaded synaptosomes by LTX.

F_{max}: the magnitude of maximal fluorescence of quin 2-loaded synaptosomes fully saturated with Ca^{2+} obtained when synaptosomes are lysed with Triton X-100 (0.1%), which exposes the intracellular quin 2 to the extracellular Ca^{2+}.

F_{min}: the magnitude of the minimum fluorescence signal, when Mn^{2+} in a concentration of 0.5 mM is added to the Triton-lysed synaptosomes. Quin 2 binding affinity of Mn^{2+} is so much higher than that of Ca^{2+} that addition of Mn^{2+} is capable of completely quenching the Ca^{2+}-dependent fluorescence in the presence of millimolar Ca^{2+} concentration.

According to Tsien et al. (15), the concentration of $[Ca^{2+}]_i$ can be calculated by the equation:

$$[Ca^{2+}]_i = \frac{(1.15 \times 10^{-7} M)(F_{max} - F)}{(F - F_{min})}$$

where $1.15 \times 10^{-7} M$ is the K_D of quin 2 for Ca^{2+} under conditions generally thought to be similar to those of cytosol.

Amount of Basal $[Ca^{2+}]_i$ and Response to α-Latrotoxin

Basal $[Ca^{2+}]_i$ in quinn 2-loaded synaptosomes suspended in a medium containing 1 mM CaCl$_2$ is 97 $\pm$ 4 nM. The increase of Ca^{2+} concentration in a medium up to 5 mM results in a rise of resting $[Ca^{2+}]_i$ to 134 $\pm$ 6 nM.

When adding LTX to quin 2-loaded synaptosomes the rise in the fluorescent signal is registered. The amount of Ca^{2+} and the rate of its accumulation are dependent on LTX concentration. When concentrations of LTX are 0.1–2.0 nM, a certain lag period precedes the variation of fluorescent signal. The duration of lag period decreases from 140 sec at 0.1 nM toxin to 20 sec at 2 nM toxin (16). Five to 10 nM LTX induces the maximal rise of $[Ca^{2+}]_i$ from a starting level of 90–100 nM to a plateau level of approximately 400 nM. At these concentrations of LTX no lag period is observed and a new equilibrium level is reached in 2 min.

Influx of Ca^{2+} in synaptosomes induced by LTX is not blocked by 10^{-4} M D-600, but in a manner similar to voltage-sensitive calcium channels it may be inactivated by a previous increase of $[Ca^{2+}]_i$ resulting from a preliminary depolarization of the plasmalemma. Inactivation of Ca^{2+} influx by LTX is not due to the change in potential of the membrane. The blockage of voltage-sensitive calcium channels by D-600 potassium depolarization does not influence the LTX effect on Ca^{2+} permeability.

If LTX is added to quin 2-loaded synaptosomes resuspended in a Ca^{2+}-free medium, obtained by replacing the omitted Ca^{2+} with 1 mM EGTA, no rise in fluorescent signal intensity is recorded. It is thought that LTX may affect the Ca^{2+} permeability of synaptosomal plasmalemma and does not induce release of Ca^{2+} from the intracellular compartments.

Properties of Channels Produced by α-Latrotoxin in Bilayer Lipid Membranes

Bilayer lipid membranes are formed by the Mueller *et al.* technique across 0.6 mm diameter holes in a Teflon cup placed in a glass cell. The membranes are made from a mixture of phosphatidylcholine and cholesterol containing the lipids at a weight ratio of 2 : 1. Heptane is used as solvent with a lipid concentration of 20 mg/ml. Phosphatidylcholine is isolated from egg yolk according to Ref. 17. Cholesterol is from Serva (Westbury, NY). Electrolyte solutions bathing the membrane contain 10 mM Tris-HCl, pH 7.4, and the required quantities of chloride salts of different metal cations.

Two Ag|AgCl electrodes connected with both compartments are used to transmit current through the system under standard voltage-clamp conditions. Current-versus-time plots and current–voltage curves are made on an Endim 620.02 *X–Y* recorder.

To remove toxin not bound to the membrane and to change ionic composition of the solution at the cis side of the membrane we apply a perfusion procedure (18). In all experiments toxin is added at the cis side of bilayer lipid membrane at a concentration of 1 p*M*. The potential at the trans side of the membrane is taken as zero. All experiments are carried out at room temperature (20–22°C).

After addition of the toxin to the solution at the cis side of bilayer lipid membrane, we observe a large increase of transmembrane current. Usually, discrete changes of conductance are observed. The amplitude histogram for these unit events has a single sharp maximum corresponding to unitary conductance of 100 pS in the solution containing 10 m*M* $CaCl_2$.

Current–voltage curves recorded for these channels are usually concave. The decrease of their steepness for negative potentials is connected, probably, with the closure of the channels. Making the membrane potential more negative, we observe some increase of channel closing frequency. We could not study these phenomena qualitatively because of the extremely long duration of the mean open time for these channels.

Our experimental data confirm the observations made by Grasso and coworkers (19) about asymmetric incorporation of LTX in planar bilayer membrane. This can be illustrated by the fact that after introduction of the venom at the cis side of the bilayer lipid membrane its introduction at the trans side of the membrane transforms the concave current–voltage curve into an essentially linear one.

The elevation of Ca^{2+} concentration at the cis side of the membrane increases the current at positive potentials. This effect is accompanied by a shift of the reversal potential, the values of which coincide within ±1 mV of the Nernst equilibrium potential for Ca^{2+}. From this we may conclude that the channels formed by LTX in bilayer lipid membranes are permeable only to Ca^{2+}, whereas $Tris^+$ and Cl^-, also present in the bathing solution, are not permeable.

Fusion Assay

α-Latrotoxin-Induced Fusion of Negatively Charged Phospholipid Vesicles

Membrane fusion is of fundamental importance in the process of neurosecretion. Phospholipid vesicles (as a relatively simple model system) are being used extensively in the study of the molecular mechanisms of membrane fusion. Recently, it has been demonstrated that presynaptic neurotoxin LTX can trigger the fusion of negatively charged phospholipid vesicles (20).

There are many methods of monitoring fusion (21–23). These assays monitor the mixing of membrane lipids and the aqueous content of two groups of vesicles. The assay presented here is performed as described by Wilschut *et al.* (21) and relies on the formation of the fluorescent Tb^{3+}/dipicolinic acid (DPA) complex on mixing of the vesicle contents. The fluorescence intensity of Tb^{3+} on its own is very low but is enhanced 10^4-fold by its interaction with DPA. In the fusion assay $TbCl_3$ is encapsulated in one group of vesicles and DPA in another. Fusion of the vesicles would then be registered as an increase of the fluorescence intensity due to the formation of the Tb^{3+}–DPA complex. The most important advantage of the assay is the fast rate of Tb^{3+}–DPA complex formation, which makes the method particularly suitable for kinetic analyses of vesicle fusion. Formation of the Tb^{3+}–DPA complex is reversible, which implies that under the experimental conditions (the presence of EDTA) the reaction is prevented from occurring outside the vesicle and also that fluorescent quenching occurs on release of Tb^{3+}–DPA. The assay is sufficiently sensitive to allow the use of low concentrations of vesicles.

For the LTX-induced fusion experiments large unilamellar vesicles are used. It should be emphasized that LTX induces no fusion of the sonicated small unilamellar vesicles. The acidic phospholipids are an essential requirement for the fusogenic activity of the neurotoxin to liposomes.

Large unilamellar vesicles consisting of a ternary mixture of phosphatidylcholine (PC), phosphatidylethanolamine (PE), and cardiolipin (CL) in a molar ratio of 2 : 3 : 5, respectively, are prepared by a reversed-phase evaporation method (24). Three populations of vesicles are prepared in (1) 5 mM $TbCl_3$, 50 mM sodium citrate, 5 mM HEPES, pH 7.4, (2) 50 mM DPA, 20 mM NaCl, 5 mM HEPES, pH 7.4, and (3) 2.5 mM $TbCl_3$, 25 mM DPA, 10 mM NaCl, 25 mM sodium citrate, 5 mM HEPES, pH 7.4, followed by filtration through 0.1-μm Nucleopore filters. Vesicles of types (1) and (2) are used for the fusion assay. Leakage of type (3) vesicle contents is determined by measuring the decrease in fluorescence (initially set at 100%) when fusion is induced by LTX.

Vesicles (1 ml) are separated from nonencapsulated material by gel filtration on Sephadex G-75 (column size, 1.0 × 25 cm); elution buffer consists of 100 mM NaCl, 1 mM EDTA, 5 mM HEPES, pH 7.4.

A typical reaction mixture (1 ml) consists of Tb^{3+} and DPA vesicles at a 1 : 1 ratio (each 50 μM in lipid) together with 0.1 mM EDTA, 100 mM NaCl, 5 mM HEPES, pH 7.4. Before use in fusion experiments vesicles are kept at 4°C. α-Latrotoxin and other additives are added as concentrated solutions directly to the cuvette. The solution in the cuvette is continually stirred. The measurements are carried out at room temperature (20–22°C) in a fluorescence spectrophotometer at an excitation of 276 nm and an emission of 545 nm, employing a cutoff filter (>530 nm) to eliminate contribution to the signal from light scattering.

In a fusion experiment, the maximum fluorescence would be reached if all of the encapsulated Tb^{3+} were chelated by DPA and the percentage of the maximal fluorescence for fusion (denoted $\%F_{max}$) was just the percentage of the encapsulated Tb^{2+} that was complexed by DPA. In the absence of EDTA, 50 μM DPA is added to Tb^{3+} vesicles [at a concentration identical to the concentration of Tb^{3+} vesicles in the fusion assay (50 μmol of lipid/ml)]. Subsequently, sodium cholate (0.5%, w/v) is added to release the contents from the vesicles. The fluorescence observed after cholate addition is taken as a maximal (100%) value.

Some experiments were made with vesicles containing Tb^{3+}–DPA in order to test the ability of LTX to provoke leakage of liposomes.

It was shown that the LTX-induced fusion was dependent on the concentration of neurotoxin. The rate of membrane fusion increased dramatically from 2% F_{max} to 35% F_{max} during 10 min at LTX concentrations of 10^{-8} and 5×10^{-7} M, respectively. α-Latrotoxin promoted fusion of other negatively charged phospholipid vesicles containing PS or PC/CL (1 : 1 molar ratio). It is unclear whether the presence of acidic phospholipids is needed for toxin binding or if it is also important for successive stages of the fusion.

When LTX and Ca^{2+} were simultaneously added to the suspension of vesicles, the scope of fusion significantly increased at nonfusogenic levels of Ca^{2+}. Enhancement of the LTX-induced fusion of acidic liposomes by other divalent cations was also observed. However, the extent of fusion in the presence of Ca^{2+} was higher than that with other divalent cations.

Fusogenic activity of LTX was markedly affected by acid media. The scope of fusion increased and was two times more effective at pH 6.0 than at pH 7.4. At low pH, LTX exhibited a hydrophobic region that was cryptic at pH 7.4, which could be responsible for the interaction with lipid membranes. It is reasonable to suppose that in the near future a molecular understanding of the correlation between structure and lipid-binding properties will provide new information regarding the region of neurotoxin responsible for its anchorage into lipid bilayer.

α-Latrotoxin-Induced Fusion of Liposomes with Bilayer Lipid Membranes

Liposomes are formed by sonication of 45 mg of PC, 5 mg of cholesterol, and 0.5 mg of amphotericin B in 1 ml of solution containing 100 mM KCl, 0.5 mM EDTA, and 10 mM Tris-HCl, pH 7.4. Sonication is carried out in a

UZDN-2T ultrasonic desintegrator at 22-kHz frequency for 10 min. The liposomes are added to the membrane surrounding the solution at a final concentration of 1 mg of lipid/ml.

After LTX addition at the cis side of the compartment the membrane conductance is increased as a result of toxin insertion into the phospholipid bilayer. During perfusion of the cis side of the membrane by the same toxin-free solution its conductance is gradually stabilized. It is necessary to point out that after perfusion by toxin-free solution the lipid bilayer conductance becomes stable due to irreversible incorporation of toxin molecules into the bilayer membrane. Next, the perfusion of the cis side is performed using a solution containing 10 mM KCl, 0.5 mM EDTA, and 10 mM Tris-HCl. Under these asymmetric conditions the current amplitude and reversal potential are subject to change. The value of the reversal potential in these conditions (10/100 mM KCl) is 55–58 mV. From this we may conclude that LTX-induced channels possess practically ideal cationic selectivity.

To investigate the interaction between liposomes and the bilayer lipid membrane we use amphotericin B incorporated into liposomal membranes as an ionophoric marker (25). In comparing the amplitude of single amphotericin channels (26) and LTX channels, we had to conclude that contribution of amphotericin-induced channels to the conductance of membrane containing a large number of latrotoxin channels must be negligible. In this case the changes in membrane selectivity can indicate its fusion with liposomes. Amphotericin B was chosen because of its predominant anion selectivity (26). It is known that amphotericin B can form ionic channels in planar bilayers when applied to both sides simultaneously. We apply amphotericin-containing liposomes only to one side of the bilayer lipid membranes in each experiment. Thus we avoid the effects of non-liposome-bound amphotericin B on the bilayer conductance.

After adding liposomes with amphotericin B at the cis side of the membrane we did not observe marked changes in the current amplitude and the reversal potential. Introduction of the liposomes at the trans side of the membrane caused a gradual increase of current amplitude and a shift of the reversal potential, which amounted to 10–15% and 10–12 mV, respectively, at 10–30 min after addition of liposomes. Addition of 2 mM Cd^{2+}, which is an effective blocker of LTX channels (27), led to significant inhibition of the current amplitude and to a shfit of the reversal potential to the anionic permeability side. The resulting value of the reversal potential was still cationic but this was explained by incomplete inhibition of LTX-induced cation permeability.

Completely analogous results were obtained when we inhibited the amphotericin-containing liposome-induced gain of membrane conductance by means of an amphotericin B channel blocker, tetraethylammonium (28). Administration of 5 mM tetraethylammonium at the cis side of the membrane causes a decrease of current and a shift of the reversal potential to the values that they had before liposome administration to the membrane trans side.

Similar results were obtained when we studied the interaction of amphotericin-containing liposomes with the planar bilayer treated by LTX when its channels were blocked with Cd^{2+}. The addition of LTX at the cis side of the membrane was followed by an increase in membrane current. Stepwise current jumps were recorded. The amplitudes of these steps corresponded to those obtained by Robello *et al.* (19) under similar conditions. Further, while the toxin-free solution was perfused, the conductance of the membrane became stable. Addition of Cd^{2+} at the cis side of the membrane decreased the conductance practically to the baseline. Trans-side application of amphotericin-containing liposomes caused a slow increase in bilayer membrane conductance. The gain in conductance was not inhibited by Cd^{2+}, but addition of tetraethylammonium was accompanied by a decrease in the membrane conductance gain. It is necessary to point out that addition of the liposomes at the cis side of the membrane did not produce any changes in its conductance under similar conditions.

We can conclude that the planar bilayer modified by LTX shows increased conductance and acquires the anionic constituent of the permeability due to the fusion with amphotericin-containing liposomes. The validity of using amphotericin B as an ionophoric marker in experiments on the fusion of bilayer lipid membranes with liposomes was shown (25). Because we carried out all the control experiments described: (1) application of amphotericin B to one side of the membrane, (2) administration of amphotericin-containing liposomes to the unmodified membrane, and (3) the above-mentioned experiments, in which amphotericin-containing liposomes added to the cis side of the membrane modified by LTX did not produce any changes in membrane conductance or in reversal potential, we can state that the observed changes in current amplitude and reversal potential are due to the incorporation of amphotericin B into the bilayer lipid membrane as a result of their interaction with the liposomal membranes. Under our experimental conditions this observation provides evidence for liposome fusing with the bilayer membrane, as other ways by which amphotericin B might insert into the bilayer membrane were excluded by control experiments. The absence of effects in control experiments, and especially the asymmetry effect of LTX, have led us to the conclusion that fusion of liposomes with the planar bilayer is due to the α-latrotoxin inserted into the planar bilayer.

It was shown that LTX molecules incorporate into phospholipid bilayers in an oriented fashion (19). Experiments with pronase acting on the trans side of the planar bilayer proved that a segment of the LTX molecule protrudes into the trans side. These observations can explain the specific effect of "fusogenic," i.e., protruding, segments of the LTX molecules. According to this suggestion one concludes that the orientation of the LTX molecule in artificial and presynaptic membranes is similar. In this case the fusogenic segment of the LTX molecule can penetrate into the nerve ending and cause the fusion of synaptic vesicles with the presynaptic membrane without the participation of calcium ions in this process.

References

1. M. C. Tzeng and P. Siekevitz, *Brain Res.* **139,** 190 (1978).
2. N. Frontali, B. Ceccarelli, A. Gorio, A. Mauro, P. Siekevitz, M. C.Tzeng, and W. P. Hurlbut, *J. Cell Biol.* **68,** 462 (1976).
3. A. Gorio, L. Rubin, and A. Mauro, *J. Neurocytol.* **7,** 193 (1978).
4. A. Grasso and M. I. Senni, *Eur. J. Biochem.* **102,** 337 (1979).
5. E. I. Grebinozhko and A. N. Nikolaenko, *Ukr. Biokhim. Zh.* **59,** 93 (1987) (in Russian).
6. B. Z. Dalimov, S. K. Kasymov, and S. I. Salikhov, *Khim. Prir. Soedin.* **5,** 679 (1988) (in Russian).
7. Y. A. Ushkaryov and E. V. Grishin, *Bioorg. Khim.* **12,** 71 (1986) (in Russian).
8. H. E. Longnecker, W. P. Hurlbut, A. Mauro, and A. W. Clark, *Nature (London)* **225,** 701 (1970).
9. C. W. Cotman, *in* ''Methods in Enzymology'' (S. Fleisher and L. Packer, eds.), Vol. 31, p. 445. Academic Press, New York, 1974.
10. W. P. Hurlbut and B. Ceccarelli, *Adv. Cytopharmacol.* **3,** 87 (1979).
11. V. K. Lishko, E. V. Nikolishina, and N. G. Himmelreich, *Biokhimiya (Moscow)* **55,** 1375 (1990) (in Russian).
12. R. Snelling and D. Nichols, *Biochem. J.* **226,** 225 (1985).
13. R. Y. Tsien, *Biochemistry* **19,** 2396 (1980).
14. R. H. Ashley, M. I. Brammer, and R. Marchbanks, *Biochem. J.* **219,** 149 (1984).
15. R. Y. Tsien, T. Pozzan, and T. Y. Rink, *J. Cell Biol.* **94,** 325 (1982).
16. N. G. Himmelreich, E. A. Saichenko, L. G. Storchak, and V. K. Lishko, *Ukr. Biokhim. Zh.* **62,** 38 (1990) (in Russian).
17. D. M. Small and M. C. Bourges, *Biochem. Biophys. Acta* **125,** 566 (1966).
18. E. M. Egorova, L. V. Chernomordik, I. G. Abidor, and Y. A. Chizmadzhev, *Biofizika* **26,** 145 (1981) (in Russian).
19. M. Robello, R. Rolandi, S. Alema, and A. Grasso, *Proc. R. Soc. London Ser. B* **220,** 477 (1984).
20. V. K. Lishko, Y. T. Terletskaya, and I. O. Trikash, *FEBS Lett.* **266,** 99 (1990).
21. J. Wilschut, N. Duzgunes, R. Fraley, and D. Papahadjopoulos, *Biochemistry* **19,** 6011 (1980).
22. D. K. Struck, D. Hoekstra, and R. E. Pagano, *Biochemistry* **20,** 4093 (1983).
23. H. Ellens, J. Bentz, and F. C. Szoka, *Biochemistry* **24,** 3099 (1985).
24. F. C. Szoka and D. Papahadjopoulos, *Proc. Natl. Acad. Sci. U.S.A.* **75,** 3194 (1978).

25. M. Moore, *Biochim. Biophys. Acta* **426,** 765 (1976).
26. L. N. Ermishkin, K. M. Kasumov, and V. M. Potseluyev, *Nature (London)* **262,** 698 (1976).
27. S. L. Mironov, Y. V. Sokolov, A. N. Chanturiya, and V. K. Lishko, *Biochim. Biophys. Acta* **862,** 185 (1986).
28. M. P. Borisova, L. N. Ermishkin, and A. Y. Silberstein, *Biochim. Biophys. Acta* **553,** 450 (1979).

[21] Natural Toxins in Study of Degeneration and Regeneration of Skeletal Muscle

John B. Harris

Introduction

Muscle is a complex tissue that is subject to continuous work. Damage to skeletal muscle is common but not usually considered of great significance because of its ability to repair itself very rapidly. A number of diseases result in prolonged periods of muscle degeneration and, in some conditions, repair is incomplete or ineffective. It is difficult to study the biological processes involved in muscle degeneration/regeneration *in situ* in humans, because it is unacceptable to subject victims of degenerative diseases to sequential biopsy, unless the biopsy is directly related to diagnosis or treatment. It is clear, however, that an effective and rational treatment of such conditions requires a good understanding of degeneration and regeneration. For this reason a number of experimental procedures have been devised to allow research workers to address the problems of the development, growth, degeneration, and regeneration of skeletal muscle. The purpose of this chapter is to review briefly the techniques available and to describe in more detail the special characteristics and availability of myotoxic toxins isolated from the crude venoms of snakes. A guide to tissue processing is also provided, and key references are identified. The suggested readings at the end of the text are not intended to be complete. Rather, they should allow the reader easy access to the wider literature.

In Vitro or *in Vivo*?

There is considerable pressure from both regulatory authorities and voluntary organizations to study basic biological processes *in vitro* in either tissue or organ culture, and a great deal of work on the molecular, cellular, and developmental biology of muscle is made in tissue culture. There are, however, serious limitations to the use of such techniques in the study of the degeneration and regeneration of muscle: skeletal muscle does not grow to full maturity in culture. Under normal conditions the tissue requires an adequate vascular supply, a functional innervation, and exposure to a variety of hormones, growth factors, and autacoids for normal development, and

Methods in Neurosciences, Volume 8

mechanical work is involved in the growth and maturation of muscle. These conditions cannot easily be satisfied *in vitro*. The advantages of working *in vivo* are overwhelming.

What Pattern of Damage Is Required?

Assuming that the decision is made to work *in vivo,* it is necessary to consider whether the question being asked requires that the whole muscle or only a few individual muscle fibers be destroyed. It should also be asked whether the destruction of small segments of a few muscle fibers is appropriate.

Segmental necrosis is the term used to describe the situation where a small segment of a muscle fiber is destroyed in such a way that regions of the fiber on either side of that segment remain intact. It is a particularly useful form of damage for studies on the biology of inflammatory cell invasion, satellite cell activation and movement, and myofilament assembly and integration. It also has some potential for the study of the involvement of gene regulation *in vivo*. Typical techniques used for the induction of segmental necrosis are the application of hot or cold probes to the surface of muscle fibers, superficial transverse cuts across the fibers, and the local application of noxious substances such as aldehydes and alcohol. A useful introduction to some of the techniques and the problems that can be answered by studying segmental necrosis may be found in the report by Papadimitriou *et al.* (1). Similar techniques, suitably modified, can be used to produce damage to the entire length of limited numbers of superficial muscle fibers.

In many cases, the investigator will need to study the regeneration of an entire muscle, and this raises a number of specific questions.

Which Muscle Should Be Used?

If a whole muscle is to be used, it is clearly ideal to investigate a muscle sufficiently small to allow easy processing. This consideration limits the size of animal used to the smaller vertebrates such as amphibia, small reptiles, and small rodents such as rats and mice. Within such species, muscles that can be used for physiological as well as morphological and biochemical studies are ideal (it is often advantageous to make multidisciplinary studies) and so muscles that can be removed with a point of origin and attachment are preferred. The muscles also need to be accessible in the living, anesthetized animal. Typical choices of muscle would include the fourth lumbrical, soleus, extensor digitorum longus, and levator auris longus muscles of rodents, the toe muscles and sartorius muscle of amphibia, and the scale muscles of reptiles. The soleus and extensor digitorum longus muscles of rodents are particularly useful because of their differing fiber-type populations, and the fourth lumbrical muscle of the rat is useful because it has very few motor units and can be used to study with ease a number of functional problems associated with degeneration and regeneration. A particularly significant advantage of using the muscles of small rodents is that a very large number of previous studies is available for information and guidance.

How Should Muscles Be Damaged?

A number of mechanical and chemical methods have been used to initiate skeletal muscle damage. Of the mechanical methods, crushing, mincing, grafting, freezing, and burning have been commonly used. Most of the mechanical methods share the problem that they involve the destruction of the basal lamina, the microvasculature, and the innervation of the muscle fibers. The loss of the basal lamina is particularly important because it acts as a scaffold for the regeneration of muscle fibers (2).

Ischemia has also been used by several workers. The ligation of the primary blood supply to a muscle results in the onset of degeneration within hours; the ischemic muscle, however, tends not to regenerate properly and is usually replaced with scar tissue.

Several chemical methods have also been used to initiate degeneration and regeneration. The most commonly used agents are hypertonic saline (i.e., NaCl), local anesthetics such as bupivicaine, and snake venoms and toxins. For many purposes, bupivicaine is ideal. It is easily available from commercial sources, it causes the rapid degeneration of skeletal muscle without causing damage to basal lamina, satellite cells, or, apparently, the microvasculature. It may damage the terminal innervation, but the damage is limited and does not appear to affect the intramuscular nerves. Its principal disadvantage is that it is extremely difficult to effect the destruction of an entire muscle and muscle fibers within the central core of a muscle are often spared. This can be overcome by making intramuscular injections of the drug but this is a disadvantage because intramuscular injections clearly introduce an element of mechanical damage to the tissue.

The remainder of this chapter will be concerned exclusively with the use of myotoxic toxins in muscle research.

Myotoxic Toxins Isolated from Snake Venoms

Toxins capable of causing damage to skeletal muscle fall into two principal classes. The most potent are the myotoxic phospholipases. These toxins (of which approximately 25 have been identified) hydrolyze phospholipids at the ester bond of the C_2 chain of 3-*sn*-phosphoglycerides, liberating fatty acids and leaving the lysophosphatide as the reaction product. They are therefore classified as phospholipases A_2 (PLA_2). Calcium ion is an essential cofactor, and will activate the phospholipases at concentrations below 1.0 mM. Several detailed reviews of the chemistry and biological activity of snake venom PLA_2 are available and the reader is advised to consult them for further information (3–5).

A less potent class of myotoxins is that represented by myotoxin A, a short-chain peptide of 42 amino acids isolated from the venom of *Crotalus viridis viridis*. To date seven related toxins have been identified.

The various myotoxins of both classes have recently been tabulated by Mebs and Ownby (4), who provide primary references documenting the source and isolation of the toxins. The biological activities of the two classes of toxin differ quite significantly and there are also differences between toxins of the same general class. The characteristics of the two classes of toxin are therefore briefly discussed.

Myotoxic Phospholipases

The myotoxic phospholipases exhibit considerable variation in structure (see, e.g., Ref. 5). Many are single-chain polypeptides of approximately 120 amino acids cross-linked by 7 disulfide bridges. Others are a complex of two subunits, noncovalently linked. Characteristically, these latter toxins contain a single particularly toxic subunit that is basic, and a second, smaller acidic subunit. The acidic subunit tends to inhibit the PLA_2 activity of the toxic subunit, but enhance its myotoxicity. Yet another group of toxins (typified by taipoxin) consists of a complex of three subunits (5). Because little is known of the interaction of the subunits of complex toxins *in vivo*, it is clearly preferable to use single-chain toxins such as notexin as experimental tools.

Potency of Myotoxic Phospholipases

The myotoxins are highly variable in potency. The most toxic are probably notexin and notechis II-5. These have an LD_{50} (intravenous, iv) in the mouse of 0.2–0.5 mg/kg, and the injection of as little as 1–2 μg of pure toxin into a rat soleus muscle will destroy the entire population of muscle fibers (6). In contrast, the myotoxic phospholipases isolated from the venoms of *Pseudechis colletti* and *Bitis caudalis* are 25–50 times less potent (4). Unfortunately, many of the toxins identified as myotoxic have not been studied in detail and no single investigator has studied in depth, using standardized techniques, the range of myotoxic phospholipases. Much comparative information is therefore missing. Most data have been compiled as a result of studies on notexin, notechis II-5, and crotoxin (summarized in Ref. 5).

Variations in Sensitivity to Myotoxic Phospholipases

There are consistent reports that oxidative and oxidative/glycolytic muscle fibers are more susceptible to the toxic effects of the phospholipases than are the glycolytic fibers. Notexin, for example, will destroy the entire population of muscle fibers in the soleus muscle of the rat (this muscle is 60–80% oxidative and 20–40% oxidative/glycolytic) but will result in the checkerboard destruction of fibers in the extensor digitorum longus muscle (EDL), a muscle that is virtually identical in bulk to the soleus. The reason seems to be that the very large population of glycolytic fibers in EDL is largely insensitive to the toxins (6, 7). The biochemical basis for this difference in sensitivity is not known, but it has the obvious and important implication for those wishing to study muscle damage that the toxins cannot be easily used if muscles of mixed fiber type are to be studied.

A second generalization, but one made with fewer firm data available, is that immature muscle, and particularly muscle growing in tissue culture, is relatively insensitive to the toxins. Because tissue culture is such an important technique in the study of the regulation of gene activity in muscle development, it would be of great value if a suitable screening procedure could be established in the hope of identifying toxins that will either destroy or modify the differentiation of muscle growing *in vitro*. This must be feasible given the amount of information already available (8).

Apart from the variable sensitivity of different muscles to the myotoxic toxins, there is a bewildering variation between species in terms of sensitivity to the myotoxins. The muscles of dogs, rats, and chickens are very sensitive to notexin and the notexin homologs, and good evidence suggests that horse and goat muscle is also very sensitive, because these species are highly sensitive to the crude venom of *Notechis scutatus* (N. J. Sharpe, personal communication). Murine muscle is remarkably resistant to notexin. On the other hand, the available evidence suggests that there is less variation in sensitivity to crotoxin. The myotoxin of *Enhydrina schistosa* (toxin VI : 5) damages guinea pig muscle (9) and, probably, murine muscle (10) but has little effect on rat muscle (unpublished observations).

Muscle Damage Caused by Myotoxic Phospholipases

The features of muscle damage caused by the myotoxic PLA_2 have been described in a number of publications. Typically, muscle damage is visible at the light microscope level within 3–6 hr. The toxins cause a hypercontraction that results in the formation of clots of hypercontracted material separated by empty muscle fiber tubes [shown in electron microscopy (EM) to be tubes of basal lamina] caused by the tearing apart of weaker sarcomeres by the contractions of adjacent stronger sarcomeres. The hypercontracted material is rapidly invaded by a variety of inflammatory and phagocytic cells. In transverse section, this pathology is represented in a variety of ways: hyaline fibers, fiber profiles filled with invading cells, fibers devoid of contractile material, etc. (2, 6, 7). It is of great significance that satellite cells, basal lamina, and microcirculation remain intact. Indeed, the satellite cells are highly activated and muscle blood flow is actually enhanced during the early stages of degeneration (2). Peripheral nerve endings are destroyed by the myotoxic toxins but they regenerate rapidly. Myelinated intramuscular nerves appear to resist the effects of the myotoxic PLA_2. The reconstruction of neuromuscular junctions involves the regeneration of acetylcholine receptor (AChR; the receptors are lost along with the sarcolemma), but acetylcholinesterase (AChE; a component of the basal lamina) is unaffected so far as is known (Harris, 1984, unpublished observations).

The regeneration of the skeletal muscle fibers proceeds as follows: new myotubes are formed within the old basal lamina at 2–3 days after inoculation of toxin. Myofibrils begin to appear at the same time and by 4 days immature muscle fibers, virtually filled with contractile material, are formed. Provided the muscle fibers are innervated, muscles regain their normal bulk by 21–28 days. The regenerated muscles are essentially normal except (1) the fibers remain centrally nucleated and (2) all fibers are slow oxidative, elaborating only slow myosins (11). Neither feature is properly understood. Central nucleation may be specific for the muscles of rodents.

Short-Chain Myotoxins

These myotoxins have so far been isolated specifically from the venom of certain species of the genus *Crotalus*, although there is immunological evidence that some species of the related genus *Sistrurus* elaborate the toxins (4). The toxins consist of between 41 and 44 amino acid residues, crosslinked by 3 disulfide bridges. They are highly homologous and are unlike any other small peptides found in natural poisons of any kind.

Potency of Short-Chain Myotoxins

The toxins have an LD_{50} of approximately 1.0–3.0 mg/kg (iv), but data are rather incomplete (4). Typically 20–30 μg of the toxins needs to be injected into a typical murine muscle to effect significant damage.

Variations in Sensitivity to Short-Chain Myotoxins

There is no evidence of great variation in the sensitivity of different species or muscle fiber types to the short-chain myotoxins.

Muscle Damage Caused by Short-Chain Myotoxins

The short-chain myotoxins cause muscle contractures both *in vitro* and *in vivo*, and vacuolation of the muscle fibers, caused by dilatation of the sarcoplasmic reticulum (SR) (4). The dilatation of the SR appears at approximately 12 hr. The basic mechanism of this dilatation is not clear. Several possibilities have been suggested: direct action of the toxins on the SR, enhancement of Na^+ entry into the cell down its concentration gradient followed by water, and inhibition of SR ATPase activity, but no theory properly explains the phenomenon (for details, see Ref. 4). A clear understanding of the dilatation would be of considerable interest because dilatation of the SR is a common feature of many myopathies.

Muscle fibers in muscles exposed to the short-chain myotoxins become necrotic at about 3 days. It is tempting to speculate that the necrotic fibers are those that were earlier vacuolated but there is no definitive evidence that this is so. It is important to note that these toxins do not destroy an entire muscle, and that the typically patchy distribution of affected muscle fibers is not understood.

Disadvantages of Using Myotoxic Toxins

Many of the disadvantages of using myotoxic toxins have been introduced above. The most significant is probably the observation that some muscle fiber types are relatively insensitive to the toxins. This has proved to be a serious problem for those wishing to study the regeneration of fast twitch glycolytic fibers. There are also variations in the sensitivity of different species, and although some relevant information on this is easily obtained from original work, there are few detailed studies of species sensitivity.

Treatment of Animals

All the procedures used to induce muscle damage will cause some discomfort to the animal, although pain does not appear to be a significant problem unless the muscles are surgically exposed. It is strongly recommended that even the most trivial procedures be made under appropriate general anesthesia. If surgery is involved, a veterinarian should be consulted and postoperative analgesia should also be provided. In addition it is essential that the animals be housed and maintained with strict regard to local, national, or international guidelines governing the use of animals in biological research.

Injection of Toxins

The toxins will usually be available as lyophilized powders. They should be made up in solution with 0.9% (w/v) NaCl at such a concentration that the required amount of toxin can be injected into the rat in a volume of 0.2 ml or less, and into the mouse in a volume of 0.1 ml or less. Larger volumes tend to cause mechanical damage and will probably leak from the site of the injection. Charcoal or an innocuous dye can be incorporated in the toxin solution so that the precise site of injection can be identified.

The injection can be made immediately over the muscle of choice or into the muscle without surgical exposure. A 25-gauge needle or smaller should be used to minimize damage caused by its insertion. In larger animals, it may be necessary to expose the muscle and to inoculate the toxin under the fascia. In such cases trials should be run using 0.9% (w/v) NaCl to determine the volume that can be appropriately injected. Contralateral muscles can be used as appropriate controls as long as systemic damage has not occurred.

Availability of Myotoxic Toxins

Relatively few of the toxins are available commercially. Individual researchers are often prepared to sell samples, but the amounts available are usually limited. Notexin is commercially available in two grades from Latoxan (Rosans, France) and the company is prepared to consider requests for other pure toxins. Venom Supplies (Tanunda, South Australia) can supply notexin, taipoxin, and other toxins from Australian snakes. The toxins are usually stable if kept in the lyophilized form below 4°C and it is advisable to buy a single large sample of toxin isolated from a single batch of venom.

If the toxin(s) of interest are to be separated from relevant crude venoms it is essential that the crude venoms be purchased from a reliable source that uses, preferably, captive snakes of known species and origin maintained in humane conditions. Many suppliers of venoms are small organizations. A representative list of suppliers and their products can be found in any current *Newsletter of the International Society on Toxinology* available at modest cost from Dr. D. Mebs (Zentrum für Rechtsmedizin, The University of Frankfurt, Frankfurt, Germany).

Assessment of Myotoxicity

Many studies require an estimate of muscle damage caused experimentally. On purely intuitive grounds, it should not be difficult: damaged muscle releases creatine kinase, myoglobin, and aspartate aminotransferase, for example. It seems reasonable that any of these could be used as the basis of a quantitative assay. There are, however, problems with each. Creatine kinase (CK) appears to be released very early after the initiation of damage. Serum levels peak at 12 hr, but then decline very rapidly. The level of CK does not appear to correlate well with muscle damage, but that may be because most studies examine muscle for evidence of damage at 24 hr (the time at which damage to muscle fibers is virtually irreversible). Serum myoglobin levels could be extremely useful. Unfortunately, the manual (spectrophotometric) method of assay is relatively insensitive. It will not, for example, detect basal levels of myoglobin and immunoassays are unavailable because the commercially available myoglobin antibody is human specific. Aspartate aminotransferase activity has been shown to be of potential value, but has so far been properly validated only for notexin. It may not be universally applicable, especially if there is any possibility of kidney or liver damage. Problems with the assessment of damage have been discussed recently by Preston *et al.* (12).

Damage within a given muscle can be assessed quantitatively using histological criteria based on the numbers of necrotic fibers (12) or vacuolated fibers (13), as appropriate. The drawbacks of these techniques are that they are laborious, demand some expertise in the assessment of muscle pathology, and are not relevant to the study of systemic poisoning.

The development of an assay procedure relevant to the study of systemic muscle damage could be of immense value. An immunological method based on myoglobin release is probably the most promising candidate, but the release of other indicators of muscle breakdown, such as 3-methylhistidine, may also be worthy of serious exploration.

Is There Any Benefit to Using Crude Venoms?

Muscle damage is caused by a large number of snake venoms as a result of both offensive bites (see Refs. 2 and 5) and the injection of crude venom (see Refs. 2 and 5). In the study of degeneration and regeneration as biological events, there is no clear advantage to the use of crude venoms over toxins.

There are, however, several disadvantages, the most significant being that crude venoms are mixtures of many toxic and nontoxic fractions, and the precise composition of venom samples varies not only between individual snakes of the same species but even between samples of venom obtained at intervals from the same snake. Standardization can therefore be a problem.

If the aim is to study the response of skeletal muscle to natural venoms, there are very strong reasons for using the crude venoms rather than isolated toxins. The most important is that many of the relevant venoms contain synergistic toxins. For example, many venoms of viperid and crotalid snakes contain myotoxic, anticoagulant, and hemorrhagic components. The combination of such toxins can ensure that muscle damage is associated with the loss of or damage to the microvasculature and blood supply. Muscle regeneration thus occurs in conditions of ischemia and is typically impaired (14). Similarly the venoms of cobras contain a number of cytolytic toxins, commonly known as cardiotoxins. These toxins are strongly potentiated by PLA_2, a component present in all snake venoms (15). The cytolytic toxins have occasionally been used to initiate muscle damage (16) but such use is uncommon.

Any study involving the assessment of antivenoms and other potential therapeutic agents on myotoxicity should include observations on both the isolated myotoxins and the crude venoms.

Processing of Tissue for Examination of Muscle Damage

Essentially there are three methods of processing tissue to prepare tissue sections: paraffin embedding, resin embedding, and the use of frozen (cryostat) sections. Preston *et al.* (12) have outlined many of the pros and cons concerning these techniques (all of which are routinely used in laboratories working on tissue organization and pathology). Some studies may involve the investigation of temporal aspects of protein loss or expression in muscle fibers during a cycle of degeneration and regeneration. Western blotting of tissue extracts or homogenates may be used for studying the presence or absence of specific structural, cytoskeletal, or functional proteins but the localization of proteins within individual muscle fibers requires the use of more sophisticated techniques, such as immunohistochemistry and immunogold labeling; the latter technique, however, has not been extensively applied to skeletal muscle.

Techniques Used in Processing of Muscle Tissue

Paraffin Embedding and Sectioning

Muscles are removed from freshly killed animals and pinned onto a thin sheet of dental wax at approximately 1.2 times their resting length. They are then immersed in formol calcium for 12 hr. At this point the fixed muscle is dehydrated in graded ethanol, washed in chloroform (twice, 1.5–2 hr each time), and immersed in paraffin wax (54–56°C, twice for 2 hr). After the tissue is impregnated it is embedded in fresh wax in a plastic mold, and the wax is allowed to set. Sections 5 μm thick can be cut on a microtome. The sections are floated onto warm water (40–45°C), collected onto glass slides, and dried (1 hr at 60°C or overnight at 37°C). Typically they will be stained with hematoxylin and eosin for histological studies.

Resin Embedding and Sectioning

Muscles are removed from freshly killed animals and pinned onto a thin sheet of dental wax at approximately 1.2 times their resting length. Larger muscles such as the soleus or extensor digitorum longus muscles of the rat should be split longitudinally into two or three segments. The muscles are then fixed by immersion in 2.5% glutaraldehyde in cacodylate buffer (pH 7.4, 0.05 M for 24 hr). The tissue is then divided into small segments of approximately 1 mm^3, and reimmersed in fixative for 24 hr. Samples are then postfixed in osmium tetroxide (1%, v/v) for 1 hr, dehydrated by passage through graded ethanol, washed in propylene oxide embedded in resin, and baked (60°C overnight). The blocks can then be used for cutting semithin sections for light microscopy after staining in toluidine blue [0.1% (v/v) in 5% (w/v) borax] or for preparing thin sections for electron microscopy.

Fixation of Tissue in Situ

It is often appropriate to begin the process of fixation *in situ*. The animal is anesthetized to a surgical level. The thorax is rapidly opened and a perfusion needle is inserted into the left ventricle. The needle should be as large as can be accommodated within the ventricle. The right auricle is then opened and perfusion started with 0.9% (w/v) NaCl containing heparin (25,000–50,000 units/liter). The perfusion is best made using a small pump at a rate of 5–7 ml/min and a perfusion pressure of 60–80 mmHg. As soon as the perfusate is clear (this will be after the passage of 20–100 ml) the perfusate is changed to 2.5% glutaraldehyde in cacodylate buffer (pH 7.4, 0.05 M). Fixation is complete when the animal is rigid and muscle tissue has a waxy and yellow appearance. It is important to ensure that no air bubbles enter the animal because even small emboli can prevent adequate fixation. The muscles are removed, divided longitudinally, and immersed in 2.5% glutaraldehyde in cacodylate buffer. The procedure is then as described for resin embedding.

Cryosectioning

Freshly frozen tissue is particularly useful because it can be used for the majority of histochemical and immunocytochemical procedures. Freshly dissected muscles are removed and placed on H_2O-dampened filter paper in a closed moist chamber on ice. The belly segment of the muscle is cut out and packed in a support of either calf liver or a synthetic material such as OCT (BDH, Ltd., Poole, England). The tissue is then frozen by immersion in isopentane and maintained at a temperature of about $-150°C$ in liquid nitrogen. The frozen stubs are mounted onto a cryostat and sections are cut at 5 μm or thereabouts.

Cryosectioning and Immunogold Labeling for Electron Microscopy

Small segments of muscle are held slightly stretched in modified sprung hair grips and fixed [2% (v/v) formaldehyde plus 0.001% (v/v) glutaraldehyde for 1 hr]. They are washed in phosphate-buffered saline (pH 7.2), cut into small pieces (about 1 mm^3), and placed in sucrose (2.3 M, overnight). The pieces are then mounted on stubs and frozen (see above). Sections are cut at a knife temperature of $-110°C$ and a block temperature of $-90°C$. The sections are collected on grids coated with iced gelatin and quenched (80 mM ammonium chloride, 10 min). The grids are washed in 0.1 M phosphate-buffered saline (PBS) containing 0.5% (w/v) bovine serum albumin (BSA) plus 15% (v/v) glycine followed by normal goat serum diluted 1 : 20 with PBS plus BSA. The sections may then be incubated with primary and secondary (gold conjugated) antibodies as appropriate. The gold-conjugated antibodies can be obtained from BioCell (Cardiff, England).

Suggested Readings

Guides to Histology/Histochemistry/Histopathology/ Electron Microscopy

J. M. Polak and S. Van Norden (eds.), "Immunocytochemistry: Practical Applications in Pathology and Biology." Wright, Bristol, England, 1983.

M. I. Filipe and B. D. Lake (eds.), "Histochemistry in Pathology," 2nd Ed. Churchill-Livingstone, Edinburgh, Scotland, 1990.

A. M. Glauert (ed.), "Practical Methods in Electron Microscopy" (published in 13 volumes). North-Holland, Amsterdam, 1972 on.

General Reference Works on Crude Venoms and Natural Toxins

Journals

Toxicon (Pergamon, Oxford, England).

Journal of Toxicology: Toxin Reviews (Dekker, New York).

Books

B. Ceccarelli and F. Clementi (eds.), "Neurotoxins: Tools in Neurobiology." Raven, New York, 1979.

J. B. Harris (ed.), "Natural Toxins: Animal, Plant and Microbial." Clarendon, Oxford, England, 1986.

J. O. Dolly (ed.), "Neurotoxins in Neurochemistry." Ellis Horwood, Chichester, England, 1988.

D. Eaker and T. Wadstrom (eds.), "Natural Toxins." Pergamon, Oxford, England, 1980.

C. L. Ownby and G. V. Odell (eds.), "Natural Toxins: Characterization, Pharmacology and Therapeutics." Pergamon, Oxford, England, 1989.

A. T. Tu (ed.), "Handbook of Natural Toxins" (6 volumes planned; Vols. I to V are currently available). Dekker, New York, 1983 on.

A. L. Harvey (ed.), "International Encyclopedia of Pharmacology and Therapeutics," Section 134, Snake Toxins. Pergamon, Oxford, England. 1991.

D. Mebs and T. Shier (eds.), "Handbook on Toxinology." Dekker. In press.

References

1. J. M. Papadimitriou, T. A. Robertson, C. A. Mitchell, and M. D. Grounds, *J. Struct. Biol.* **103,** 124 (1990).
2. J. B. Harris and M. J. Cullen, *Electron Microsc. Rev.* **3,** 183 (1990).
3. P. Rosenberg, *in* "Neurotoxins in Neurochemistry" (J. O. Dolly, ed.), p. 27. Ellis Horwood, Chichester, England, 1988.
4. D. Mebs and C. L. Ownby, *Pharmacol. Ther.* **48,** 223 (1990).
5. J. B. Harris, *in* "International Encyclopedia of Pharmacology and Therapeutics" A. L. Harvey, ed.). Pergamon, Oxford, England, 1991.
6. J. B. Harris and M. A. Johnson, *Clin. Exp. Pharmacol. Physiol.* **5,** 587 (1978).
7. J. B. Harris, M. A. Johnson, and E. Karlsson, *Clin. Exp. Pharmacol. Physiol.* **2,** 383 (1975).
8. T. A. Linkhart, C. H. Clegg, and S. D. Haushka, *Dev. Biol.* **86,** 19 (1981).
9. S. L. Geh and H. T. Toh, *Toxicon* **16,** 633 (1978).
10. G. A. Brook, L. F. Torres, P. Gopalakrishnakone, and L. W. Duchen, *Q. J. Exp. Physiol.* **72,** 571 (1987).
11. R. G. Whalen, J. B. Harris, G. S. Butler-Browne, and S. Sesodia, *Dev. Biol.* **141,** 24 (1990).
12. S. A. Preston, C. Davis, and J. B. Harris, *Toxicon* **28,** 201 (1990).
13. C. L. Ownby, J. M. Gutierrez, T. B. Colberg, and G. V. Odell, *Toxicon* **20,** 877 (1982).
14. J. M. Gutierrez, C. L. Ownby, and G. V. Odell, *Exp. Mol. Pathol.* **40,** 367 (1984).
15. A. L. Harvey, *Toxin Rev.* **4,** 41 (1985).
16. R. Couteaux, J.-C. Mira, and A. D'Albis, *Biol. Cell.* **62,** 171 (1988).

[22] Neosurugatoxin: A Probe for Neuronal Nicotinic Receptors in Adrenal Medulla, Brain, and Ganglia

A. Wada, Y. Uezono, M. Arita, K. Tsuji, N. Yanagihara, H. Kobayashi, and F. Izumi

Introduction

Nicotinic receptors in nervous tissues are pharmacologically and structurally different from those in skeletal muscle and *Torpedo* electroplax (1, 2). Myogenic nicotinic receptors are inhibited by α-bungarotoxin and composed of four subunits having the stoichiometry $\alpha_2\beta\gamma\delta$ in fetal noninnervated skeletal muscle and electroplax or $\alpha_2\beta\varepsilon\delta$ in adult innervated skeletal muscle.

In rat brain, molecular biological studies have identified at least four distinct α subunits (α_2, α_3, α_4, and α_5) (3) and three β subunits (β_2, β_3, and β_4) (4) (α and β subunits of myogenic nicotinic receptors are designated α_1 and β_1). Although we do not know the stoichiometry of these subunits and the possible existence of other subunit(s) in *in vivo* neuronal nicotinic receptors, injection into *Xenopus* oocytes of mRNA encoding for α_2, α_3, or α_4 in pairwise combination with mRNA for β_2 or β_3 leads to the expression of functional nicotinic receptors (4–6).

α-Bungarotoxin does not suppress neuronal nicotinic receptor-mediated responses and the regional distribution of the toxin binding in the brain differs from that of acetylcholine or nicotine (7). Nicotinic agonists and antagonists bind to brain with dissociation constants (K_d) that are several orders of magnitude different from those required to exert pharmacological actions (7, 8). In addition, classical nicotinic agents do not discriminate between neuronal and muscular nicotinic receptors. Identification and characterization of neuronal nicotinic receptors require probes that exhibit high affinity and high selectivity for neuronal nicotinic receptors.

Neosurugatoxin was isolated in 1981 from the Japanese ivory mollusk *Babylonia japonica* (molecular formula, $C_{30}H_{34}N_5O_{15}Br \cdot H_2O$; M_r 802) (9, 10). The usefulness of neosurugatoxin as a potent and selective antagonist of neuronal nicotinic receptors has been documented. We first introduce our studies by examining the effects of neosurugatoxin on several distinct types of ion channels and catecholamine secretion in cultured bovine adrenal medullary cells, with special references to those of histrionicotoxin from the

Colombian frog *Dendrobates histrionicus* (11) and *d*-tubocurarine. The experiments from other laboratories on neosurugatoxin in brain and sympathetic and parasympathetic ganglia are also summarized.

Adrenal Medulla

Adrenal medulla, a paraneuron embryologically derived from the neural crest, is an excellent experimental system, because a large amount of homogeneous cell population can be readily cultured and quantitated with mutually related cellular responses such as ion permeability via (1) the nicotinic receptor–ion channel complex (12–16), (2) voltage-dependent Na^+ channels (12, 14–18), (3) voltage-dependent Ca^{2+} channels (12, 14–16, 18, 19), (4) voltage-dependent K^+ channels (15, 19), and (5) Ca^{2+}-dependent K^+ channels (15, 19), as well as (6) secretion of catecholamines (12–18) in an extremely reproducible manner.

Isolation (20) *and Primary Culture* (21) *of Bovine Adrenal Medullary Cells*

Oxygenated Krebs–Ringer phosphate buffer [mM: NaCl, 154; KCl, 5.6; $MgSO_4$, 1.1; $CaCl_2$, 2.2; NaH_2PO_4, 0.85; Na_2HPO_4, 2.15; glucose, 10; and 0.5% (w/v) bovine serum albumin (BSA), pH 7.4, adjusted by NaOH] is used unless otherwise indicated. Fresh bovine adrenal glands are perfused in retrograde fashion via adrenal vein (22) with Ca^{2+}-free, BSA-free Krebs–Ringer phosphate buffer at 37°C for 10 min by peristaltic pump. The adrenal cortex is removed by blade and the medulla is sliced by Stadie-Rigg slicers (Natume, Tokyo, Japan). The slices are washed with ice-cold Ca^{2+}-free, BSA-free, Krebs–Ringer phosphate buffer and then subjected to stepwise collagenase digestion twice, each being carried out at 37°C in a water bath with shaking at 120 excursions/min under 100% O_2. The first digestion is performed for 10 min in 20 ml digestion medium [Ca^{2+}-free Krebs–Ringer phosphate buffer containing 120 units/ml collagenase S-1 (Nacalai Tesque, Kyoto, Japan) and 50 μg/ml soybean trypsin inhibitor], after which the medium is filtered through a nylon mesh and the resultant filtrate is discarded. The slices are then subjected to a second digestion that is carried out for 60 min in 120 ml digestion medium and isolated cells are obtained by filtration. Cells are then washed three times by centrifugation (600 g, 2 min at 4°C), suspended in Krebs–Ringer phosphate buffer, and finally filtered to remove aggregated cells. Our procedures yield approximately 8 × 10^8 isolated cells from 10 bovine adrenal glands.

For culture of the isolated cells, Eagle's minimum essential culture medium, tubes, and pipettes are autoclaved at 120°C for 30 min. Isolated cells are washed three times with Eagle's minimum essential medium (pH 7.4 adjusted by NaHCO$_3$) supplemented with 10% (v/v) calf serum, 3 μM cytosine arabinoside, 60 μg/ml aminobenzylpenicillin, 100 μg/ml streptomycin, and 0.3 μg/ml amphotericin B, and suspended in the same composition of culture medium. Cells are plated at a density of 4 × 10^6 cells/dish (diameter: 35 mm; Falcon, Los Angeles, CA) and cultured at 37°C in 5% CO$_2$–95% air under a humidified atmosphere in a CO$_2$ incubator. Culture medium is changed every third day and cells are used for experiments between days 3 and 7 of culture.

Secretion of Catecholamines and Influx of $^{45}Ca^{2+}$

Culture medium is aspirated and cells are washed twice with 2 ml ice-cold Krebs–Ringer phosphate buffer. Incubation is initiated by adding 2 ml prewarmed (37°C) Krebs–Ringer phosphate buffer that contains 2 μCi ^{45}CaCl$_2$ (Amersham, Arlington Heights, IL) with or without carbachol, veratridine, high concentrations of extracellular K$^+$, neosurugatoxin, histrionicotoxin, and d-tubocurarine. High K$^+$ medium is prepared by reducing NaCl to maintain the isotonicity of the solution. Neosurugatoxin is dissolved in dimethyl sulfoxide at concentrations between 20 nM and 2 mM, stored at −80°C, and diluted 200-fold in incubation medium immediately before use. Incubations are carried out at 37°C for up to 5 min with gentle shaking in an environmental incubator shaker (G24; New Brunswick Scientific Co. Inc., Edison, NJ). The reaction is terminated by adding one of the antagonists [selected depending on the secretagogue used: hexamethonium (1 mM), tetrodotoxin (1 μM), and diltiazem (1 mM), final concentration], after which the medium is immediately transferred to a test tube, and the cells are washed four times with 2 ml ice-cold Ca^{2+}-free Krebs–Ringer phosphate buffer to remove extracellular ^{45}Ca^{2+}. Catecholamines are acidified by 0.4 M perchloric acid, adsorbed to aluminum hydroxide, and estimated by the ethylenediamine condensation method (23), using a Hitachi (Tokyo, Japan) F-4010 fluorescence spectrophotometer with an excitation wavelength of 420 nm and emission wavelength of 540 nm. Cells (4 × 10^6) contain 49.2 ± 8.3 μg (n = 21) of catecholamines as epinephrine plus norepinephrine. Calcium-45 in the cells is solubilized in 1 ml Triton X-100 and radioactivity is counted in toluene base scintillator using a Beckman (Palo Alto, CA) LS-7000 liquid scintillation counter. The amount of Ca^{2+} influx is calculated from the initial specific activity of ^{45}Ca^{2+} in the incubation medium.

Influx of $^{22}Na^+$

Influx of $^{22}Na^+$ is estimated by the same procedure used to estimate $^{45}Ca^{2+}$ influx, except that cells are incubated with 2 μCi ^{22}NaCl (New England Nuclear, Boston, MA) in 1 ml Krebs–Ringer phosphate buffer.

Results and Discussion

In the stimulus–secretion coupling of adrenal medulla, the influx of Ca^{2+} via voltage-dependent Ca^{2+} channels is indispensable to trigger the secretion of catecholamines. In addition, we previously showed that either carbachol-induced Na^+ influx via nicotinic receptor–ion channel complexes or veratridine-induced Na^+ influx via voltage-dependent Na^+ channels activates voltage-dependent Ca^{2+} channels, whereas high K^+ directly gates voltage-dependent Ca^{2+} channels without increasing Na^+ influx (12, 13, 17).

Nicotinic Receptor–Ion Channel Complex

Carbachol caused rapid and transient influx of $^{22}Na^+$, $^{45}Ca^{2+}$, and secretion of catecholamines that attained a plateau at 1 min (12, 13). Carbachol (300 μM) increased Na^+ influx by 245.6 ± 15.0 nmol ($n = 10$) and Ca^{2+} influx by 5.5 ± 0.4 nmol ($n = 8$) per 4×10^6 cells, and secretion of catecholamines by 6.2 ± 0.3 μg ($n = 8$) over the basal values (Na^+ influx 10.4 ± 0.8, Ca^{2+} influx 0.5 ± 0.1, and secretion 0.6 ± 0.2) ($n = 10$) obtained in nonstimulated cells. Neosurugatoxin, histrionicotoxin, and d-tubocurarine, at concentrations higher than 0.1 nM, 0.1 μM, and 1 μM, respectively, inhibited carbachol-induced events without affecting basal responses (Fig. 1). The concentration–inhibition curves of each agent for carbachol-induced influx of $^{22}Na^+$, $^{45}Ca^{2+}$, and secretion of catecholamines were similar to each other. Our results suggest that these agents decreased catecholamine secretion by interfering with Ca^{2+} influx. Neosurugatoxin and histrionicotoxin, however, did not inhibit voltage-dependent Ca^{2+} channels (see below). Because carbachol-induced Na^+ influx contributes to Ca^{2+} influx and proceeds via nicotinic receptor–ion channel complexes (but not via voltage-dependent Na^+ channels) (12, 13), present observations suggest that the inhibition of Na^+ influx via nicotinic receptor–ion channel complexes is responsible for the reduction of Ca^{2+} influx. The IC_{50} (half-maximal inhibitory concentration) values of neosurugatoxin, histrionicotoxin, and d-tubocurarine required to suppress carbachol-induced $^{22}Na^+$ influx were 27 nM, 3 μM, and 3.9 μM, respectively. Our results agree with those by Bourke et $al.$ (24) in adrenal medulla, which showed that neosurugatoxin reversibly inhibited nicotine (5 μM)-induced

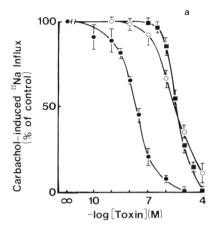

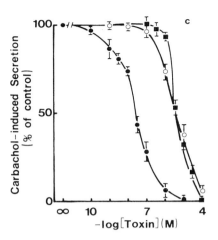

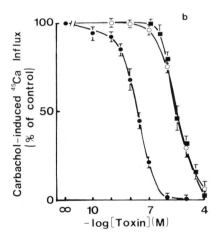

FIG. 1   Inhibitory potency of neosur-ugatoxin, histrionicotoxin, and *d*-tu-bocurarine for carbachol-induced (a) $^{22}Na^+$ influx, (b) $^{45}Ca^{2+}$ influx, and (c) catecholamine secretion in cultured bovine adrenal medullary cells. In an environmental incubator shaker, cells were incubated at 37°C for 1 min in Krebs–Ringer phosphate buffer con-taining 2 μCi $^{22}NaCl$ or $^{45}CaCl_2$ with or without 300 μM carbachol, various concentrations of neosurugatoxin (●), histrionicotoxin (○), and *d*-tubo-curarine (■). Basal values at 37°C without carbachol were subtracted and carbachol-induced responses in the absence of test compound were assigned a value of 100%. Mean ± SD from 8 to 10 separate experiments. (Reprinted with permission from Ref. 16, Pergamon Press PLC.)

catecholamine secretion with an IC_{50} value of 30 nM. The sensitivity of nicotinic receptors to neosurugatoxin in adrenal medulla is comparable with that reported in parasympathetic ganglia (25) and brain (25–27).

Inhibitory effects of neosurugatoxin on carbachol-induced influx of ^{22}Na$^+$ and ^{45}Ca^{2+} and on secretion of catecholamines were reversed by the increased concentrations of carbachol, while those of histrionicotoxin were not (Fig. 2). These results suggest that neosurugatoxin shares the common binding sites with carbachol and inhibits the interaction between carbachol and its recognition sites in a competitive manner in adrenal medulla. Pharmacological experiments in parasympathetic ganglia (25) and [^{3}H]nicotine-binding

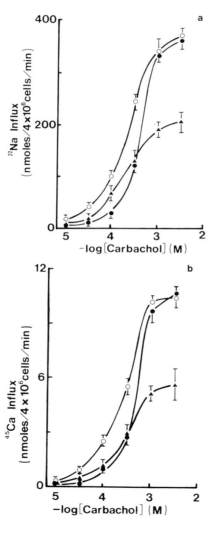

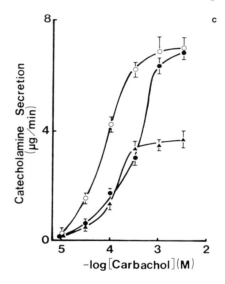

FIG. 2   Inhibitory mode of neosurugatoxin and histrionicotoxin for carbachol-induced (a) ^{22}Na$^+$ influx, (b) ^{45}Ca^{2+} influx, and (c) catecholamine secretion. In the absence (○) or presence of neosurugatoxin (30 nM; ●) and histrionicotoxin (3 μM; ▲), cells (4 × 10^6) were stimulated at 37°C for 1 min with or without 10 μM–3 mM carbachol. Values at 37°C were subtracted. Mean ± SD from four to six experiments. (Reprinted with permission from Ref. 16, Pergamon Press PLC.)

studies in brain (26, 28), on the other hand, suggested that neosurugatoxin inhibits nicotinic receptors in a noncompetitive manner. The apparent discrepancy in the inhibitory mode of neosurugatoxin on nicotinic receptors so far examined may be related to the existence of multiple subtypes of neuronal nicotinic receptors (1–6, 29).

The selectivity of neosurugatoxin for nicotinic over muscarinic receptors has been shown by the lack of effects of neosurugatoxin on muscarinic receptor-mediated phosphatidylinositol metabolism in adrenal medulla (24), contraction of ileum (25), and the binding of muscarinic drugs to brain membranes (25, 26, 28).

Voltage-dependent Na$^+$ Channels

Veratridine induced sustained influx of ^{22}Na$^+$ and ^{45}Ca^{2+} and secretion of catecholamines for at least 5 min (12, 17). During a 5-min period, veratridine (100 μM) increased Na$^+$ influx by 248.9 $\pm$ 16.3 nmol ($n = 6$), Ca^{2+} influx by 6.9 $\pm$ 0.4 nmol ($n = 7$) per 4×10^6 cells, and secretion of catecholamines by 6.4 $\pm$ 0.5 μg ($n = 7$). Neosurugatoxin did not affect veratridine-induced events, indicating that neosurugatoxin has no effect on voltage-dependent Na$^+$ channels (Fig. 3). Histrionicotoxin at concentrations higher than 10 μM reduced veratridine-induced influx of ^{22}Na$^+$ and ^{45}Ca^{2+} and secretion with an IC$_{50}$ value of 50 μM. Because histrionicotoxin did not inhibit voltage-dependent Ca^{2+} channels (see below) and veratridine-induced Na$^+$ influx is requisite for Ca^{2+} influx (12, 17), the present results suggest that histrionicotoxin inhibited Na$^+$ influx via voltage-dependent Na$^+$ channels and thereby reduced Ca^{2+} influx and catecholamine secretion.

Voltage-Dependent Ca^{2+} Channels

High K$^+$ evoked rapid and transient influx of ^{45}Ca^{2+} and secretion of catecholamines that reached a maximum at 1 min, but did not increase ^{22}Na$^+$ influx (12). In 1 min, high K$^+$ (56 mM)-induced increments in Ca^{2+} influx and secretion amounted to 6.3 $\pm$ 0.3 nmol ($n = 5$) per 4×10^6 cells and 5.9 $\pm$ 0.1 μg ($n = 5$), respectively. Neosurugatoxin (1 μM) and histrionicotoxin (100 μM) did not alter high K$^+$-induced responses (data not given) (16), indicating that both toxins do not interfere with voltage-dependent Ca^{2+} channels.

Brain

[^{3}H]Dopamine Release from Striatal Synaptosomes

In perfused rat striatal synaptosomes, in which presynaptic nicotinic receptors mediate dopamine release, Rapier et al. (30, 31) measured the ratio of second/first (S_2/S_1) evoked release of [^{3}H]dopamine. Addition of neosuruga-

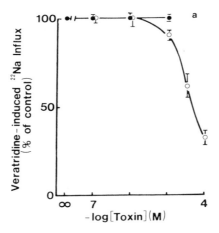

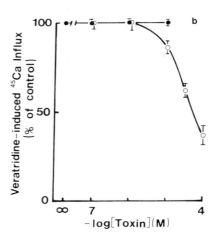

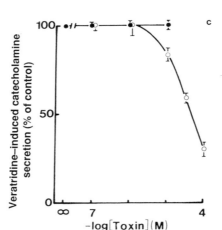

FIG. 3 Effects of neosurugatoxin and histrionicotoxin on veratridine-induced (a) $^{22}Na^+$ influx, (b) $^{45}Ca^{2+}$ influx, and (c) catecholamine secretion. Cells were stimulated at 37°C for 5 min with or without 100 μM veratridine and indicated concentrations of neosurugatoxin (●) and histrionicotoxin (○). Values at 37°C were subtracted. A value 100% represents veratridine-induced response in the absence of test compound. Mean ± SD from four experiments. (Reprinted with permission from Ref. 16, Pergamon Press PLC.)

toxin (50 nM) 10–20 min before the second stimulation reduced S_2/S_1 caused by dimethylphenylpiperazinium (1–5 μM) or nicotine (1 μM) to 59 and 46.5% of the control ratio, but had no effect on S_2/S_1 due to high K^+ (16–28 mM).

Luteinizing Hormone Secretion from Adenohypophysis

In ovariectomized rats, Billiar *et al*. (32) injected neosurugatoxin into the third ventricle and determined the concentrations of luteinizing hormone (LH) in right atrial blood. Injection of neosurugatoxin (0.2–1 μg) every 15 min for 2 hr decreased the frequency of pulsatile secretion of LH by 40–44% without affecting the amplitude of LH secretion pulses. Although the anatomical site(s) of action of neosurugatoxin is not known, coadministration of cytidine (1 μg), a nicotinic agonist, blocked the inhibitory effect of neosurugatoxin (0.2 μg).

Nicotine-Induced Antinociception

Antinociceptive responses caused by subcutaneous injection of nicotine have been suggested to be mediated via nicotinic receptors in central nervous system. Using the mouse tail-flick method, Yamada *et al.* (27) observed that subcutaneous injection of neosurugatoxin (0.4–3.8 nmol/kg) 10 min prior to nicotine administration inhibited nicotine-induced antinociception with an IC_{50} value of 0.65 nmol/kg, a value three to four orders of magnitude lower than that of nicotinic antagonists mecamylamine, pempidine, and hexamethonium.

Nicotinic Receptors Expressed in Xenopus Oocytes

Recent molecular cloning studies in rat brain have demonstrated at least seven distinct genes possibly encoding for neuronal nicotinic receptors (2). Four of these genes contain contiguous cysteine residues, at positions homologous to 192 and 193 in the *Torpedo* sequence, that seem to be important in the binding of acetylcholine; they are classified as α subunits (3). The residual three genes lacking these cysteine residues are designated β subunits (4). Although the functional role of α_5 and β_3 subunits is not known, mRNAs encoding for either α subunit in combination with either β subunit have been documented to form electrically excitable nicotinic receptors in the *Xenopus* oocyte expression system (4–6). Electrophysiological studies of oocytes by Luetje *et al.* (29) revealed that incubation with neosurugatoxin (2 nM) for 30 min almost abolished acetylcholine-induced current responses of $\alpha_2\beta_2$, $\alpha_3\beta_2$, and $\alpha_4\beta_2$, but little affected those of $\alpha_1\beta_1\gamma\delta$ (myogenic nicotinic receptors). Washing oocytes for 60 min to remove neosurugatoxin resulted in partial recovery of the responses of $\alpha_3\beta_2$ (45.7% still inhibited) and $\alpha_4\beta_2$ (36.5% still inhibited).

[^{3}H]Nicotine Binding

Brain Membranes

In Vitro Study

In rat borebrain membranes, Yamada *et al.*(26) reported that neosurugatoxin inhibited [^{3}H]nicotine binding with an IC_{50} value of 78 nM and the competition curve by the toxin was biphasic (pseudo Hill slope, 0.44). The potency of neosurugatoxin was approximately 140, 165, 1350, 2000, and 6000 times greater than that of decamethonium, d-tubocurarine, pentolinium, hexamethonium, and mecamylamine. Scatchard analysis revealed that neosurugatoxin reduced the maximal binding capacity (B_{max}) of [^{3}H]nicotine without altering its K_d, suggesting that the toxin noncompetitively inhibited nicotine binding. The inhibition by neosurugatoxin was not readily reversible. Neosurugatoxin (10 μM), on the other hand, did not suppress the binding of [^{3}H] quinuclidinyl benzylate to muscarinic receptors and of ^{125}I-labeled α-bungarotoxin, a selective ligand for myogenic nicotinic receptors, to brain membranes.

In Vivo Study

Rats injected with neosurugatoxin (3.2 μg twice, at 24-hr intervals) into the lateral ventricle were decapitated 3, 7, and 14 days after the first administration of the toxin, and [^{3}H]nicotine binding to membranes was examined in various regions of brain (28). After 3 days, [^{3}H]nicotine binding was reduced in cerebral cortex, hippocampus, and thalamus, but not in striatum, cerebellum, and brainstem. Binding of cis-[^{3}H]methyldioxolane to muscarinic receptors was not decreased in cerebral cortex and hippocampus. In cerebral cortex, Scatchard analysis showed that the B_{max} of [^{3}H]nicotine was reduced by 51.6 and 28.4% after 3 and 7 days, respectively, but the K_d was not changed. At 14 days after toxin administration, however, the B_{max} of [^{3}H]nicotine in toxin-injected rats became comparable with that of control rats.

Brain Sections

In slide-mounted tissues, neosurugatoxin inhibited [^{3}H]methylcarbamylcholine binding to rat thalamus with an IC$_{50}$ value of 338 nM, a value 259 times lower than that of hexamethonium (33).

Autoradiographic studies by Billiar et al. (32) showed that neosurugatoxin (10 μM) abolished [^{3}H]nicotine binding, but not ^{125}I-labeled α-bungarotoxin binding to medial habenular nucleus.

Sympathetic Ganglia

Surugatoxin, a compound structurally related to neosurugatoxin, was isolated along with neosurugatoxin from B. japonica. Surugatoxin was subsequently shown to be inactive as a toxin and its toxic effects previously reported seem to be attributed to the contaminating neosurugatoxin (9, 10). Hayashi and Yamada (34) found that intraarterial injection of surugatoxin (6.2–12.3 nmol/kg) into cat superior cervical ganglia suppressed the contraction of nictitating membrane caused by preganglionic, but not postganglionic, electrical stimulation of cervical nerve. Brown *et al.* (35) reported that suruga-toxin (0.1–2 μM) depressed carbachol-induced depolarization of rat superior cervical ganglia in a competitive manner. Surugatoxin (12.3 μM), on the other hand, failed to inhibit the contraction of rat diaphragm elicited by phrenic nerve stimulation (34).

Parasympathetic Ganglia

In guinea pig ileum pretreated with neosurugatoxin for 5 min, the concentra-tion–response curves for nicotine-induced contraction of smooth muscle were shifted to the right and the maximal contraction was also depressed as the concentration of neosurugatoxin was increased to 3 and 30 nM (25). It seems that neosurugatoxin inhibits nicotinic receptors at parasympathetic ganglia in a noncompetitive manner.

Acknowledgments

The authors would like to thank Dr. J. W. Daly, National Institutes of Health (Bethesda, MD) for his generous gift of histrionicotoxin. We also thank Ms. Yumiko Toyohira for line drawings.

References

1. J. Lindstrom, R. Schoepfer, and P. Whiting, *Mol. Neurobiol.* **1**, 281 (1987).
2. C. W. Luetje, J. Patrick, and P. Séguéla, *FASEB J.* **4**, 2753 (1990).
3. S. Couturier, L. Erkman, S. Valera, D. Rungger, S. Bertrand, J. Boulter, M. Ballivet, and D. Bertrand, *J. Biol. Chem.* **265**, 17560 (1990).
4. R. M. Duvoisin, E. S. Deneris, J. Patrick, and S. Heinemann, *Neuron* **3**, 487 (1989).
5. K. Wada, M. Ballivet, J. Boulter, J. Connolly, E. Wada, E. S. Deneris, L. W. Swanson, S. Heinemann, and J. Patrick, *Science* **240**, 330 (1988).
6. J. Boulter, J. Connolly, E. Deneris, D. Goldman, S. Heinemann, and J. Patrick, *Proc. Natl. Acad. Sci. U.S.A.* **84**, 7763 (1987).
7. P. B. S. Clarke, *Trends Pharmacol. Sci.* **8**, 32 (1987).
8. S. Wonnacott, *Hum. Toxicol.* **6**, 343 (1987).
9. T. Kosuge, K. Tsuji, K. Hirai, K. Yamaguchi, T. Okamoto, and Y. Iitaka, *Tetrahedron Lett.* **22**, 3417 (1981).
10. T. Kosuge, K. Tsuji, and K. Hirai, *Chem. Pharm. Bull.* **30**, 3255 (1982).

11. C. E. Spivak, M. A. Maleque, A. C. Olivera, L. M. Masukawa, T. Tokuyama, J. W. Daly, and E. X. Albuquerque, *Mol. Pharmacol.* **21**, 351 (1982).
12. A. Wada, H. Takara, F. Izumi, H. Kobayashi, and N. Yanagihara, *Neuroscience* **15**, 283 (1985).
13. A. Wada, H. Takara, N. Yanagihara, H. Kobayashi, and F. Izumi, *Naunyn-Schmiedeberg's Arch. Pharmacol.* **332**, 351 (1986).
14. M. Arita, A. Wada, H. Takara, and F. Izumi, *J. Pharmacol. Exp. Ther.* **243**, 342 (1987).
15. A. Wada, M. Arita, N. Yanagihara, and F. Izumi, *Neuroscience* **25**, 687 (1988).
16. A. Wada, Y. Uezono, M. Arita, K. Tsuji, N. Yanagihara, H. Kobayashi, and F. Izumi, *Neuroscience* **33**, 333 (1989).
17. A. Wada, F. Izumi, N. Yanagihara, and H. Kobayashi, *Naunyn-Schmiedeberg's Arch. Pharmacol.* **328**, 273 (1985).
18. A. Wada, Y. Uezono, M. Arita, Y. Yanagawa, M. Satake, and F. Izumi, *Naunyn-Schmiedeberg's Arch. Pharmacol.* **342**, 323 (1990).
19. A. Wada, H. Kobayashi, M. Arita, N. Yanagihara, and F. Izumi, *Neuroscience* **22**, 1085 (1987).
20. J. Brooks, *Endocrinology (Baltimore)* **101**, 1369 (1977).
21. D. L. Kilpatrick, F. H. Ledbetter, K. A. Carson, A. G. Kirshner, R. Slepetis, and N. Kirshner, *J. Neurochem.* **35**, 679 (1980).
22. J. L. Borowitz, *Biochem. Pharmacol.* **18**, 713 (1969).
23. H. Weil-Malherbe, *Biochem. J.* **51**, 311 (1952).
24. J. E. Bourke, S. J. Bunn, P. D. Marley, and B. G. Livett, *Br. J. Pharmacol.* **93**, 275 (1988).
25. E. Hayashi, M. Isogai, Y. Kagawa, N. Takayanagi, and S. Yamada, *J. Neurochem.* **42**, 1491 (1984).
26. S. Yamada, M. Isogai, Y. Kagawa, N. Takayanagi, E. Hayashi, K. Tsuji, and T. Kosuge, *Mol. Pharmacol.* **28**, 120 (1985).
27. S. Yamada, Y. Kagawa, N. Takayanagi, E. Hayashi, K. Tsuji, and T. Kosuge, *Brain Res.* **375**, 360 (1986).
28. S. Yamada, H. Ushijima, K. Nakayama, E. Hayashi, K. Tsuji, and T. Kosuge, *Eur. J. Pharmacol.* **156**, 279 (1988).
29. C. W. Luetje, K. Wada, S. Rogers, S. N. Abramson, K. Tsuji, S. Heinemann, and J. Patrick, *J. Neurochem.* **55**, 632 (1990).
30. C. Rapier, R. Harrison, G. G. Lunt, and S. Wonnacott, *Neurochem. Int.* **7**, 389 (1985).
31. C. Rapier, G. G. Lunt, and S. Wonnacott, *J. Neurochem.* **54**, 937 (1990).
32. R. B. Billiar, J. Kalash, V. Romita, K. Tsuji, and T. Kosuge, *Brain Res. Bull.* **20**, 315 (1988).
33. S. Yamada, D. R. Gehlert, K. N. Hawkins, K. Nakayama, W. R. Roeske, and H. I. Yamamura, *Life Sci.* **41**, 2851 (1987).
34. E. Hayashi and S. Yamada, *Br. J. Pharmacol.* **53**, 207 (1975).
35. D. A. Brown, J. Garthwaite, E. Hayashi, and S. Yamada, *Br. J. Pharmacol.* **58**, 157 (1976).

[23] Neurotoxins as Tools in Characterization of γ-Aminobutyric Acid-Activated Chloride Channels

Frank Zufall

Introduction

γ-Aminobutyric acid (GABA) is the major inhibitory transmitter in the central nervous system of both vertebrates and invertebrates (crustacea, insects). In addition, it plays a key role in peripheral inhibition at the neuromuscular junction of invertebrates. Vertebrate GABA receptors have been subdivided into two major classes: $GABA_A$ receptors directly operate chloride channels, are activated by muscimol, and are selectively and reversibly inhibited by the plant alkaloid bicuculline, whereas $GABA_B$ receptors couple to Ca^{2+} and K^+ channels via GTP-binding proteins and are activated by baclofen (1). The $GABA_A$ receptor of mammalian brain has been extensively characterized by the application of biochemical and molecular cloning techniques. It is a heterooligomeric protein composed of at least four subunits (α, β, γ, δ) (reviewed in Ref. 2) and can be purified from the cow cerebral cortex by using benzodiazepine affinity chromatography. These studies have also established that the $GABA_A$ receptor, together with nicotinic acetylcholine receptors and glycine receptors, is a member of the superfamily of ligand-gated receptor–ion channel complexes (3). In invertebrates, most GABA receptors resemble the vertebrate $GABA_A$ subtype in that they operate chloride channels and are activated by muscimol (4, 5). However, because most invertebrate GABA receptors are insensitive to bicuculline (5), the plant alkaloid picrotoxin, which has a strong convulsant action in vertebrates and invertebrates, became an important tool as antagonist. A $GABA_B$ receptor has not been found in arthropods so far.

Particular interest in the GABA receptor–chloride channel complex is based on the fact that this protein is a major molecular target for many clinically important drugs such as sedative barbiturates and anxiolytic benzodiazepines, as well as drugs of abuse such as alcohol (6). It has also been recognized as an important target contributing to the neurotoxicity of some groups of insecticides (7) and naturally occurring toxins such as certain mycotoxins (7).

When neurotoxins are used as tools in the characterization of neurotransmitter receptors, e.g., for binding studies, it is desirable to know the exact molecular mode of action of these substances. This chapter is focused on electrophysiological mode of action studies and describes two examples of toxin tools for the GABA receptor. The first part deals with the action of picrotoxin, and the second part describes the effect of an important mycotoxin, avermectin B_{1a}, on GABA-activated chloride channels. The work reported here was done using patch-clamp recordings from crustacean muscles.

Picrotoxin

Picrotoxin, found in the shrub *Anamirta cocculus,* consists of two components, picrotoxinin and picrotin, in a 1:1 molar ratio (8). The chemical structure of picrotoxinin, the active component, is shown in Fig. 1A. Picrotoxin played an important role in the pioneering work of establishing GABA as an inhibitory transmitter at the crustaceen neuromuscular junction because of its antagonistic effect on inhibitory postsynaptic potentials at this synapse (9–11). The mechanism by which picrotoxin exerts its action has been discussed and is a subject of controversy. Historically, picrotoxin has been classified as a channel blocker. Using the patch-clamp technique it can be shown that picrotoxin does not block the open chloride channel but most probably acts as an allosteric antagonist.

Intrinsic gm6b stomach muscles (12) from crayfish (*Austropotamobius torrentium*), which are not innervated by inhibitory axons (13), were isolated and treated with 2 mg/ml collagenase (1A; Sigma, St. Louis, MO) for 30 min at 18°C in order to remove connective tissue. Outside-out patches were established as described (14–17) and moved to a recording chamber that could be perfused separately. A special concentration step technique, the "liquid filament switch," (18) was used for applying concentration steps of various drugs: A liquid filament of 30-μm diameter is ejected into the superfusing solution from a small tube that can be shifted by a piezocrystal to hit the outside-out patch at the tip of a stationary patch electrode. This technique allows an electrically triggered and ultrafast application of test solutions within 200 μsec. The modified van Harreveld solution used for the preparation and the patches contained the following (mM): NaCl, 220; KCl, 5.4; CaCl$_2$, MgCl$_2$, 2.5; and Tris–maleate buffer, 10, at pH 7.6. The high-chloride intracellular solution contained the following (mM): KCl, 150; NaCl, 5; MgCl$_2$, 2; CaCl$_2$, 1; Tris–maleate buffer, 10, at pH 7.2. Recording and evaluation of the patch-clamp data have been described in detail (14–19).

Figure 1B shows an example of the current evoked by the pulsed application of 1 mM GABA. An outside-out patch was held under voltage clamp at

-85 mV, near the reversal potential of potassium. The application of GABA (for 2 sec) elicited a chloride current of about -400 pA, accompanied by an increase in the noise level of the current trace due to fluctuations in the number of open channels. The GABA-activated current rose to a maximum within 100 msec and receptor desensitization occurred with a time constant of minutes (20). This current is due to the simultaneous activation of about 100 single chloride channels, as calculated from the single-channel amplitude at this potential (14). This striking channel density was found regularly in these patches and offered the possibility of whole cell-like experiments at excised patches. When 1 mM GABA and 10 μM picrotoxin were applied simultaneously, the current reached only 59% of the control. Neither rise time nor desensitization time constant of the current seemed to be affected by picrotoxin. A reapplication of GABA after a washing period of 7 sec resulted in an inward current of the same amplitude as in the control, indicating that picrotoxin was no longer bound. In Fig. 1C, the same membrane patch was first exposed only to picrotoxin, which did not result in any channel activation. Then it was rapidly switched to a solution containing 1 mM GABA. In this case, the GABA-activated current was not markedly reduced compared to the control in Fig. 1A. Unbinding of picrotoxin was virtually complete within the rise time of the GABA response.

Using the same type of experiment as in Fig. 1B, a dose–response curve for the antagonistic action of picrotoxin with an apparent inhibitory constant K_i of 15 μM was obtained (17).

In a second step, the action of picrotoxin on single-channel kinetics was investigated. For this purpose, patches with a low channel density were selected and low agonist concentrations were used in order to avoid superpositions of channel openings. In these measurements the test solutions were applied continuously for several minutes. Figure 1D shows an example of single chloride channel openings gated by GABA (1 μM) in control solution (upper trace) and in the presence of 10 μM picrotoxin (lower trace). It is obvious that the main conductance of these channels, which is 44 pS, was unaltered by the toxin. Also the distribution of single-channel open times was not affected by picrotoxin (not shown). The open time distribution both in control solution and in the presence of picrotoxin could be fitted by a single exponential of about 2.5 msec, representing the apparent mean open time (14, 17). However, as can also be seen in the original recordings of Fig. 1D, the rate of openings was markedly reduced by picrotoxin. Therefore, the main effect of picrotoxin on single chloride channels is a stabilization of the closed states.

These results allow several conclusions concerning the usefulness for picrotoxin as a tool in the characterization of GABA-activated chloride channels and its molecular mode of action. Since binding and unbinding of picrotoxin

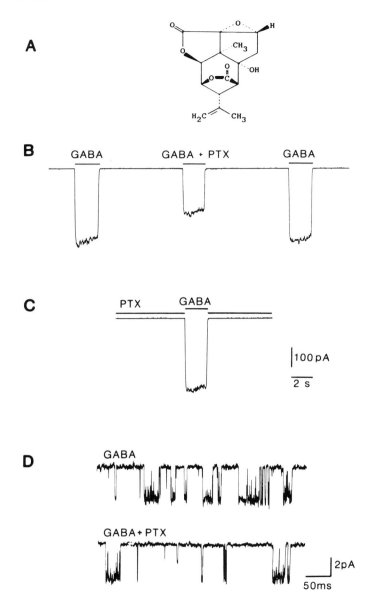

FIG. 1 (A) The chemical structure of picrotoxinin, the active component of picrotoxin. (B and C) Inward chloride currents produced by the pulsed application of 1 mM GABA for 2 sec to an outside-out patch from crayfish muscle under voltage clamp. (B) Effect of 10 μM picrotoxin (PTX) on GABA-activated current as obtained by simultaneous application of PTX and GABA. Same calibration as in (C). (C) 10 μM

is fast, occurring within the rise time of the current (about 100 msec), picrotoxin does not seem to be a satisfactory ligand for biochemical studies. A slow channel block of picrotoxin ($\tau_{block} > 100$ msec) can also be excluded, therefore. A physical blocking of the opened chloride channel, a so-called open channel block, can be excluded because picrotoxin had no effect on the lifetime of individual chloride channel openings. Short interruptions of channel openings, which are typical for open channel block (21), were not detected in the evaluation of single-channel kinetics. Thus, picrotoxin most probably seems to act via an allosteric site stabilizing the closed states of the channel and this confirms previous conclusions concerning the action of picrotoxin on the GABA receptor–channel complex (14, 22, 23). It should be noted that picrotoxin is not specific for GABA-activated chloride channels but has also been reported to inhibit other ligand-gated chloride channels (24).

Avermectin

The avermectins compose a class of polycyclic lactones from *Streptomyces avermitilis* (25, 26) that are extremely toxic against a broad spectrum of nematodes and arthropods, whereas their toxicity for mammals is relatively low. The structure of avermectin B_{1a} (AVM), one of the major components of the avermectin complex, is shown in Fig. 2A. Previous mode of action studies revealed a reduction in input resistance of muscle membranes by AVM caused by an increase of chloride permeability (27). It has also been shown that AVM is not specific for ligand-gated chloride channels but can also affect voltage-dependent chloride channels (28). Here the effect of AVM was investigated for the first time at the single-channel level to gain some insights on its molecular mode of action.

The methods for this study were the same as described for the picrotoxin experiments. The lipophilic AVM was kindly donated by Merck, Sharp & Dohme (Rahway, NJ). A stock solution of 0.1 mM AVM in dimethyl sulfoxide

---

PTX is applied before and after, but not during, the GABA response. Holding potential, -85 mV; bandwidth of recording, 0–2.0 kHz. (D) Recordings of single chloride channel openings from an outside-out patch as obtained by the continuous application of 1 μM GABA (upper trace) and 1 μM GABA in the presence of 10 μM picrotoxin. The records were filtered with an eight-pole bessel filter, bandwidth 0–1.5 kHz, and sampled at 10 kHz. The holding potential was -85 mV. [(B and C) Reprinted with permission from Ref. 16.]

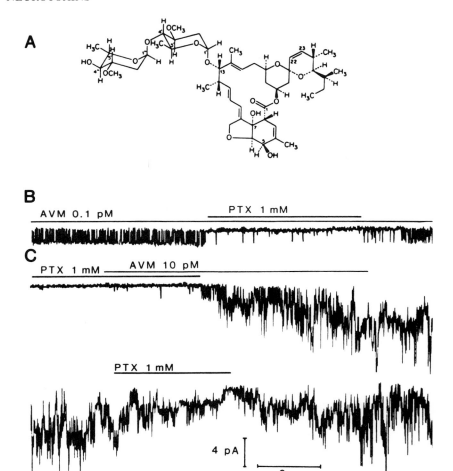

FIG. 2   (A) Structure of the avermectin B_{1a} (AVM) molecule. (B and C) Recordings from an outside-out patch at low time resolution. (B) Openings of the GABA-activated chloride channel in response to 0.1 pM AVM. During the application of 1 mM picrotoxin (PTX) the channel activity was almost completely inhibited. (C) PTX (1 mM) was added first, followed by 10 pM AVM. As long as PTX was present no channel opening appeared. After the end of PTX application, AVM elicited superimposed channel activity with no obvious desensitivation. Even after the end of AVM application, the channel activation continued. If PTX was added again, the channel activity decreased, but then increased again without any further adding of AVM. Bandwidth: 0–500 Hz. Reprinted with permission from Ref. 15.

(DMSO) was stored frozen, and dilutions of that solution were made fresh every day with a final maximal DMSO concentration of 0.001% (v/v). After each experiment, the tubing and recording chamber were washed with saline containing 10% DMSO.

When AVM was applied at the low concentration of 0.1 pM to an outside-out patch from crayfish stomach muscle, openings of the GABA-activated chloride channel could be detected (Fig. 2B). Avermectin was not found to activate channels on patches that did not respond to GABA, suggesting that AVM did not act as an ionophore. Furthermore, the effect of AVM was specific for chloride channels; glutamate-activated cation channels, which are frequently present in these patches (19), were not affected by AVM. When picrotoxin (1 mM) was added to the superfusing solution, the activity of the AVM-activated channel was almost completely inhibited (Fig. 2B). This effect was reversible. In Fig. 2C (continuous recording) picrotoxin was applied first and then a higher concentration of AVM (10 pM) was added, which normally led to an irreversible activation of single-channel currents. No channel activation was seen. However, when the picrotoxin superfusion was stopped, the typical irreversible effect of 10 pM AVM associated with a high rate of channel openings was found. The amplitude distribution of single-channel currents during this high rate of activation revealed the same unitary conductance as after stimulation with subpicomolar concentrations of AVM, suggesting that the same type of channel was activated by reversible and irreversible stimulation with AVM (16). After termination the AVM application channel activity continued. When picrotoxin (1 mM) was then added again, the rate of channel opening was reduced as long as the drug was present. It increased again after removal of picrotoxin without any additional application of AVM.

Another series of experiments was aimed at describing more precisely the location of the binding site of AVM at the receptor channel complex. Chloride channels were first activated in the cell-attached mode by a low dose of AVM (0.1 pM) inside the patch pipette. Subsequently, inside-out patches were formed and AVM at a higher concentration (100 pM) was applied to the cytoplasmic side of these patches. This additional AVM application did not enhance the rate of channel openings. Thus, a direct action of AVM on the cytoplasmic side of these channels seems to be ruled out under the conditions employed. Our results suggest that the channel is activated by AVM at a site facing the extracellular space.

These experiments show that AVM is a powerful agonist at a certain class of ligand-gated chloride channels. In the nanomolar concentration range irreversible activation of chloride channel openings was induced, probably due to irreversible binding of AVM to the receptor channel complex. Thus AVM appears to be a valuable tool both for biochemical studies and also for electrophysiological experiments in which a drug-induced increase of chloride permeability is desirable. However, it should be kept in mind that AVM does not seem to be specific for ligand-gated chloride channels because it has also been reported to induce the opening of voltage-dependent chloride channels (28).

Conclusions

Pharmacological tools like picrotoxin and avermectin have proved to be valuable in establishing the involvement of specific transmitters at certain synapses. In view of a great diversity of transmitter receptors discovered in recent years, it seems important to characterize the pharmacological profile of different receptors. This is another useful application of neurotoxins. Particularly in combination with the patch-clamp technique, the application of specific neurotoxins provides an additional tool to enhance the information about receptors gained from biochemical and molecular biology studies.

References

1. N. Bowery, G. W. Price, A. L. Hudson, D. R. Hill, G. P. Wiekin, and M. J. Turnbull, *Neuropharmacology* **23**, 219 (1984).
2. H. Betz, *Neuron* **5**, 383 (1990).
3. G. Grenningloh, A. Rienitz, B. Schmitt, C. Methfessel, M. Zensen, E. D. Gundelfinger, and H. Betz, *Nature (London)* **328**, 215 (1987).
4. H. L. Atwood, *in* "Biology of Crustacea" (H. L. Atwood and D. C. Sandeman, eds.), Vol. 3, p. 105. Academic Press, New York, 1982.
5. J. J. Rauh, S. C. R. Lummis, and D. B. Sattelle, *Trends Pharmacol. Sci.* **11**, 325 (1990).
6. A. T. Eldefrawi and M. E. Eldefrawi, *FASEB J.* **1**, 262 (1987).
7. M. E. Eldefrawi and A. T. Eldefrawi, *in* "Neurotox '88: Molecular Basis of Drug and Pesticide Action" (G. G. Lunt, ed.), p. 207. Elsevier, Amsterdam, 1988.
8. L. A. Porter, *Chem. Rev.* **67**, 441 (1967).
9. K. A. C. Elliott and E. Florey, *J. Neurochem.* **1**, 181 (1956).
10. A. Takeuchi and N. Takeuchi, *J. Physiol. (London)* **177**, 225 (1965).
11. A. Takeuchi and N. Takeuchi, *J. Physiol. (London)* **205**, 377 (1969).
12. D. M. Maynard and M. R. Dando, *Philos. Trans. R. Soc. London, B* **268**, 161 (1974).
13. C. K. Govind, H. L. Atwood, and D. M. Maynard, *J. Comp. Physiol.* **96**, 185 (1975).
14. C. Franke, H. Hatt, and J. Dudel, *J. Comp. Physiol. A* **159**, 591 (1986).
15. F. Zufall, C. Franke, and H. Hatt, *J. Comp. Physiol. A* **163**, 609 (1988).
16. F. Zufall, C. Franke, and H. Hatt, *J. Exp. Biol.* **142**, 191 (1989).

17. F. Zufall, C. Franke, and H. Hatt, *Brain Res.* **503,** 342 (1989).

18. J. Dudel, C. Franke, and H. Hatt, *Biophys. J.* **57,** 533 (1990).

19. C. Franke, H. Hatt, and J. Dudel, *J. Comp. Physiol. A* **159,** 579 (1986).

20. J. Dudel, C. Franke, and H. Hatt, *in* "Neurotox '88: Molecular Basis of Drug and Pesticide Action" (G. G. Lunt, ed.), p. 405. Elsevier, Amsterdam, 1988.

21. E. Neher and J. H. Steinbach, *J. Physiol. (London)* **277,** 153 (1978).

22. T. G. Smart and A. Constanti, *Proc. R. Soc. London, B* **227,** 191 (1986).

23. M. A. Simmonds, *in* "Actions and Interactions of GABA and Benzodiazepines" (N. G. Bowery, ed.), p. 27. Raven, New York, 1984.

24. E. Marder, *in* "The Crustacean Stomatogastric System" (A. I. Selverston and M. Moulins, eds.), p. 263. Springer-Verlag, Berlin, 1987.

25. R. W. Burg, M. Miller, E. E. Baker, J. Birnbaum, S. A. Currie, R. Hartman, Y. L. Kong, R. L. Monaghan, G. Olsen, I. Putter, J. B. Innac, H. Wallick, E. O. Stapley, R. Diwa, and S. Omura, *Antimicrob. Agents Chemother.* **15,** 361 (1979).

26. D. J. Wright, *in* "Neuropharmacology and Pesticide Action" (M. G. Ford, G. G. Lunt, R. C. Reay, and P. N. R. Usherwood, eds.), p. 174. Ellis Horwood, Chichester, England, 1986.

27. L. C. Fritz, C. C. Wang, and A. Gorio, *Proc. Natl. Acad. Sci. U.S.A.* **76,** 2062 (1979).

28. I. M. Abalis, A. T. Eldefrawi, and M. E. Eldefrawi, *J. Biochem. Toxicol.* **1,** 69 (1986).

[24]   Palytoxin: Characterization of Mode of Action in Excitable Cells

Martin-Pierre Sauviat

Introduction

Palytoxin (PTX) is a powerful water-soluble toxin produced by coelenterate species belonging to the genus *Palythoa*. The toxin has a unique structure and produces multiple effects on both nonexcitable and excitable cells that have already been reviewed. The most outstanding effects of the toxin can be summarized in the following points. Palytoxin induces release of potassium and is hemolytic in erythrocytes (1, 2). It depolarizes excitable cells (3) and increases the intracellular calcium content in both heart (4, 5) and smooth (6) muscles. Palytoxin also belongs to the non-TPA (12-*O*-tetradecanoylphorbol-13-acetate) type of tumor promoters and stimulates arachidonic acid metabolism (7).

Although the molecule was discovered over 20 years ago, its mode of action has not yet been established. The aim of the present chapter is to examine the possible mode of action of palytoxin on the basis of recent electrophysiological data.

Electrophysiology of Palytoxin

A common effect of palytoxin in excitable tissues is depolarization of membranes (3, 5, 8–10) as illustrated in Fig. 1A. The depolarization induced by PTX is abolished when Na^+ is removed from the extracellular medium (Fig. 1A). It is thus assumed to be carried by Na^+. Under voltage-clamp conditions, the toxin induces an inward current (8, 9) that fails to inactivate and is also sensitive to external Na^+ concentration (Fig. 1B). The observation that the depolarization and the current induced by palytoxin were resistant to voltage-dependent Na^+ channel inhibitors (tetrodotoxin and saxitoxin) suggested that palytoxin does not activate this channel to depolarize the membrane but instead induces a nonselective channel (8). Patch-clamp experiments gave evidence that single ion channels are associated with the application of PTX in heart (11, 12) and neuroblastoma (13) cells. These observations question the nature of the membrane receptor involved in the toxin action and of the mechanism by which the toxin opens membrane

Methods in Neurosciences, Volume 8

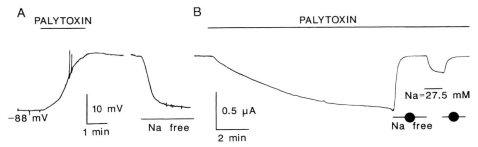

FIG. 1 Effect of PTX on the resting membrane potential and resting current of frog sartorius skeletal muscle fibers. (A) Palytoxin (200 nM) in Ringer's solution irreversibly depolarized the resting membrane potential recorded in a whole, cleaned, skeletal muscle using an intracellular microelectrode. The depolarization induced by the toxin was abolished when external Na$^+$ was replaced by mannitol (Na$^+$ free). Interruption of the trace: 3 min of continuous record has been omitted. (B) Palytoxin (37 nM) induced an inward current that was suppressed when Na$^+$ was removed from the Ringer's solution. A subsequent application of 27.5 mM Na$^+$ induced an inward resting current of smaller magnitude than in normal Ringer's solution. (●) Na$^+$-free solution. The membrane was held at -80 mV. [Redrawn with permission from Ecault and Sauviat (9). Copyright © 1991, The Macmillan Press, Ltd.]

channels. Does palytoxin transform the Na$^+$, K$^+$-ATPase or its vicinity into a channel, as suggested on erythrocyte membranes (2)? Does it modify existing voltage-dependent Na$^+$ channels or induced its own channel? In the light of recent findings concerning the characteristics of the conductance induced by PTX a partial answer can be given to these questions and a possible model for PTX action suggested.

Characterization of Palytoxin-Induced Channel

This section deals with the main pharmacological and electrical properties of the PTX-induced conductance in excitable membranes, leading to the building of a model that could account for the mode of action of PTX.

External Na$^+$ Concentration Dependence

The amplitude of the current induced by PTX is a function of the external Na$^+$ concentration ([Na$^+$]$_o$). The current does not present an [Na$^+$]$_o$-dependent saturation and a first order relation exists between [Na$^+$]$_o$ and the current amplitude (8, 9). This suggests the existence of a monomolecular reaction between the cation and the toxin-induced channel.

Dose–Response Effect

The effects of PTX are dose dependent. The concentration of toxin that produces the half-development of PTX action is 60 nM in frog heart (8), about 50 nM in frog sciatic nerve (10), and 0.23 nM in neuroblastoma cells (13). The stoichiometry of the reaction between PTX and the membrane, 2.35 in frog heart and 1.82 in neuroblastoma cells, suggests that at least two molecules of toxin interact with the membrane.

Electrical Properties

The PTX-induced channel appears to flicker between a closed and open state (Fig. 2A). The number of open channels in a patch seems to be dependent on the concentration of PTX (11). The decay of the open time distribution is exponential with a time constant of about 235 msec, while the closed state is composed of a short-duration (time constant 3.9 msec) and a long-duration component (time constant 2.65 sec) (12). Palytoxin-induced opening of channels at various membrane potentials is shown in Fig. 2B. The current induced by PTX exhibits an ohmic dependence on the voltage axis (Fig. 2C).

Selectivity of Palytoxin-Induced Channel

The channel is not only permeable to Na$^+$ but also accepts various other cations. In Table I the slope conductances measured from current–voltage curves from different ionic species on different tissues are summarized. Three main observations can be drawn from Table I: (i) Li$^+$, generally considered a good substitute for Na$^+$ as far as the voltage-dependent Na$^+$ channel is concerned, presents a lower conductance than Na$^+$ through the PTX-induced pore. Lithium ion also supports less PTX-induced depolarization than Na$^+$ in the membrane of frog heart (8) and nerve (10); (ii) large cations such as K$^+$, Cs$^+$, ammonium, and guanidinium present a relatively high conductance; (iii) Ca^{2+} was able to carry an inward current through the PTX channel.

Permeability of Palytoxin-Induced Channel

The permeability ratios (P_x/P_{Na}) between the tested ion (X^+) and Na$^+$, calculated for various ionic species in different tissues for both the PTX-induced conductance and the voltage-gated sodium channel, are summarized

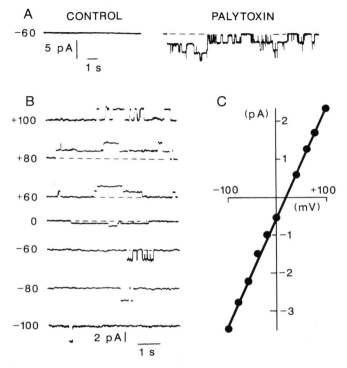

FIG. 2   Palytoxin-induced single channels were recorded from an inside-out membrane patch for cultured mouse neuroblastoma cells. Pipette and bath solutions were, respectively, a standard external solution [(mM): NaCl, 140; KCl, 5; CaCl$_2$, 2; MgCl$_2$, 2; HEPES (NaOH) buffer, 10; glucose, 11; pH 7.3] and an internal solution [(mM): KCl, 140; MgCl$_2$, 2; HEPES (NaOH) buffer, 10; pH 7.3]. Palytoxin at a final concentration of about 1.9 nM had been added to the pipette medium. (A) Current traces recorded at −60 mV about 1 min (left) and 10 min (right) after formation of the gigaohm seal. Three PTX-induced channels of the same amplitude were recorded. (B) Palytoxin-induced single channels recorded at various potentials (indicated in millivolts to the left of each trace). (C) Amplitude of the PTX-induced single-channel current shown in (B) as a function of voltage. The straight line was obtained from linear regression through the points. The reversal potential and the slope conductance were +18 mV and 28 pS, respectively. [Redrawn with permission from Rouzaire-Dubois and Dubois (13). Copyright © 1991, Pergamon Press PLC.]

TABLE I   Slope Conductance of the Palytoxin-Induced Channel Obtained from
Current–Voltage Relationships

| Tissue source | [PTX] (nM) | Unit | Ions tested | | | | | | | Refs.[a] |
			Na	Li	K	Cs	Ammonium	Guanidinium	Ca	
Rat Myocytes	0.5	pS	9.1	3.1	9.6	9.4	—	—	—	11
Guinea pig Myocytes	1.0	pS	9.5	9.2	—	11.0	16.5	—	—	12
Neuroblastoma cells	19	pS	26.0	—	—	—	—	—	—	13
Frog skeletal muscle fibers	37	μS	8.9	5.0	7.9	—	—	7.0	1.2	9

[a] References 11, 12, and 13 correspond to unitary conductance measured on patch-clamped cells and Ref. 9 to macroscopic conductance measured on voltage-clamped fibers.

in Table II. The permeability sequence, which comes from Table II and from data obtained on PTX-depolarized frog sciatic nerve (10), is then $Ca^{2+} = Ba^{2+} < TMA < $ choline $< K^+ < Li^+ = $ hydroxylamine $< $ methylhydroxylamine $< Cs^+ < $ methylamine $< Na^+ < $ ammonium $< $ guanidinium. Such a permeability sequence differs from the sequence of the voltage-dependent Na^+ channel of the frog muscle and the squid giant axon (14). Nevertheless, in frog muscle, the PTX-induced channel shares some common points with the end-plate Na^+ channel, in which ammonium and guanidinium are highly permeable. But these channels are different, because although Na^+ and K^+ are able to cross the membrane with nearly equal ease at the end plate (14), K^+ is only weakly permeant in the PTX-induced channel.

Size of Palytoxin-Induced Channel

The size of the PTX-induced pore must correspond to at least the size of the largest cation that crosses the channel. Therefore the PTX-induced pore possesses at least the diameter of guanidinium (9), which is estimated to be 4.8 Å (14). However, the channel might certainly be larger than this, because dimethylguanidinium was also found to cross it in frog skeletal fibers (unpublished observations, 1990). Such a pore size might account at least in part for a certain lack of specificity.

Block by Guanidinium Molecules

Because guanidinium ions pass through the PTX-induced channel (9, 15) the effects of tetrodotoxin (TTX), saxitoxin (STX), and amiloride, molecules in which a guanidinium group is involved in the blocking action on Na^+ currents,

TABLE II Relative Permeability Ratio of the Palytoxin-Induced Channel to Cations[a]

Tissue source	Permeability ratio (P_x/P_{Na})									Refs.
	Na+	Li+	K+	Cs+	NH4+	Gua	Chol	TMA	Ca2+	
Palytoxin-induced channel										
Squid axon	1	0.62	—	0.75	1.45	—	—	—	—	15
Guinea pig myocytes	1	0.93	—	0.95	1.21	—	—	—	—	12
Crayfish axon	1	—	—	—	1.72	1.11	—	0.0	—	15
Neuroblastoma cells	1	—	0.7	—	—	—	0.16	0.089	0.011	13
Frog skeletal muscle	1	0.69	0.019	—	—	2.09	—	—	—	9
Voltage-dependent sodium channel										
Squid axon	1	1.1	0.083	0.016	0.27	—	—	—	—	14
Frog node	1	0.93	0.08	<0.023	0.16	0.3	—	<0.005	—	14
Frog muscle	1	0.96	0.086	—	—	0.093	—	<0.08	—	14
Frog end plate	1	0.87	1.11	1.42	1.79	1.59	—	—	—	14
Crystal radius (Å)										
	0.9	0.6	1.33	1.69	1.5	2.4	—	—	0.99	14

[a] The permeability ratio (P_x/P_{Na}) between the tested ion (X^+) and Na+ was calculated from the apparent reversal potential determined from current–voltage relationships, according to the Goldman–Hodgkin–Katz equation $dE_{rev} = RT/ZF \ln[(P_x [X^+]_o)/(P_{Na}[Na^+]_o)]$, in which dE_{rev} is the reversal potential difference between the two ions, $[X^+]_o$ and $[Na^+]_o$, the external concentration of both ions; T, the absolute temperature; F, the Faraday constant; Z, the valency of the ion; R, the perfect gas constant. Gua, Chol, and TMA are guanidinium, choline, and tetramethylammonium ions, respectively. For comparison, similar values obtained from the voltage-dependent sodium channel have been reported.

have been examined on PTX-induced conductance. Tetrodotoxin $(0.2 \mu M)$, which entirely inhibits the voltage-dependent Na+ channel of the giant axon of cockroach, only partially inhibits the depolarization induced by PTX $(3 \mu M)$ and then only when applied before PTX (16, 17). In frog skeletal muscle, 10 μM TTX, a concentration about 17 times greater than the concentration that entirely blocks the Na+ channel (18), again only slightly and reversibly reduces the magnitude of the inward resting current induced by 37 nM PTX (8). Saxitoxin (30 nM), the structural analog of TTX, has little or no effect on the maintained depolarization induced by 10 nM PTX on frog nerve (10). Amiloride, on the other hand, dose dependently and reversibly blocks the PTX-induced conductance of frog skeletal muscle. The block occurs with an apparent dissociation constant of 0.3 mM and a stoichiometry of 1, which indicates a one-to-one relationship between the amiloride molecule and the PTX-induced channel (9).

It is tempting to think that it is the guanidinium group in each these molecules that is responsible for their blocking effect. The rapid inhibitory effect and recovery from block of TTX and amiloride suggests that these molecules do not bind to a specific site or receptor at the PTX channel input but that they behave as a simple cationic molecule (9), as has been proposed for amiloride blockage of the Na^+ channel in epithelial membrane (19).

Sensitivity to External pH

Change in external pH in the range 6.2 to 8.4 does not apparently affect the PTX-induced depolarization in frog nerve (10). In frog skeletal muscle, acidic pH solution blocks the palytoxin-induced current, whereas basic pH facilitates the conducting properties of the toxin pathway (9). In chick embryonic ventricular cells, PTX increases or decreases the intracellular pH, depending on the value of extracellular pH, suggesting that the toxin opens a preexisting hydrogen-conducting pathway (20) or that conductance is permeable to protons. The observation that the PTX-induced conductance decreases with the proton concentration might suggest that the toxin activates the Na^+/H^+ antiporter, the Na^+ flux of which is known to be amiloride sensitive. Although the antiporter can be activated by the toxin via a mechanism that is distinct from that of phorbol ester (20), it cannot be considered as the only process responsible for the Na^+ influx induced by the toxin, because the ionic selectivity of the exchanger (21) differs from the selectivity of the PTX-induced channel as far as Li^+ and Cs^+ are concerned. On the other hand, the perfect reversibility of the effect of external pH change suggests that pH might induce changes in the molecular configuration around a pK_a value. Palytoxin exhibits a chromophore absorbing at 263 nm, reversibly acid and base labile, involved in the toxicity of the molecule (22). External pH might modulate the chemical structure of the chromophore, leading to the passage of one ionic form to the other. Other possible explanations to account for the block of the PTX-induced conductance are that acidic pH might modify the availability of negative surface charges and displaced Ca^{2+} from phospholipids phosphate and carbonyl groups (23), altering the amount of Ca^{2+} bound to the membrane.

Ouabain Sensitivity

Experiments with ouabain on erythrocyte membranes have suggested that the toxin binds to the Na^+, K^+-ATPase and converts the enzyme or its close vicinity into an open channel (2). In frog nerve (10), 100 μM ouabain and 30 nM cyamarin (an aglycon of strophanthidin) block the depolarizing action of 30 nM PTX, which is resistant to 1 mM strophanthidin. The difference between cyamarin and strophanthidin was attributed to the absence of sugar in the strophanthidin molecule. It has thus been suggested that there may be some overlap between the sugar residues of PTX and cardiac glycoside and the sugar-binding domain of the ATPase. These observations are supported by recent findings concerning the structure of the Na^+, K^+-ATPase, which is composed of two different subunits (24). The α subunit, sensitive to cardiac glycosides, shows affinity for Na^+ and K^+ and contains the phosphorylation site and the ATP-binding site. The β subunit, the cytoplasmic domain of which contains three to four glycosylation sites, functions as a receptor for the α subunit to be anchored in the membrane. The sugar moiety of the β subunit could be the common region at which PTX, ouabain, and cyamarin overlap, whereas strophanthidin (devoid of sugar) occupies only the glycoside site located on the α subunit. If this is so, this means that PTX does not directly act on the α subunit, at which the catalytic and transport processes occur. Nevertheless this hypothesis of the binding of PTX to the β subunit of the Na^+, K^+-ATPase needs further experiments to be clearly demonstrated.

Role of External Calcium

Figure 3A shows that external Ca^{2+} plays an important role in the development of the PTX-induced conductance in frog skeletal muscle. In Ca^{2+}-free solution PTX induces a low-conductance state, characterized by the development of an inward current of weak amplitude with a slow kinetic of establishment. The addition of 2 mM Ca^{2+} to the Ca^{2+}-free solution leads to the development of a current of larger magnitude with a fast kinetic of establishment (9). This suggested that the PTX effect occurs in two steps: first, PTX binds to a membrane receptor (R) and makes a complex (R–PTX) that is responsible for the development of an inward current of small amplitude; second, in regard to the stoichiometry of toxin action (8, 13), two nearby complexes are associated or activated by external Ca^{2+}, which behaves as a cofactor to induce a high-conductance state (2R–PTX):

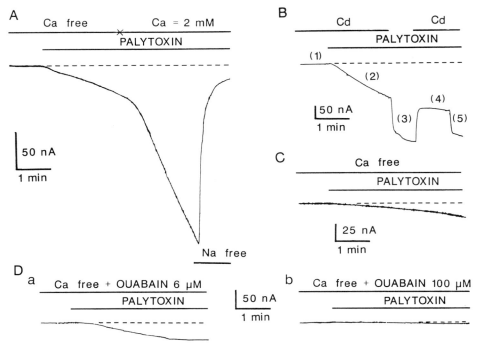

FIG. 3   Effect of PTX (37 nM) on the resting inward Na$^+$ current recorded at -80 mV holding potential in voltage-clamped cut-end frog skeletal fibers. (A) The fiber had been bathed for 5 min in a Ca^{2+}-free Ringer's solution before the toxin was added. After 2 min 30 sec, 2 mM Ca^{2+} was added to the control solution containing the toxin. A further application of an Na$^+$-free solution reversed the action of the toxin. (B) Effect of PTX on the inward current in the presence of 20 mM Cd^{2+} in Ringer's solution. (1) The membrane was bathed 5 min in a Ringer's solution containing Cd^{2+}. (2) Palytoxin was added to the control solution. (3) Cd^{2+} was removed from the solution containing the toxin, added again in (4), and removed in (5). (C) Effect of palytoxin on a Ca^{2+}-free and La^{3+}-loaded membrane. The membrane had been bathed for 5 min each in a Ca^{2+}-free Ringer's solution, Ca^{2+}-free solution containing 10^{-4} M ethylene glycol tetraacetic acid, Ca^{2+}-free solution containing La^{3+} (2 mM), Ca^{2+}-free solution, and finally Ca^{2+}-free solution containing PTX. (D) Effect of PTX in a Ca^{2+}-free Ringer's solution containing 6 μM ouabain (a) and 100 μM ouabain (b). The membrane was successively bathed for 10 min each in a Ca^{2+}-free Ringer's solution and a control solution containing ouabain before addition of palytoxin. Dashed line represents the zero current in the control solution. [(B and C) Redrawn from Ecault and Sauviat (9). Copyright © 1991, The Macmillan Press Ltd.]

Both states can be pharmacologically characterized. The high-conductance state, which develops in the presence of Ca^{2+}, is reversibly inhibited by Cd^{2+} and La^{3+} (8). Cadmium ion inhibits durably the resting inward current induced by PTX, which recovers immediately after Cd^{2+} removal. The inhibition induced by Cd^{2+} is dose dependent and exhibits saturation at concentrations larger than 10 mM. The half-inhibitory effect is reached at about 3 mM. Pretreatment with Cd^{2+} does not protect the membrane against PTX action but lengthens the kinetic of development of the current; Cd^{2+} removal leads to an immediate increase of the current amplitude, which is reversibly inhibited by a subsequent application of Cd^{2+} (Fig. 3B). Cadmium ion and La^{3+} are known to bind to the membrane and to replace Ca^{2+}. Cadmium ion might be able to occupy anionic sites on phospholipid head groups of the membrane, which would otherwise be occupied by Ca^{2+} (25, 26). Lanthanum ion is known to displace Ca^{2+} and to bind firmly and almost irreversibly to phospholipids and proteins of the membrane (27). Although it is difficult to determine the part linked to the occupation of membrane negative surface charges by the cations, the reversibility of their action strongly suggests that they replace Ca^{2+} on the high-conducting PTX complex. It should be noted that Sr^{2+} is able to replace Ca^{2+} to induce a high-conductance state (5).

The low-conductance state might probably be the state in which PTX binds to a membrane receptor. Experiments in which the frog muscle membrane is successively depleted in Ca^{2+} by treatment with a Ca^{2+}-free solution containing ethylene glycol tetraacetic acid and loaded with La^{3+} show that the amplitude of the PTX-induced current is decreased and its kinetic of establishment is lengthened (Fig. 3C). Pretreatment of frog muscle fiber with 6 μM ouabain, a concentration that blocks Na^+, K^+-ATPase and depolarizes frog skeletal muscle membrane by 10 mV, had almost no effect on the amplitude of inward current induced by PTX in a Ca^{2+}-free solution (Fig. 3D). In other experiments, pretreatment with 100 μM ouabain almost entirely inhibits the inward current induced by the toxin (Fig. 3D).

These observations show that La^{3+} prevents the binding of the toxin. This might suggest that PTX requires free negative surface charges to bind to the membrane. However, ouabain also inhibits the low-conductance state induced by PTX. This favors the Na^+, K^+-ATPase hypothesis, inasmuch as the enzyme activity has been found to be sensitive to Cd^{2+} (25) but is not inhibited by La^{3+}. Further experiments are required to elucidate this point.

Mode of Palytoxin Action

Whatever the nature and identity of the membrane receptor involved in PTX action, the mechanism by which PTX associates with that receptor, resulting in the opening or formation of ion channels, remains unknown.

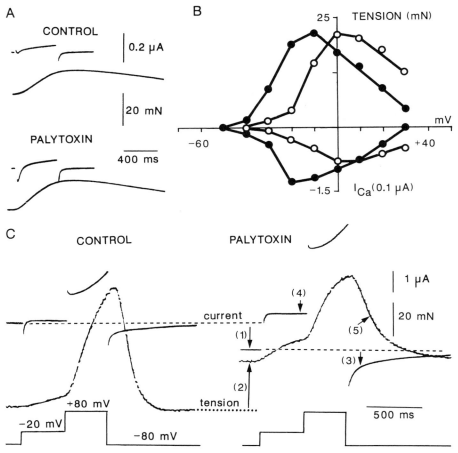

FIG. 4 Effect of 37 nM PTX on the calcium current and the mechanical activity of frog heart recorded in Na$^+$-free Ringer's solution containing tetrodotoxin, Cs$^+$, tetraethylammonium, and 4-aminopyridine. (A) Effect of 5 min of PTX application on the Ca^{2+} current (I_{Ca}; upper traces) and the phasic tension (lower traces) responses elicited by a depolarizing step to -20 mV applied from a -80-mV holding potential. (B) Current–voltage (lower curves) and tension–voltage (upper curves) relationships. Holding potential was -80 mV. Na$^+$-free Ringer's solution before (○) and after (●) PTX application. (C) Membrane currents and the mechanical activity recorded simultaneously in normal Ringer's solution. The membrane potential was held at -80 mV. A 60-mV depolarizing step followed by a 180-mV depolarizing step elicited the phasic and tonic components of the tension, respectively. In the presence of PTX,

Experimental data have shown that (i) PTX does not form a channel when applied to lipid bilayers (28) and thus does not appear to act by itself as an ionophore; (ii) lipids may participate in formation of the PTX-binding site. Artificial liposomes are unable to fix the toxin while liposomes made from lipids of human erythrocytes and rat brain do (29); (iii) the action of PTX cannot be attributed to the liberation of a soluble internal messenger (13).

Palytoxin does not use any one of the voltage-dependent Na^+ channels and binds to the membrane even in the absence of external Ca^{2+}; it does, however, require external Ca^{2+} to develop its depolarizing action. Without any assumptions concerning the nature of the membrane structure borrowed by PTX to exert its toxicity, a model has been proposed for the PTX action on neuroblastoma cell membranes (13). Dose–response curves indicate a stoichiometry of two for the toxin effect (8, 13). Moreover, kinetic analysis of the toxin effect has suggested that the action of PTX on the membrane is cooperative (13). An interpretation is that the formation of ion channels results from the association of at least two molecules of toxin. Palytoxin binds to a receptor membrane (R) and forms a complex (R–PTX) that associates with one free PTX molecule to induce a conducting channel (R–PTX$_2$):

$$R + PTX \longleftrightarrow R\text{–}PTX + PTX \longleftrightarrow R\text{–}PTX_2 \longleftrightarrow R\text{–}PTX_2^*$$

The receptor–toxin complex (R–PTX$_2^*$) can leave or reincorporate into the membrane from the outer or the inner face and might account for the internalization of the molecule, which could then react with different cellular constituents and induce secondary effects.

Palytoxin also alters, directly or indirectly, the voltage-dependent Na^+ and K^+ conductances (8, 17, 30) as well as the Ca^{2+} conductance, the alteration of which is the subject of the last section.

Effect of Palytoxin on Calcium Current and Mechanical Activity

Palytoxin increases Ca^{2+} uptake (4, 6). Although Ca^{2+} has been shown to enter via the PTX-induced channel in the absence of Na^+ (9, 13), this cannot account for the increase in internal Ca_i^{2+} content observed under physiological condi-

---

an inward resting current (1), an outward current (4), and a tonic contracture (2) developed while the amplitude of the tail current increased (3). The phasic tension was increased and the tonic tension was reduced. The time course of the relaxation phase was lengthened (5). [(A and B) Redrawn from Sauviat (5). Copyright © 1989, The Macmillan Press Ltd.]

tions. Palytoxin increases transiently the Ca^{2+} current and the phasic tension of frog heart muscle recorded in Na^+-free solution (Fig. 4A) and shifts the apparent reversal potential for Ca^{2+} toward more negative membrane potentials (Fig. 4B), suggesting that the internal Ca^{2+} content increases (5). In embryonic chick ventricular cells, PTX increased Ca_i^{2+} in a manner that was dependent on the presence of extracellular Ca^{2+} (31). As would be expected during Ca^{2+} loading, current–voltage, time to peak–voltage, and inactivation time constant–voltage as well as tension–voltage curves are all shifted toward more negative membrane potentials. In the presence of Na^+ in the control solution, PTX has multiple effects. It induces an inward resting current associated with the development of a tonic contracture (Fig. 4C) and increases the amplitude of the phasic component of the tension while the tonic component is reduced. The time constant of the relaxation phase is markedly lengthened (Fig. 4C). In frog heart, the tonic component of the tension depends on Ca^{2+} entry via Na^+–Ca^{2+} exchange, which may also be the major mechanism leading to relaxation. The effect of PTX on tonic tension and relaxation is therefore probably linked to alteration of the Na^+–Ca^{2+} exchange. A fundamental feature of Na^+–Ca^{2+} exchange is that an elevation in internal Na^+ (Na_i^+) will promote an exchange of Na_i^+ for external Ca^{2+}. Palytoxin increases the tail current, which is identified as a Ca^{2+} current generated by the Na^+–Ca^{2+} exchange under depolarization (Fig. 4C). From this point of view, the toxin should behave like an Na^+ ionophore such as ionomycin and monensin, which have been used as tools to depolarize the membrane by increasing the internal Na^+ content to study the role of Na^+–Ca^{2+} exchange in contributing to the depolarization-induced increase in internal Ca^{2+} content of heart muscle. The cardiotoxicity of palytoxin has been attributed to the contribution of its actions on Ca_i^{2+}, on the internal pH and the resulting action on Na^+/H exchange and possibly on Na^+/Ca^{2+} exchange (31).

A last point concerning the toxin action is the development of an outward current (Fig. 4C), which appears at the same time as the inward resting current. This current is activated in the presence of Ca^{2+} and is not present when Ca^{2+} is replaced by Sr^{2+}. It has been identified as a Ca^{2+}-dependent K^+ current (5, 32).

Conclusion

Palytoxin is a unique type of cytolysin with complex action. The first step of the toxin action would be the binding of the toxin to a membrane receptor, which lead to the formation of cationic pores principally permeable to Na^+. The conductance induced by the toxin would then play a key role in a cascade of events that affect other membrane conductances and induce metabolic alterations by which PTX may promote tumors.

Acknowledgments

The author thanks Doctor Jean-Marc Dubois for reading the manuscript and making suggestions, and Doctor Ian Findlay for helpful comments, discussions, and grammatical improvements.

References

1. L. Beress, *in* "Toxins as Tolls in Neurochemistry" (F. Hucho and Y. A. Ouchinnikov, eds.), p. 83. de Gruyter, Berlin, 1983.
2. E. Habermann, *Toxicon* **27,** 1171 (1989).
3. A. R. Ibrahim and W. T. Shier, *J. Toxicol. Toxin Rev.* **6,** 159 (1987).
4. M. D. Rayner, B. J. Sanders, S. M. Harris, Y. C. Lin, and B. E. Morton, *Res. Commun. Chem. Pathol. Pharmacol.* **11,** 55 (1985).
5. M.-P. Sauviat, *Br. J. Pharmacol.* **98,** 773 (1989).
6. H. Ozaki, J. Tomono, H. Nagase, and N. Urakawa, *Jpn. J. Pharmacol.* **33,** 1155 (1983).
7. H. Fujiki and T. Sugimura, *Adv. Cancer Res.* **49,** 699 (1987).
8. M.-P. Sauviat, C. Pater, and J. Berton, *Toxicon* **25,** 695 (1987).
9. E. Ecault and M.-P. Sauviat, *Br. J. Pharmacol.* **102,** 523 (1991).
10. N. A. Castle and G. R. Strichartz, *Toxicon* **26,** 941 (1988).
11. M. Ikeda, K. Mitani, and K. Ito, *Naunyn-Schmiedeberg's Arch. Pharmacol.* **337,** 591 (1988).
12. I. Muramatsu, M. Nishio, S. Kigoshi, and D. Uemura, *Br. J. Pharmacol.* **93,** 811 (1988).
13. B. Rouzaire-Dubois and J.-M. Dubois, *Toxicon* **28,** 1147 (1990).
14. B. Hille, "Ionic Channels of Excitable Membranes." Sinauer, Sunderland, Massachusetts, 1984.
15. C. H. Wu and T. Narahashi, *Annu. Rev. Pharmacol. Toxicol.* **28,** 141 (1988).
16. M.-P. Sauviat and Y. Pichon, *J. Physiol. (Paris)* **73,** 56A (1977).
17. Y. Pichon, *Toxicon* **20,** 41 (1982).
18. C. Pater and M.-P. Sauviat, *Gen. Physiol. Biophys.* **6,** 305 (1987).
19. D. C. Eaton and K. L. Hamilton, *in* "Ion Channels" (T. Narahashi, ed.), Vol. 1, p. 251. Plenum, New York, 1988.
20. C. Frelin, P. Vigne, and J.-P. Breittmayer, *FEBS Lett.* **264,** 63 (1990).
21. R. L. Mahnensmith and P. S. Aronson, *Circ. Res.* **56,** 773 (1985).
22. R. Moore and P. J. Scheuer, *Science* **172,** 495 (1971).
23. B. Hille, *in* "Membranes: A Series of Advances" (G. Eisenmann, ed.), Vol. 3, p. 255. Dekker, New York, 1975.

24. K. Geering, *J. Membr. Biol.* **115,** 109 (1990).
25. S. J. Kopp, *Handb. Exp. Pharmacol.* **80,** 195 (1986).
26. E. M. B. Sorensen, D. Acosta, and D. G. Nealon, *Toxicol Lett.* **25,** 319 (1985).
27. R. B. Martin and F. S. Richardson, *Q. Rev. Biophys.* **12,** 181 (1979).
28. L. Laufer, S. Stengelin, L. Beress, and F. Hucho, *Biochim. Biophys. Acta* **818,** 55 (1985).
29. E. Habermann, *Naunyn-Schmiedeberg's Arch. Pharmacol.* **323,** 269 (1983).
30. J.-M. Dubois and J. B. Cohen, *J. Pharmacol. Exp. Ther.* **201,** 148 (1977).
31. C. Frelin, P. Vigne, and J. P. Breittmayer, *Molec. Pharmacol.* **38,** 904 (1990).
32. M.-P. Sauviat, *Pfluegers Arch.* **414** (Suppl. 1), S178 (1989).

[25] Palytoxin: Mechanism of Acidifying Action in Excitable Cells

Christian Frelin and Jean-Philippe Breittmayer

The distribution of H^+ across the plasma membrane of eukaryotic cells is such that the internal pH (pH_i) is almost 1 pH unit lower than expected if H^+ were passively distributed. For an average membrane potential of -60 mV and for an external pH value of 7.4, a pH_i value of 6.4 would be expected if H^+ were in electrochemical equilibrium across the plasma membrane. In most cells, including excitable cells, pH_i is maintained at a value of 7.0–7.4 by membrane H^+ extrusion mechanisms (1) such as the Na^+/H^+ antiporter and the Na^+-dependent Cl^-/HCO_3^- antiporter. The biochemical properties and physiological roles of these pH_i-regulating mechanisms have been reviewed recently (2, 3). They will not be considered here.

Because H^+ is not passively distributed across the plasma membrane, an increase in the membrane permeability to H^+ is expected to produce an intracellular acidification and to lead to secondary changes in the activity of pH_i-regulating mechanisms. Evidence for the physical reality and the possible functions of membrane H^+ "channels" is, however, still weak. The observation that, in many cells, the pH_i value is relatively insensitive to changes in the membrane potential (see, e.g., Ref. 4) suggests that, under normal conditions, membrane electrogenic H^+ movements are of small amplitude or that the changes in pH_i consecutive to these movements are strongly buffered. Yet there may be circumstances or specific cell types in which such movements may play a significant role (5, 6) and we previously suggested that palytoxin (PTX) may be a probe for identifying and studying such channels in excitable cells (7). This chapter defines the methods used for analyzing the action of PTX. Experimental protocols that allow one to distinguish primary from secondary actions of the toxin are discussed in detail.

Properties of Palytoxin

Palytoxin (Fig. 1) is one of the most potent toxins known. It has been isolated from marine coelenterate and consists of a long, aliphatic, partially unsaturated chain with interspersed cyclic ether, hydroxyl, and carboxyl groups (8, 9). Its pharmacological properties have been reviewed recently (10). A general action of PTX is to depolarize excitable cells, including

Methods in Neurosciences, Volume 8

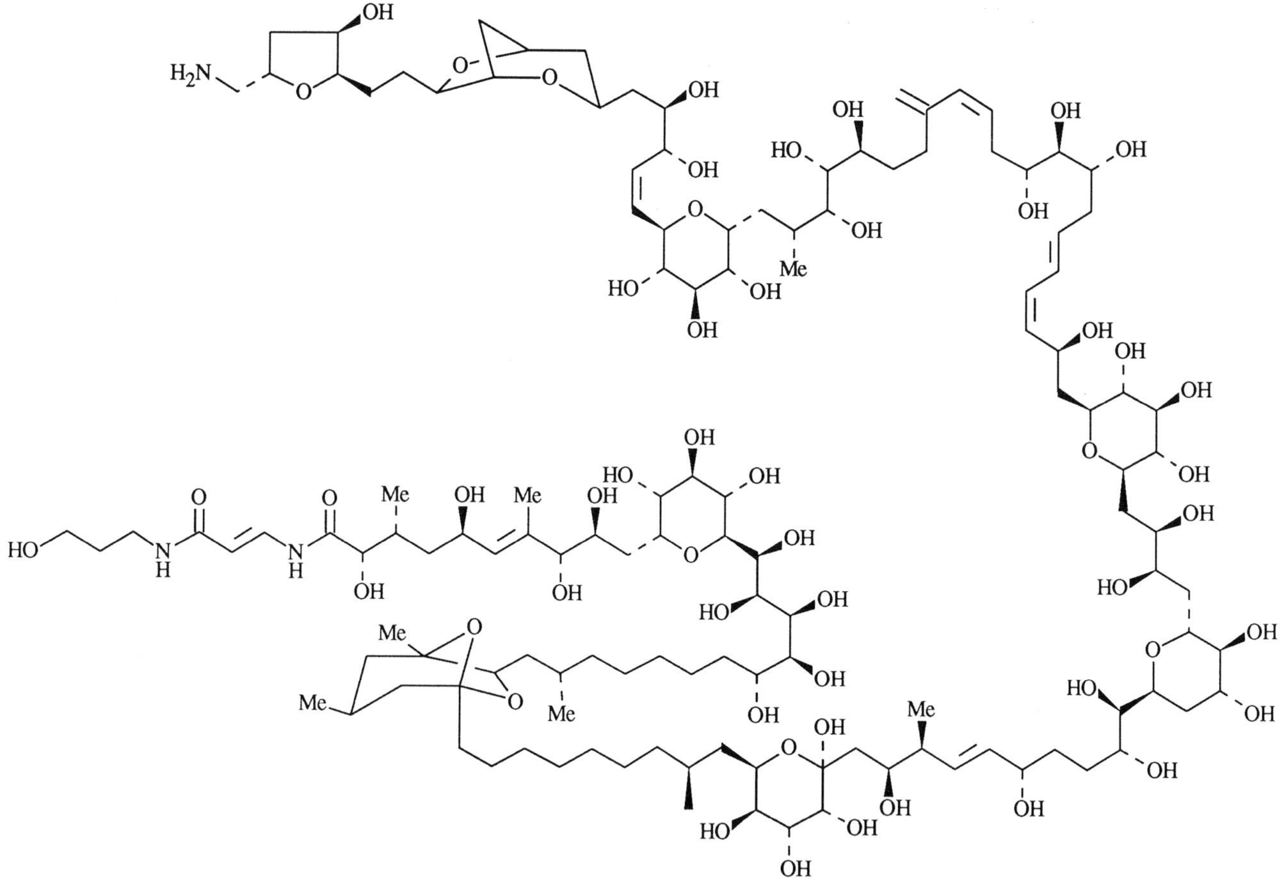

Fig. 1   The structure of palytoxin.

neuronal cells, cardiac cells, skeletal muscle cells, and vascular smooth muscle cells, in a manner that is dependent on extracellular Na^+ and that is insensitive to tetrodotoxin. Toxicity is mainly due to a profound vasoconstrictor effect via a direct action on smooth muscle cells and via the release of norepinephrine by sympathetic nerve terminals (11).

Palytoxin from *Palythoa caribaeorum* used in our experiments was kindly provided by Dr. E. Habermann (Liebig University, Giessen, Germany). Solutions are prepared in 1% bovine serum albumin (BSA) and stored at $-20°C$. Palytoxin is now available from Calbiochem (San Diego, CA).

Action of Palytoxin on $^{22}Na^+$ Uptake

Experiments are performed using cultured cells plated into 24-well tissue culture clusters. The culture medium is aspirated off by suction and cells rinsed with a K^+-free Earle's salt solution (145 mM NaCl, 1.8 mM CaCl$_2$, 0.8 mM MgSO$_4$ buffered at pH 7.4 with 25 mM HEPES–Tris). Cells are then incubated for 3 min at 37°C in 200 μl of prewarmed K^+-free Earle's salt solution supplemented with 1 μCi/ml $^{22}Na^+$ (0.5 Ci/mg, Amersham, Arlington Heights, IL) and the desired concentration of agonist. At the end of the incubation period, cell layers are rapidly washed three times with cold 0.1 M MgCl$_2$, digested in 0.1 N NaOH, and the cell-associated radioactivity is determined using a γ counter. A K^+-free incubation solution is used to prevent $^{22}Na^+$ efflux mediated by the Na^+,K^+-ATPase. This may also be achieved with ouabain. The rate of $^{22}Na^+$ uptake measured under these conditions represents the activity of a number of known membrane Na^+ transport systems (e.g., the Na^+/H^+ antiporter and the $Na^+/K^+/Cl^-$ cotransporter) and of unknown transport systems. Under the conditions used, voltage-dependent, tetrodotoxin-sensitive Na^+ channels do not contribute to the measured $^{22}Na^+$ flux unless an open conformation of the channel is stabilized by neurotoxins. The contribution of the Na^+/H^+ antiporter to the measured flux is evaluated using a highly potent inhibitor of the system: ethylisopropylamiloride (EIPA) (12). At an external Na^+ concentration of 140 mM, complete inhibition of Na^+/H^+ exchange activity is achieved using 10 μM EIPA (13).

The addition of PTX to chick heart cells produces a large increase in the rate of $^{22}Na^+$ uptake, which is similar in amplitude to the increase produced by opening voltage-dependent Na^+ channels but which is insensitive to 1 μM tetrodotoxin (7). The PTX-activated $^{22}Na^+$ flux can be divided into two pharmacologically distinct components. A first component (20–30% of the total PTX-activated ^{22}Na$^+$ flux) is suppressed by 10 μM EIPA. The concentration of EIPA that produced half-maximum inhibition (IC$_{50}$) of the PTX-activated flux component is 0.5 μM, a value close to the IC$_{50}$ value for EIPA inhibition of the rate of ^{22}Na$^+$ uptake by acidified cardiac cells (0.2 μM) (13). The close correspondence between the two values indicates that the action of PTX probably involves an increased activity of the Na$^+$/H$^+$ antiporter. The remaining component of the PTX-activated ^{22}Na$^+$ flux is prevented by another derivative of amiloride: 3,4-dichlorobenzamil (IC$_{50}$ 8μM), which is known to inhibit the Na$^+$/Ca^{2+} exchange system although it should not be considered as specific (14, 15). One possible mechanism could be that by loading cells with Ca^{2+}, PTX promotes Na$^+$ influx by the Na$^+$/Ca^{2+} exchanger. If this is true, then an incubation of cells in a low-Ca^{2+} (50 nM) solution, which prevents intracellular Ca^{2+} accumulation, should prevent the PTX-activated, 3,4-dichlorobenzamil-inhibitable ^{22}Na$^+$ flux component. Experiments performed so far indicate that the PTX-activated ^{22}Na$^+$ flux component is dependent on external Ca^{2+} in chick cardiomyocytes (16) but not in rat aortic myocytes. This indicates that, at least in aortic myocytes, 3,4-dichlorobenzamil blocks PTX-activated ^{22}Na$^+$ uptake by a mechanism that does not involve Na$^+$/Ca^{2+} exchange.

Thus at least two Na$^+$ permeation pathways are involved in the action of PTX on chick cardiac cells: (1) the Na$^+$/H$^+$ antiporter and (2) a 3,4-dichlorobenzamil-inhibitable pathway. It is uncertain whether the latter is the Na$^+$/Ca^{2+} antiporter.

Intracellular pH Measurements Using Flow Cytometry

An increased rate of ^{22}Na$^+$ uptake by the Na$^+$/H$^+$ antiporter can be achieved by two types of mechanisms: (1) a modification of the kinetic properties of the system and (2) a primary intracellular acidification (2). The only way to distinguish between these two possibilities is to perform pH$_i$ measurements. The development of pH-sensitive fluorescent probes that can be loaded into living cells has greatly improved the simplicity and accuracy of the methods used to measure the pH$_i$ in living cells. Cardiac cells are loaded with biscarboxyethylcarboxyfluorescein (BCECF) using the following procedure. Freshly dissociated heart cells from 12-day-old chick embryo are pelleted by centrifugation (15 min at 1000 g and room temperature) and resuspended in Eagle's minimum essential medium supplemented with 10% (v/v) fetal bovine serum and a 10 μM concentration of the acetoxymethyl ester of BCECF (Calbiochem). After 1 hr of incubation at 37°C, cells are collected by centrifugation (15 min at 1000 g and room temperature), resuspended in an Earle's salt solution (140 mM NaCl, 5 mM KCl, 1.8 mM CaCl$_2$, 0.8 mM MgSO$_4$

buffered at pH 7.4 with 25 mM HEPES–Tris), and kept in the dark at room temperature until analysis. Freshly dissociated cells may also be plated on culture dishes and maintained in culture for a few days. Cells are loaded with 10 μM BLECF/AM in complete culture medium while still attached to their plates. Cells are then rinsed twice with serum-free culture medium and quickly dispersed using a Ca^{2+}-free, balanced salt solution supplemented with 5 mM EDTA and 0.05% (v/v) trypsin. Time of exposure to the trypsin solution should be kept to a minimum (<5 min). Cells are then diluted with complete culture medium containing 10% fetal bovine serum, collected by centrifugation (15 min at 1000 g and room temperature), resuspended in an Earle's salt solution, and left in the dark at room temperature for at least 1 hr to allow cells to recover. The same procedure is used for vascular smooth muscle cells and endothelial cells.

Flow cytometric analysis of the BCECF fluorescence is performed using an ATC 3000 cell sorter (Odam, Bruker, Wissembourg, France) equipped with an argon laser (Coherent, Innova, 90, Auburn, CA) tuned at 488 nm. Fluorescence emission is detected at 520–550 nm and 610 nm, using the filter settings shown in Fig. 2. The two fluorescence emissions, their ratio, the electric volume, and the wide-angle scatter are collected cell by cell in real time. Data are gated using the electric volume and wide-angle light scatter to exclude dead cells and debris from the analysis. A detailed account of the gating procedure and of the advantages of flow cytometry over other fluorimetric techniques can be found elsewhere in this volume (17).

For calibrating the BCECF fluorescence, aliquots of the cell suspension are incubated for 30 min at room temperature in an Na^+-free, 145 mM KCl–Earle's salt solution buffered at different pH values using mixtures of HEPES, Tris, and 2-(N-morpholino)ethanesulfonic acid (MES) buffers and supplemented with 1 μM nigericin. These conditions ensure an equilibration of pH_i and pH_o (18). Figure 3 shows a plot of the BCECF fluorescence as a function of pH_o obtained using chick cardiac cells. It indicates an apparent pK_a value for intracellularly trapped BCECF of 6.95. This value is close to the pK_a value for BCECF in simple aqueous buffers (6.97–6.99) (19).

Action of Palytoxin on pH_i under Polarized Membrane Conditions

The addition of PTX to chick cardiac cells incubated in a physiological salt solution induces a 0.2- to 0.3-pH unit cellular acidification (7). It is well known that the major function of the Na^+/H^+ antiporter is to protect cells against excessive intracellular acidification (2). This suggests (1) that the primary action of PTX is to acidify cells and (2) that the activation of the Na^+/H^+ antiporter observed in $^{22}Na^+$ uptake experiments is secondary to

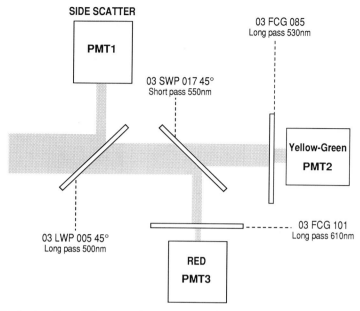

FIG. 2   Optical path and filters used to measure BCECF fluorescence by flow cytometry. Side scatter, yellow-green, and red fluorescences are detected by three photomultiplier tubes (PMT). Red fluorescence (>610 nm) is detected by PMT3. Yellow-green fluorescence (520–550 nm) is detected by PMT2. Filters were from Melles-Griot (Irvine, CA).

the acidification. Independent evidence for such a mechanism is provided by the observation that Na^+-free conditions and EIPA, which prevents H^+ extrusion by the Na^+/H^+ antiporter, potentiate the acidifying action of PTX (7).

A variety of hormones, phorbol esters, and growth-regulating substances also increase Na^+/H^+ exchange activity (2). Their action is achieved via a modification of the kinetic properties of this system, probably consecutive to a phosphorylation of the antiporter protein (20). Direct activations of the Na^+/H^+ antiporter by growth factors are clearly distinct from the activation produced by PTX. They lead to a cellular alkalinization (instead of a cellular acidification produced by PTX) and this action on pH_i is prevented by Na^+-free conditions and by amiloride derivatives (rather than being potentiated in the case of PTX). This is interesting because PTX, like phorbol esters, has tumor-promoting activity. However, unlike phorbol esters, PTX does not bind to or activate protein kinase C (21). Palytoxin and phorbol esters produce

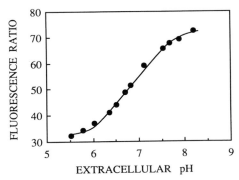

Fig. 3 Calibration of BCECF fluorescence. Dispersed chick cardiac cells that have been loaded with BCECF are diluted into a 145 mM KCl solution buffered at different pH values in the presence of 1 μM nigericin to equilibrate pH_i and pH_o. The fluorescence of BCECF is measured 30 min later and plotted as a function of pH_o values. The line shows the theoretical titration curve obtained using a pK_a value of 6.95.

opposite changes in pH_i, and so it is unlikely that their tumor-promoting activity is related in some way to their action on pH_i.

Action of Palytoxin under Depolarized Membrane Conditions

Sodium ion-free conditions and EIPA, which both completely block Na^+/H^+ exchange activity, should potentiate the acidifying action of PTX to the same extent. In fact, a greater acidifying action of PTX is observed under Na^+-free conditions than in the presence of Na^+ and of EIPA. This indicates that the inhibition of H^+ extrusion by the Na^+/H^+ antiporter is not the only mechanism by which Na^+-free conditions potentiate the acidifying action of PTX. An involvement of the Na^+-dependent Cl^-/HCO_3^- exchanger, which usually acts in parallel to the Na^+/H^+ exchanger to protect cells against intracellular acidifications (2), can be ruled out for experiments performed in the absence of bicarbonate. One possible mechanism could be that Na^+-free conditions prevent the depolarizing action of PTX (10, 22) and increase the driving force for H^+ entry through electrogenic pores in the plasma membrane.

This possibility can be tested by using depolarizing membrane conditions. When the membrane potential is close to zero, the driving force for electrogenic H^+ movements across the plasma membrane is determined only by the intra- and extracellular H^+ concentrations. If care is taken to reduce the activity of pH_i-regulating mechanisms, an opening of an H^+-conductive pathway should lead to a simple equilibration of pH_i with pH_o. Figure 4 shows the results of a typical experiment performed with aortic smooth muscle cells of the A7r5 cell line. Cells are incubated in an Na^+-free, 145 mM K^+–Earle's salt solution to ensure (1) that pH_i-regulating mechanisms are not operating for their substrates (Na^+ for the Na^+/H^+ exchanger and HCO_3^- for the Cl^-/HCO_3^- exchanger) and are not present in the incubation solution and (2) that the membrane potential is close to zero (for $[K^+]_o = [K^+]_i$). Figure 4 shows that the addition of 0.1 μM PTX to the cells leads to rapid changes in pH_i, the magnitude and direction of which are dependent on the value of pH_o. When pH_o is 7.4, no change in pH_i is observed. When pH_o is 8.3, a cellular alkalinization to a value of 7.95 is observed. Finally, when pH_o is 5.7, a large cellular acidification to pH_i 5.9 is observed. Thus, PTX treatment of K^+-depolarized cells simply leads to an equilibration of pH_i with pH_o. The fact that PTX produces opposite changes in pH_i depending on the value of pH_o also rules out the possibility that PTX acidifies cells by stimulating the metabolic production of H^+. It is known, for instance, that in neutrophils the chemotactic peptide formylmethionyllysylproline (fMLP) induces a cellular acidification that is potentiated by Na^+-free conditions and by amiloride derivatives. An increased activity of the Na^+/H^+ antiporter occurs secondarily to the primary acidification and limits its extent. The acidification pro-

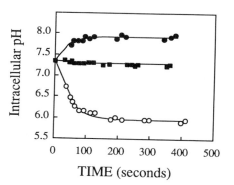

FIG. 4   The action of PTX on the pH_i of K^+-depolarized smooth muscle cells. Aortic myocytes (A7r5 line) loaded with BCECF are diluted into a 145 mM KCl solution (containing 1.8 mM $CaCl_2$ and 0.8 mM $MgSO_4$) and buffered at pH_o 8.3 (●), 7.4 (■), or 5.7 (○) appropriate mixtures of HEPES, Tris, and MES buffers and 0.1 μM PTX added at time zero. Changes in the fluorescence of BCECF are then monitored by flow cytometry. Each point shown represents the average of 3000 single-cell measurements.

duced by fMLP is consecutive to the production of reactive oxygen species by NADPH oxidase (23).

The acidifying action of PTX was first described in chick cardiac cells (7). It was also observed in rat aortic smooth muscle cells (Fig. 4) and in endothelial cells from brain microvessels (data not shown). No action of PTX on pH_i was reported in 3T3 fibroblasts (24). This may be evidence that PTX interacts with a membrane structure that is expressed in a cell-specific manner. Palytoxin has no ionophore properties by itself (10).

Relationships between Palytoxin-Induced Changes in pH_i and Changes in $[Ca^{2+}]_i$

In excitable cells that respond to PTX by a cellular acidification, PTX also opens a Ca^{2+} uptake pathway in the plasma membrane that leads to an increase in the cytoplasmic concentration of Ca^{2+} (16). This raises the possibility that the acidification induced by PTX is not a primary effect of the toxin but is consecutive to its action on $[Ca^{2+}]_i$. Intracellular acidifications are often associated with increases in $[Ca^{2+}]_i$, as first described in cardiac cells (25). In fibroblasts, the rise in cytoplasmic $[Ca^{2+}]_i$ that follows an activation of phospholipase C and the release of Ca^{2+} from intracellular stores is accompanied by an intracellular acidification (26). Coupled changes in pH_i and in $[Ca^{2+}]_i$ may be due to the existence of intracellular buffering sites that are common to H^+ and Ca^{2+} (25).

Three types of evidence indicate that the action of PTX on the pH_i of chick cardiac cells is not secondary to changes in $[Ca^{2+}]_i$. First we observed, thanks to the flow cytometry technique, that all cells respond to PTX by a change in pH_i. Yet PTX increases $[Ca^{2+}]_i$ in only about one-third of the cells analyzed (16). The obvious conclusion is that there must be cells in which PTX produced a change in pH_i without producing a parallel change in $[Ca^{2+}]_i$ and, at least in these cells, changes in pH_i cannot be consecutive to changes in $[Ca^{2+}]_i$. More evidence is that under depolarizing membrane conditions and at variable pH_o values, PTX always increases $[Ca^{2+}]_i$ although opposite changes in pH_i are observed (16). Finally, we observed that when cardiac cells are incubated in an acidic, 145 mM K^+ solution containing 50 nM Ca^{2+}, PTX still produced a cellular acidification. Under these conditions, PTX had no action on $[Ca^{2+}]_i$ (16). The obvious conclusion of these experiments is that most of the PTX-induced cellular acidification is not consecutive to the changes in $[Ca^{2+}]_i$ and therefore represents a primary action of the toxin. Changes in pH_i secondary to PTX-induced changes in $[Ca^{2+}]_i$ may also contribute to the acidifying action of PTX.

All evidence obtained so far indicates that a primary action of PTX is to produce an intracellular acidification in a manner that is independent of Na^+ and Ca^{2+} and that is consistent with the opening of a membrane H^+-conducting pathway. The acidification then leads to a secondary activation of the Na^+/H^+ antiporter, which reduces the extent of the acidification but loads cells with Na^+. Both a decrease in pH_i and an intracellular Na^+ load are well known to alter cardiac contractility and may contribute to the toxic action of PTX.

Membrane leakage pathways for H^+ have been observed in *Axolotl* oocytes (27), in snail neurons (5), in brain synaptosomes (28), and in various epithelial cells (6). Whether these pathways are targets for PTX is not currently known.

The acidifying action of PTX is not the only mechanism by which the toxin acts on excitable cells. In chick cardiac cells (16) and in rat aortic myocytes, PTX also opens a Ca^{2+}-uptake pathway that is unrelated to L-type or T-type Ca^{2+} channels or to Na^+/Ca^{2+} exchange and that seems to be independent of changes in pH_i. Recent patch-clamp experiments peformed on guinea pig and rat cardiomyocytes indicated that PTX opens a voltage-independent, nonselective cationic channel that is permeable to Na^+ and K^+ but not to Ca^{2+} (29, 30). The permeability of this channel to H^+ has not been determined. It could be that, in fact, PTX stabilizes an open conformation of several related forms of nonspecific ionic channels (possibly "receptor-operated channels"). A tissue-specific expression of these channels may further explain the diversity of the actions of the toxins in different cell types.

Acknowledgments

This work was supported by the CNRS and the Association pour la Recherche sur le Cancer. We are grateful to Dr. P. Vigne for helpful discussions.

References

1. A. Roos and W. Boron, *Physiol. Rev.* **61**, 296 (1981).
2. C. Frelin, P. Vigne, A. Ladoux, and M. Lazdunski, *Eur. J. Biochem.* **174**, 3 (1988).
3. S. Grinstein, "Na/H Exchange." CRC Press, Boca Raton, Florida, 1989.
4. P. Vigne, C. Frelin, and M. Lazdunski, *EMBO J.* **3**, 1865 (1984).
5. R. C. Thomas and R. W. Meech, *Nature (London)* **299**, 826 (1981).
6. A. S. Verkman, *J. Bioenerg. Biomembr.* **19**, 481 (1987).
7. C. Frelin, P. Vigne, and J.-P. Breittmayer, *FEBS Lett.* **264**, 63 (1990).
8. R. E. Moore, G. Bartolini, J. Barchi, A. A. Bothner-By, J. Dadok, and J. Ford, *J. Am. Chem. Soc.* **104**, 3776 (1982).

9. J. K. Cha, W. J. Christ, J. M. Finan, H. Fujioka, Y. Kishi, L. L. Klein, S. S. Ko, J. Leder, W. W. McWhorter, K. P. Pfaff, M. Yonega, D. Uemura, and Y. Hirata, *J. Am. Chem. Soc.* **104,** 7369 (1982).
10. E. Habermann, *Toxicon* **27,** 1171 (1989).
11. H. Nagase and H. Karachi, *J. Pharmacol. Exp. Ther.* **242,** 1120 (1987).
12. P. Vigne, C. Frelin, E. J. Cragoe, and M. Lazdunski, *Biochem. Biophys. Res. Commun.* **116,** 86 (1983).
13. C. Frelin, P. Vigne, and M. Lazdunski, *J. Biol. Chem.* **259,** 8880 (1984).
14. D. Kim and T. W. Smith, *Mol. Pharmacol.* **30,** 164 (1986).
15. M. Floreani, M. Tessari, P. Debetto, S. Luciani, and F. Carpenedo, *Naunyn-Schmiedeberg's Arch. Pharmacol.* **336,** 661 (1987).
16. C. Frelin, P. Vigne, and J.-P. Breittmayer, *Mol. Pharmacol.* **38,** 904 (1990).
17. C. Frelin and J.-P. Breittmayer, this volume [17].
18. J. A. Thomas, R. N. Buchsbaum, A. Zimniak, and E. Racker, *Biochemistry* **18,** 2210 (1979).
19. T. J. Rink, R. Y. Tsien, and T. Pozzan, *J. Cell Biol.* **95,** 189 (1982).
20. C. Sardet, L. Counillon, A. Franchi, and J. Pouyssegur, *Science* **247,** 723 (1990).
21. H. Fujiki, M. Suganuma, M. Nakayasu, H. Hakii, T. Horiucki, S. Takayama, and T. Sugimura, *Carcinogenesis* **7,** 707 (1986).
22. M.-P. Sauviat, C. Pater, and J. Berton, *Toxicon* **25,** 695 (1987).
23. S. Grinstein, W. Furuya, and W. D. Biggar, *J. Biol. Chem.* **261,** 512 (1986).
24. E. V. Wattenberg, K. L. Byron, M. L. Villereal, H. Fujiki, and M. R. Rosner, *J. Biol. Chem.* **264,** 14668 (1989).
25. R. D. Vaughan Jones, W. J. Lederer, and D. A. Eisner, *Nature (London)* **301,** 522 (1983).
26. H. E. Ives and T. O. Daniel, *Proc. Natl. Acad. Sci. U.S.A.* **84,** 1950 (1987).
27. M. E. Barish and C. Baud, *J. Physiol. (London)* **352,** 248 (1984).
28. T. Jean, C. Frelin, P. Vigne, P. Barbry, and M. Lazdunski, *J. Biol. Chem.* **260,** 9678 (1985).
29. I. Muramatsu, M. Nishio, S. Kigoshi, and D. Uemara, *Br. J. Pharmacol.* **93,** 811 (1988).
30. M. Ikeda, K. Mitani, and K. Ito, *Naunyn-Schmiedeberg's Arch. Pharmacol.* **337,** 591 (1988).

[26] Pertussis Toxin in Analysis of Receptor Mechanisms

Terry Reisine and Susan F. Law

Introduction

Guanine nucleotide regulatory (G) proteins are cell membrane-associated proteins that have an important role in the signal transduction process (1–3). They have been shown to couple cell-surface receptors to different effector systems such as the adenylate cyclase complex and ionic conductance channels. Multiple G proteins are expressed in mammalian cells (4–6) and recent studies have shown that more than one G protein can couple with a given receptor (7–9). Conceivably, different G proteins may link a given receptor to different cellular effector systems. This complexity of receptor–G protein interaction may provide the stuctural basis for an individual neurotransmitter or hormone to independently regulate multiple cellular effector systems.

A number of biochemical and pharmacological tools have been developed to study the structural and functional roles of G proteins. Recently, cDNA encoding the different subunits of G proteins have been cloned, which has allowed for the investigation of the factors controlling the expression of G proteins in mammalian cells as well as the elucidation of domains in G proteins involved in their coupling to receptors and cellular effector systems (4–6). Furthermore, availability of peptide-directed antisera against different G proteins has allowed for studies to better understand the selectivity of the physical association of G proteins with different cellular components as well as the cellular localization of G proteins (8–11). However, before cDNA encoding G proteins was cloned and the amino acid sequence of the G proteins elucidated, G protein structure and function had been primarily investigated through the use of bacterial toxins. These agents are still extensively employed to elucidate functional roles of G proteins in different biological systems. The two major toxins employed for G protein analysis are cholera and pertussis toxin. Cholera toxin has been used extensively to examine the stimulatory G protein (G_s) (1–3, 12). Pertussis toxin has been employed to investigate the functions of the inhibitor of adenylate cyclase activity, G_i, as well as a G protein expressed in high levels in brain termed G_o (1–3, 12). This chapter will be directed at describing methodologies employing pertussis toxin to elucidate the biochemical properties and functions of G_i and G_o.

Methods in Neurosciences, Volume 8

Selectivity for α subunits of G_i and G_o

Pertussis toxin is isolated from the bacteria *Bordetella pertussis* (12). It has been shown to modify the function of G proteins by catalyzing the ADP-ribosylation of a cysteine residue on the carboxy terminal of the α subunit of G_i and G_o (13). Previous studies have shown that G_{ia} is more sensitive to the actions of pertussis toxin than G_{oa} (14). However, the α subunit of G_s does not contain the recognition site of pertussis toxin and therefore is not modified by it. Furthermore, a recently identified G protein from brain, G_z, does not contain the cysteine residue acceptor for ADP-ribosylation and therefore is not affected by pertussis toxin (15). The selective chemical modification of the α subunit of G_i (G_{ia}) and G_o (G_{oa}) is the basis for the specificity of pertussis toxin for inactivating these G protein subunits.

Pertussis toxin catalyzes the transfer of an ADP-ribose group from NAD to either G_{ia} or G_{oa} (12). By using [^{32}P]NAD as a donor, pertussis toxin can be employed to selectively direct the covalent incorporation of [^{32}P]ADP-ribose into these G protein α subunits. As a result, it is possible to specifically tag either G_{ia} or G_{oa} with a radioactive label. By subjecting the radioactive G protein α subunit to gel electrophoresis and autoradiography, it is possible to identify the presence of either G_{ia} or G_{oa} in different tissues and to examine their physical properties.

ADP-ribosylation of G_i or G_o causes their uncoupling from membrane-associated receptors, thereby inactivating the receptors (1–3, 12). In contrast, pertussis toxin does not prevent G_s from associating with receptors involved in the stimulation of adenylate cyclase or other G proteins insensitive to pertussis toxin from coupling with receptors mediating hormone and neurotransmitter stimulation of phospholipase C activity. The ability of pertussis toxin to selectively uncouple G_i and G_o from receptors has resulted in the identification of those signal transduction pathways in which these G proteins serve a critical biological role.

Biochemical Analysis of G Proteins Using Pertussis Toxin

Numerous studies have utilized the ability of pertussis toxin to catalyze the [^{32}P]ADP-ribosylation of G_{ia} and G_{oa} to detect the presence of these G proteins in the membranes of a variety of cells (12). The conditions of the pertussis toxin reaction may vary depending on the tissue source of the G proteins. In studies to detect pertussis toxin-sensitive G proteins in the mouse anterior pituitary cell line AtT-20, which expresses both G_{ia} and G_{oa}, selective [^{32}P]ADP-ribosylation of these G protein subunits can be accomplished by reacting 25 μg of cell membranes with preactivated pertussis toxin (20

μg/ml) at 30°C for 60 min in a solution containing 1 mM ATP, 1 mM EDTA, 1 mM dithiothreitol, 10 mM thymidine and 5 μM [^{32}P]NAD (20,000 cpm/ pmol) (16). The reaction is terminated by diluting the reactants with sample buffer for gel-electrophoretic analysis. For these studies, pertussis toxin is activated by its incubation in a solution of 50 mM 4-(2-hydroxyethyl)-1-piperazine-ethanesulfonic acid (HEPES; pH 8), 20 mM dithiothreitol, 1 mg/ml bovine serum albumin, and 0.125% (w/v) sodium dodecyl sulfate (SDS) at 30°C for 30 min. Radiolabeled material is analyzed by SDS-polyacrylamide gel electrophoresis (SDS-PAGE) and autoradiography. Under the conditions used, proteins of 40–41 kDa are selectively [^{32}P]ADP-ribosylated in AtT-20 cell membranes. Incorporation of radiolabel into these proteins is a linear function of the amount of membrane in the reaction between 10 and 100 μg of membrane protein (16, 17). The radiolabeled material most likely represents G_{ia} and/or G_{oa} because it exhibits electrophoretic mobility similar to immunoreactive G_{ia} and G_{oa} detected with antisera selective for these proteins as analyzed by Western blotting (18).

The selective [^{32}P]ADP-ribosylation of G_{ia} and G_{oa} catalyzed by pertussis toxin allows these proteins to be monitored under various experimental procedures such as in studies to immunoprecipitate G proteins, either with antisera directed against the G protein or with antisera directed against proteins associated with G_{ia} or G_{oa}. The utility of covalently tagging the G protein α subunit with [^{32}P]ADP-ribose is that it allows for a relative quantification of the immunoprecipitation of the G protein by various antisera. For example, in studies examining solubilized G_{ia} from rat brain, it is possible to immunoprecipitate G_{ia} with a peptide-generated antiserum (antiserum 8730) that is directed to the C-terminal region of all G_{ia}s (9). Immunoprecipitation of brain G_{ia} can be shown by reacting solubilized G_{ia} with antiserum 8730 followed by addition of protein A-Sepharose and centrifugation. To demonstrate that G_{ia} has been immunoprecipitated, the immunoprecipitate is reacted with pertussis toxin and [^{32}P]NAD and the labeled material subjected to SDS-PAGE and autoradiography. As shown in Fig. 1A, significantly greater levels of [^{32}P]ADP-ribosylated 41-kDa material are present in the antiserum 8730 immunoprecipitate than in preimmune controls. The material immunoprecipitated is most likely G_{ia}, since analysis of the antiserum 8730 immunoprecipitate by SDS-PAGE and Western blotting revealed that the 41-kDa proteins were immunoreactive to antiserum 8730 (Fig. 1C), which selectively interacts with G_{ia} on immunoblots (19). To determine the relative degree of immunoprecipitation of G_{ia}, solubilized G_{ia} was reacted with pertussis toxin, 0.4 M thymidine, and [^{32}P]NAD and the radiolabeled G protein was immunoprecipitated with antiserum 8730. Analysis of the immunoprecipitate by SDS-PAGE and autoradiography revealed that antiserum 8730 immunoprecipitated significantly greater levels of [^{32}P]ADP-ribo-

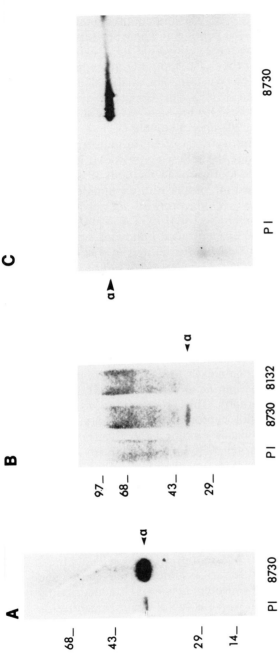

FIG. 1 Immunoprecipitation of $G_{i\alpha}$ using a peptide-directed antisera. To immunoprecipitate $G_{i\alpha}$, peptide-generated antisera directed against $G_{i\alpha}$ (8730) were added to solubilized proteins from rat brain, allowed to incubate, and then reacted with protein A–Sepharose. Precipitation of the immune complex was facilitated by centrifugation. The immunoprecipitate was washed extensively and then reacted with pertussis toxin and [^{32}P]NAD to induce the [^{32}P]ADP-ribosylation of $G_{i\alpha}$. The labeled proteins were subjected to SDS-PAGE and autoradiography to visualize the labeled G protein. In (A) is the autoradiogram showing the [^{32}P]ADP-ribosylated G_{α} subunit in the antiserum 8730 immunoprecipitate (8730) and preimmune (PI) control. Arrowhead points to the 41-kDa radiolabeled material. Size markers ($\times 10^{-3}$) are presented to the left of the autoradiogram. In (B), solubilized rat brain proteins were first reacted with pertussis toxin and [^{32}P]NAD, exposed to GTPγS to dissociate $G_{i\alpha}$ from G_{b} subunit, and then immunoprecipitated with either antiserum 8730, or antiserum 8132, which is a peptide-generated antiserum directed against G_{b36}. The immunoprecipitates were extensively washed and subjected to SDS-PAGE and autoradiography. The autoradiogram is presented with size markers ($\times 10^{-3}$) to the left. To further show that antiserum 8730 immunoprecipitated $G_{i\alpha}$, the antiserum 8730 immunoprecipitate was washed extensively, subjected to SDS-PAGE, and the proteins transferred to nitrocellulose paper and Western blotted with antiserum 8730. Stained protein is presented in (C).

sylated G_{ia} than preimmune controls (Fig. 1B). The immunoprecipitation was specific because it could be blocked by the peptide to which antiserum 8730 was generated (not shown) and, furthermore, antiserum 8132, which is a peptide-directed antiserum selective for the β_{36} subunit of G_i and which does not directly interact with G_{ia}, based on Western blot analysis, does not immunoprecipitate [^{32}P]ADP-ribosylated G_{ia} (Fig. 1B). Using these immunoprecipitation procedures, previous studies (19) have shown that antiserum 8730 can maximally immunoprecipitate 30–40% of soluble G_{ia}.

Pertussis toxin-catalyzed [^{32}P]ADP-ribosylation of G_{ia} in antiserum 8730 immunoprecipitates was conducted using the following protocol: rat brain proteins were solubilized using previously described methods (9, 20) employing a solubilization buffer composed of 20 mM 3-[(3-cholamidopropyl) dimethylammonio]-1-propane sulfonate (v/v) glycerol, 0.5 μg aprotinin/μl, diluted in 50 mM Tris-HCl (pH 7.8) containing 1 mM EGTA, 5 mM MgCl$_2$, 10 μg leupeptin, 2 μg pepstatin, and 200 μg bacitracin. Following solubilization, the samples are centrifuged at 100,000 g for 60 min at 4°C and the supernatant is then applied to an Ultrogel AcA 34 gel-exclusion column. (IBF, Vielleneuve, France). The running buffer consists of 50 mM Tris-HCl (pH 7.8), 1 mM EGTA, 5 mM MgCl$_2$, 10% (v/v) glycerol, and 5 mM CHAPS. The column dimensions are 70 $\times$ 1.6 cm with a flow rate of 6.0 ml/hr at 4°C. This sample preparation was employed because studies in our laboratory not only involve an investigation of the properties of G proteins but also their coupling with somatostatin receptors (9, 20) and attempts to immunoprecipitate somatostatin receptor–G protein complexes using G protein-directed antisera are best obtained by this partial purification of receptor–G protein complexes by gel-exclusion chromatography. Thus, eluted fractions are examined for the presence of somatostatin receptors in a high-affinity, G protein-coupled conformation using a radioligand-binding assay (20, 21). Eluted fractions containing peak receptor–G protein activity are combined, concentrated, and used in immunoprecipitation studies as previously described (9).

To immunoprecipitate G proteins, solubilized G proteins derived from rat brain are incubated with an aliquot of G protein-specific antiserum for 4–6 hr, and as with all subsequent steps, the samples are placed on a rotator at 4°C. One hundred microliters of 50% (w/v) protein A-Sepharose beads (CL-4B; Sigma, St. Louis, MO), three times washed and diluted in a buffer of 50 mM Tris-HCl (pH 7.8), 1 mM EGTA, 5 mM MgCl$_2$, 10 μg leupeptin, 2 μg pepstatin, and 200 μg bacitracin (buffer A), is added to the sample and incubated overnight. Another aliquot of G protein antiserum is added, bringing the total antiserum dilution to 1 : 20, which is the optimal concentration of antiserum for immunoprecipitation of G proteins. The samples are incubated for three more hours and then centrifuged at 10,000 rpm for 2 min. The supernatant is removed, the immunoprecipitate washed several times with buffer A, and then washed three more times with a buffer containing 50 mM NaCl and 0.1% (v/v) Tween 20 (buffer B). Then the α subunits of G_i and/or G_o (depending on which α subunit has been immunoprecipitated) are reacted with [^{32}P]NAD and pertussis toxin to ^{32}P-ADP-ribosylate the G protein. The procedures used to [^{32}P]ADP-ribosylate immunoprecipitated G_a subunits involve reacting the immunoprecipitated G_{ia} subunit with activated pertussis toxin in a buffer containing 0.1 M EDTA, 0.1 M dithiothreitol (DTT), 0.2 M thymidine, and 0.1 mM [^{32}P]NAD. Pertussis toxin is activated by its reaction with a buffer containing 0.2 M HEPES (pH 8.0), 0.1 M DTT, 10 mg/ml bovine serum albumin (BSA), and 1% (w/v) SDS. To further quantify the relative amount of G_a subunit immunoprecipitated, solubilized G_{ia} or G_{oa} is first reacted with [^{32}P]NAD and pertussis toxin and then immunoprecipitated with G_a-directed antiserum. Analysis of the immunoprecipitated [^{32}P]ADP-ribosylated G_a and the soluble [^{32}P]ADP-ribosylated G_a remaining in the supernatant by SDS-PAGE and autoradiography followed by excision of the gel slice containing the labeled G protein and determination of the radioactivity in each gel slice by liquid scintillation spectroscopy can reveal the relative efficiency of the immunoprecipitation of the pertussis toxin-sensitive G_a under study. Such quantification can be confirmed by metabolically labeling G_a subunits in cell lines with [^{35}S]methionine, solubilizing the G proteins, and immunoprecipitating the ^{35}S-labeled G proteins with peptide-directed antisera.

Pertussis toxin-catalyzed [^{32}P]ADP-ribosylation of G_a subunits is an important approach to detect G_a subunits that may be coprecipitated with other cellular proteins. For example, G_{ia} is associated with β subunits of G proteins (G_b) (1–3). The ability of pertussis toxin to catalyze the [^{32}P]ADP-ribosylation of G_{ia} in antiserum 8730 immunoprecipitates indicates that G_b was coimmunoprecipitated, because the β–δ complex is required for the ADP-ribosylation of α subunits (22). In preliminary studies we have observed that antisera directed against a subtype of G_b, referred to as G_{b36}, are able to immunoprecipitate both G_{b36} and pertussis toxin-sensitive G_a subunit (Fig. 2). This was shown by immunoprecipitating soluble G_{b36} subunit from rat brain with peptide-directed antiserum selective for G_{b36} (antiserum 8132) and reacting the immunoprecipitate with pertussis toxin and [^{32}P]NAD to catalyze the [^{32}P]ADP-ribosylation of G_{ia} that was coimmunoprecipitated. Analysis of the radiolabeled G_{ia} by SDS-PAGE and autoradiography revealed that G_{b36}-directed antiserum was able to coimmunoprecipitate G_{ia}. Furthermore, anti-G_{b36} antiserum was able to immunoprecipitate similar levels of pertussis toxin-sensitive G protein as anti-G_{ia} antiserum (Fig. 2). Coimmunoprecipitation of the G protein subunits did not occur if G_{ia} and G_{b36} were uncoupled by the presence of GTPγS as shown in Fig. 1B. GTPγS has been shown to bind to G_{ia} that has been ADP-ribosylated and the interaction of this guanine nucleotide with the G protein complex dissociates the α and β subunits (14).

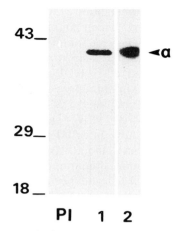

FIG. 2 G_{ia}/G_{b36} complexes can be immunoprecipitated with antisera directed against G_{b36}. For these studies, solubilized rat brain proteins were reacted with either antiserum 8730 (lane 1) or antiserum 8132 (lane 2). G proteins complexed with these antisera were immunoprecipitated with protein A-Sepharose and the immunoprecipitated material was washed extensively and then reacted with pertussis toxin and [^{32}P]NAD. The labeled proteins were subjected to SDS-PAGE and autoradiography. The autoradiogram is presented with size markers ($\times 10^{-3}$) to the left. PI refers to preimmune control and the arrowhead points to the ^{32}P-labeled G_a subunit.

Besides G_{b36}, G_{ia} is also coupled with the somatostatin receptor, because antiserum directed against G_{ia} (antiserum 8730) was able to immunoprecipitate solubilized somatostatin receptors from rat brain and the pituitary tumor cell line AtT-20 (8, 9). These studies and others have shown that G_{ia} can form a complex with G_{b36} and the somatostatin receptor and further supports a role for G_{ia} in mediating the physiological actions of somatostatin.

Use of Pertussis Toxin to Study Functional Roles of G Proteins

In addition to its use in studies to examine the biochemical properties of G proteins, pertussis toxin has been employed to investigate the functional role of G proteins (1–3, 12). Pertussis toxin was first identified by its ability to activate pancreatic islets by facilitating hormone secretion from this tissue (23). This facilitory action appears to be due in part to pertussis toxin blocking the inhibitory influence of somatostatin on glucagon and insulin release from these cells (24). The results from these investigations were the first evidence that somatostatin acted through an inhibitory G protein to induce its biological actions. This hypothesis was supported by experiments conducted in the tumor cell line cyc$^-$ S49 lymphoma, which lacks G_s, but expresses G_{ia}, which was shown to couple somatostatin receptors to adenylate cyclase in an inhibitory manner (25, 26).

In addition to revealing that somatostatin receptors are linked to adenylate cyclase via G_{ia}, pertussis toxin has been used to reveal that G_{ia} and/or G_{oa} couple the somatostatin receptor to ionic conductance channels. A number of studies have reported that pretreatment of neurons or pituitary cells in culture with pertussis toxin blocks the facilitation of K^+ currents by somatostatin (27–30). In these studies, cells are either exposed to pertussis toxin or pertussis toxin is injected directly into the cells or applied to excised patches of cell membranes containing K^+ channels. In elegant studies by Yatani *et al.* (27), it was reported that exposure of the pituitary cell line GH$_3$ to pertussis toxin abolished the potentiation by somatostatin of a voltage-dependent K^+ conductance. Actions of somatostatin could be reconstituted with a purified G protein that the authors referred to as G_K, and which was later shown to correspond to a subtype of G_{ia}. This was the first direct evidence that G_{ia} couples somatostatin receptors to K^+ channels and reveals that somatostatin receptors are linked to divergent cellular effector systems, such as the adenylate cyclase complex and K^+ channels via G_{ia}. In more recent studies, evidence has also been provided that somatostatin receptors are also linked to Ca^{2+} channels via pertussis toxin-sensitive G protein, indicating that G proteins can greatly diversify the cellular actions of a given neurotransmitter (31).

In addition to amplifying the biological actions of a given neurotransmitter, G proteins have also been shown to provide the means by which different neurotransmitters can converge to regulate the same biological response. Thus in recent electrophysiological studies by North and colleagues (32), it has been shown that opiate, α_2-adrenergic, and somatostatin receptors are expressed on the same neurons in the locus coeruleus and that activation of any of these receptors results in the simulation of the same K^+ channel. These investigators have proposed that these different receptors are linked to the same K^+ channels and have also shown that pertussis toxin uncouples each receptor from K^+ channels in these cells. These findings suggest that the same pertussis toxin-sensitive G protein may link all of these receptors to the same effector system and may provide the basis for convergence of the actions of different neurotransmitters on a common cellular effector system.

Conclusions

Pertussis toxin has been a useful tool to study the molecular mechanisms by which G protein-linked receptors mediate the biological actions of neurotransmitters. Together with recently developed agents such as G protein-directed antisera and cDNA encoding G proteins, pertussis toxin may be expected to be employed to further investigate the structure–function relationship of receptor, G protein, and cellular effector system interactions. Future directions will involve studies to elucidate the binding sites within receptors, G proteins, and effector systems involved with their coupling. Furthermore, attempts will be made to determine whether different G proteins link receptors to different cellular effector systems. Such studies will greatly advance our understanding of the molecular mechanisms of the signal transduction process.

Acknowledgment

This work was supported by NIMH Grant MH 45533.

References

1. A. Gilman, *Annu. Rev. Biochem.* **56,** 615 (1987).
2. E. Neer and D. Clapham, *Nature (London)* **333,** 129 (1988).
3. T. Reisine, *Biochem. Pharmacol.* **39,** 1499 (1990).
4. H. Itoh, T. Kozasa, S. Nagat, S. Nakamura, T. Katada, M. Ui, S. Iwai, E. Ohtsuka, H. Kawasaki, K. Suzuki, and Y. Kaziro, *Proc. Natl. Acad. Sci. U.S.A.* **83,** 3776 (1986).
5. D. Jones and R. Reed, *J. Biol. Chem.* **262,** 14241 (1987).
6. J. Robishaw, M. Smigel, and A. Gilman, *J. Biol.Chem.* **261,** 9587 (1986).
7. S. Sengoles, A. Spiegel, E. Padrell, R. Iyengar, and M. Caron, *J. Biol. Chem.* **265,** 4507 (1990).
8. S. F. Law, S. Rens-Domiano, D. Manning, and T. Reisine, *J. Biol. Chem.* **266,** 17,885 (1991).
9. T. Reisine, S. Rens-Domiano, S. F. Law, and J.-M. Martin, *Methods Neurosci.* **5,** 215 (1991).
10. D. Matesic, D. Manning, B. Wolfe, and G. Luthin, *J. Biol. Chem.* **264,** 21645 (1989).
11. A. Williams, M. Woolkalis, M. Poncz, D. Manning, A. Gerwitz, and L. Brass, *Blood* **76,** 721 (1990).
12. R. Sekura, J. Moss, and M. Vaughan, "Pertussis Toxin." Academic Press, Orlando, Florida, 1985.
13. R. West, J. Moss, M. Vaughan, T. Lius, and T. Y. Liu, *J. Biol. Chem.* **260,** 14428 (1985).
14. R. M. Huff and E. Neer, *J. Biol. Chem.* **261,** 1105 (1986).
15. H. Fong, K. Yoshimoto, P. Eversole-Cire, and M. Simon, *Proc. Natl. Acad. Sci. U.S.A.* **85,** 3066 (1988).

16. N. Mahy, M. Woolkalis, K. Thermos, K. Carlson, D. Manning, and T. Reisine, *J. Pharmacol. Exp. Ther.* **246,** 779 (1988).
17. M. Woolkalis, M. Nakada, and D. Manning, *J. Biol. Chem.* **261,** 3408 (1986).
18. N. Mahy, M. Woolkalis, D. Manning, and T. Reisine, *J. Pharmacol. Exp. Ther.* **247,** 390 (1988).
19. K. Carlson, L. Brass, and D. Manning, *J. Biol. Chem.* **264,** 13298 (1989).
20. H. T. He, S. Rens-Domiano, J.-M. Martin, S. F. Law, S. Borislow, M. Woolkalis, D. Manning, and T. Reisine, *Mol. Pharmacol.* **37,** 614 (1990).
21. K. Raynor and T. Reisine, *J. Pharmacol. Exp. Ther.* **251,** 510 (1989).
22. E. Neer, J. Lok, and L. Wolf, *J. Biol. Chem.* **259,** 14224 (1984).
23. T. Katada, J. Northup, G. Bokoch, M. Ui, and A. Gilman, *J. Biol. Chem.* **259,** 3578 (1984).
24. T. Katada and M. Ui, *J. Biol.Chem.* **254,** 469 (1979).
25. K. Jakobs, K. Aktories, and G. Schultz, *Nature (London)* **303,** 177 (1983).
26. K. Jakobs and G. Schultz, *Proc. Natl. Acad. Sci. U.S.A.* **80,** 3899 (1983).
27. A. Yatani, J. Codina, R. Sekura, L. Birnbaumer, and A. Brown, *Mol. Endocrinol.* **1,** 283 (1987).
28. H. L. Wang, C. Bogen, T. Reisine, and M. Dichter, *Proc. Natl. Acad. Sci. U.S.A.* **86,** 9616 (1989).
29. M. Inoue, S. Nakajima, and Y. Nakajima, *J. Physiol. (London)* **407,** 177 (1988).
30. T. Jacquin, J. Champagnat, S. Mandamba, M. Denavit-Saubie, and G. Siggins, *Proc. Natl. Acad. Sci. U.S.A.* **85,** 948 (1988).
31. H. L. Wang, T. Reisine, and M. Dichter, *Neuroscience* **38,** 355 (1990).
32. R. A. North, *Br. J. Pharmacol.* **98,** 13 (1989).

[27] Resiniferatoxin

Arpad Szallasi and Peter M. Blumberg

Introduction

Vanilloids, the best known example of which is capsaicin, are the pungent constituents in "hot" peppers. The vanilloids provide a unique probe for a well-defined population of small-diameter primary afferent neurons subserving chemogenic pain, warm sensation, neurogenic inflammation, and a variety of physiological reflexes and local regulatory functions (1, 2). Capsaicin-induced excitation of these neural pathways is followed by functional impairment, which, in a dose-dependent manner, may be either reversible (desensitization) or irreversible (1). The ability of vanilloids to induce blockade of these pathways has led to their therapeutic use as nonnarcotic analgesics (3), and development of improved agents in this class represents an ongoing objective.

The biochemical mechanisms underlying vanilloid action remain unknown. It appears, however, that the initial excitation is a result of the opening of a ligand-gated nonspecific cation channel provoking a tetrodotoxin-resistant membrane depolarization and release of inflammatory neuropeptides; the functional impairment is thought to be due to a combination of intracellular calcium accumulation, the osmotic shock associated with cation influx, and block of intraaxonal transport of trophic factors (2). The identification of the capsaicin receptor, which might be either the channel itself or a closely associated modulatory subunit, had proven problematic due to the lipophilicity of capsaicin and its relatively low potency (2).

An exciting recent advance in the vanilloid field has been our discovery that resiniferatoxin (RTX), a naturally occurring diterpene combining structural features of the phorbol ester tumor promoters and of capsaicin (see structures in Fig. 1), functions as an ultrapotent capsaicin analog (4–6) and that the esterification of other phorbol-related diterpenes with homovanillic acid at the C-20 position yields synthetic vanilloids of the RTX class with unique spectra of action (7). Resiniferatoxin, for example, displays a 100- to 10,000-fold greater potency than capsaicin for most of the responses tested but shows only equal potency for induction of pain (5, 8). Other differences between RTX and capsaicin include different pharmacokinetics (a slower tissue penetration for RTX) (9) and unique actions, such as the acute desensitization in the rat of the pulmonary chemoreceptors by RTX without induc-

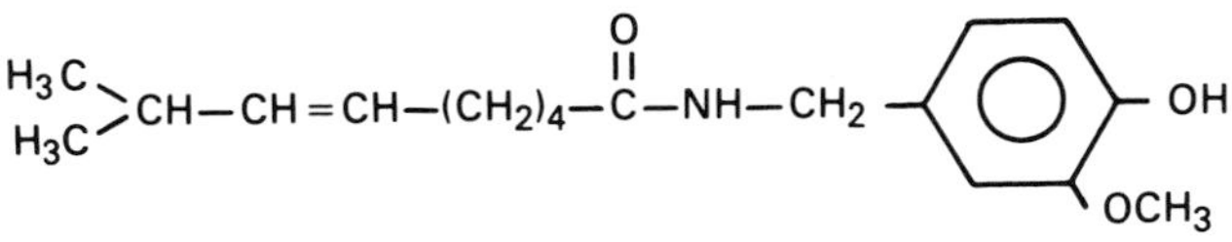

Capsaicin

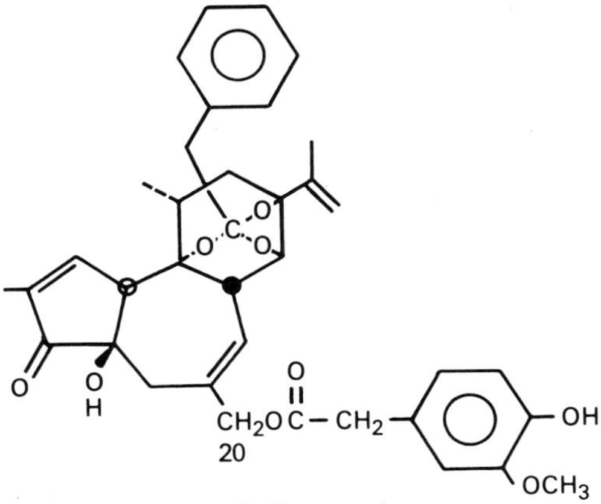

Resiniferatoxin

FIG. 1 Structure of resiniferatoxin and capsaicin.

tion of the triad of the pulmonary chemoreflex, which is a major limiting factor for the *in vivo* use of capsaicin (10). The high lipophilicity of capsaicin and its moderate potency had confounded efforts to demonstrate and characterize the postulated capsaicin receptor (2). The much higher potency of RTX, together with our extensive experience in the behavior of diterpene esters in binding assays, has now resolved this problem (8, 11). We describe here the approaches for measurement of the specific binding of [^{3}H]RTX, thought to represent a vanilloid receptor (8, 11). This binding assay contributes a powerful new tool for the analysis of the pharmacology of the receptor, for its isolation, and for the detection of putative endogenous analogs.

Methodology

Radioligand

^{3}H-Labeled RTX (37 Ci/mmol) is synthesized by esterification of resiniferonol 9,13,14-ortho-phenylacetate (Chemicals for Cancer Research, Inc., Chaska,

MN), the parent diterpene of RTX, with [^{3}H]homovanillic acid (Chemical Synthesis and Analysis Laboratory, NCI-FCRF, Frederick, MD). The labeled compound is purified on high-performance liquid chromatography (HPLC) using a reversed-phase column (5 μm, 4.6 mm i.d. × 25 cm, ALTEX Ultrasphere-ODS; Rainin, Woburn, MA) eluted with 80% methanol. The [^{3}H]RTX is cochromatographed with authentic RTX. [In our experiments RTX was purchased from Chemicals for Cancer Research, but it is also available from LC Services Corporation (Woburn, MA) and from Fluka Chemical Corporation (Ronkonkoma, NY).] The biological activity of [^{3}H]RTX is confirmed in two assays: induction of hypothermia in CD-1 mice (10^{-5} g/kg, subcutaneous) (4) and induction of ear edema in Sprague-Dawley rats (2×10^{-7} g/ear) (5).

Tissue Preparation

General Considerations

Although several brain areas and vegetative neural pathways may play a role in some vanilloid actions (1), the best characterized capsaicin-sensitive pathway remains a nociceptive pathway that involves cell bodies of small diameter in sensory (dorsal root and trigeminal) ganglia with a peripheral unmyelinated axon and a central fiber with arborization in the dorsal horn (rexed laminae I and II) of the spinal cord (1). Physiological experiments indicate that vanilloid receptors are distributed throughout this pathway (1). Experimentally, we can demonstrate receptor binding in membranes obtained from sensory ganglia and from dorsal horn, whereas our efforts to observe specific [^{3}H]RTX binding in the periphery (in cornea, ureter, or tooth pulp, tissues with dense sensory innervation) have not yet been successful. Specific [^{3}H]RTX binding is found in sensory ganglia of rats, mice, guinea pigs, pigs, cows, and sheep but not in chickens (11), in keeping with mammals being the only group susceptible to the pungency of capsaicin (1).

Preparing Rat Dorsal Root Ganglion Membranes

Here we give a detailed protocol for obtaining membranes from rat dorsal root ganglia (DRG); this protocol can easily be modified for other tissues or species.

To make a rat DRG membrane preparation the following solutions and tools are needed:

Dissecting microscope; 16× magnification is adequate
Scissors and forceps, including microdissection scissors (e.g., Roboz RS-5600 or RS-5630, Roboz Surgical Instruments Co., Washington D.C.) and watchmaker's forceps
Brinkmann Polytron tissue homogenizer (Brinkmann Instruments, Inc.,

Westbury, NY), or, alternatively, a motor-driven Potter–Elvehjem
homogenizer (Harvard Apparatus, Inc., South Natick, MA)

Refrigerated centrifuge with an SS34 Sorvall (Du Pont Co., Wilmington,
DE) or similar rotor

Ultracentrifuge with an SW27 (Beckman Instruments, Inc., Palo Alto,
CA) or similar rotor

Phosphate-buffered saline (PBS), 0.02 M, pH 7.4: this is prepared by
dissolving 0.2 g KCl, 8.0 g NaCl, 1.15 g Na_2HPO_4, and 0.2 g KH_2PO_4
in 1 liter distilled water

Disrupting buffer, containing (in mM): KCl, 5; NaCl, 5.8; $MgCl_2$, 2;
glucose, 12; sucrose, 137; HEPES, 10; dithiothreitol (DTT), 5; EGTA,
2; pH 7.4

Assay buffer (same as the disrupting buffer but omitting DTT and EGTA
and including 0.75 mM $CaCl_2$): this is prepared by dissolving 0.363 g
KCl, 0.407 g $MgCl_2 \cdot 6H_2O$, 0.339 g NaCl, 0.110 g $CaCl_2 \cdot 2H_2O$, 2.378
g glucose, 46.9 g sucrose, and 2.383 g HEPES in distilled water; adjust
pH to 7.4 by adding 5 M NaOH, bring the final volume to 1 liter, filter
sterilize, and keep at 4°C.

Procedure

1. Sacrifice rats (we usually use Sprague-Dawley rats, females, 200–250 g)
by decapitation under CO_2 anesthesia; it can readily be done by placing the
rat in a closed chamber containing a layer of dry ice pellets (the CO_2 generated
by the dry ice quickly renders the rat unconscious) and then severing the
neck with sharp scissors.

2. Dissect the spinal column by cutting the ribs, free its ventral surface of
musculature, and then make two ventrolateral incisions to permit removal of
the vertebral bodies in one continuous strip. Collect the opened spinal columns in ice-cold phosphate-buffered saline.

3. Ganglia are removed under a dissecting microscope (we recommend
placing the spinal column on a Petri dish filled with ice while the dissections
are made): tease the ganglia from the intervertebral foramina using watchmaker's forceps and cut both dorsal and ventral roots as well as the spinal
segmental nerve with the aid of microdissection scissors as close to the
ganglia as possible. Collect the dissected ganglia in ice-cold disruption buffer.

4. Homogenize ganglia with the aid of a Polytron tissue homogenizer
(setting 8, 20–30 sec) or a motor-driven Potter–Elvehjem homogenizer (approximately 20 strokes). Cool the samples with ice/water mixture during the
homogenization.

Note: We usually collect DRG from the cervical and the upper thoracical
spinal segments; from an average of 20 ganglia/rat we obtain 200–300 μg of
membrane protein. Generally, we kill 15 rats and pool the dissected ganglia
in 4 ml of disrupting buffer.

5. Centrifuge homogenized samples in a refrigerated centrifuge (4°C) for 15 min at 8000 rpm (SS34 rotor) to remove nuclei and mitochondria (neither contains specific [³H]RTX-binding sites); the resulting supernatant is further centrifuged at 23,000 rpm (SW27 rotor) for 60 min at 4°C; the pellet represents the plasma membrane-enriched microsomal fraction.

6. Resuspend the pellet in assay buffer (approximately 1 mg membrane protein/ml assay buffer); distribute aliquots of the membrane suspension into 1.5-ml microfuge tubes and freeze them quickly on dry ice. Aliquots can be kept at −70°C without noticeable loss of activity for up to 6 months until assayed.

A possible shortcut is to use a total particulate fraction. Homogenized samples are filtered over surgical gauze to remove tissue fragments and membranes are then washed twice with the disrupting buffer (a Beckman or similar microfuge, 12,500 g_{max} for 15 min at 4°C).

Membranes can also be obtained from dorsal root ganglia or the dorsal horn of the spinal cord of large mammals (pigs, cows, etc.) by a similar procedure. Spinal columns can be purchased from slaughterhouses; they should be cooled on ice as soon as possible. We use pig spinal cords, cool them on ice, and then freeze them on dry ice. Frozen spinal cords are cut into approximately 0.5-cm long disks and both dorsal horns are dissected from each disk with a warm razor blade (place the spinal cord disks on a Petri dish filled with dry ice pellets to prevent thawing while the dissections are made). Finally, the dorsal one-third of the dorsal horn is removed and kept on dry ice until it is homogenized.

Unlike rat DRG, pig DRG or dorsal horn membranes can be satisfactorily prepared in a 20 mM Tris-HCl or a 10 mM HEPES buffer (pH 7.4) containing 0.25–0.32 M sucrose (see Comments on Buffers, pH, and Ions).

Binding Assay

Here we give a basic protocol for measuring [³H]RTX binding in rat DRG membranes. The reader is referred to sources such as Ref. 12 for theoretical considerations regarding membrane receptor assays and for standard procedures to do saturation, inhibition, and kinetic experiments.

The following supplies are needed:

Assay buffer (see above)
Assay buffer containing 10 mg/ml bovine serum albumin (fraction V; Sigma, St. Louis, MO)

A 20 mM Tris-HCl buffer (pH adjusted to 7.4 at 4°C) containing 10 mg/
   ml bovine serum albumin for presoaking filters
A 20 mM Tris-HCl wash buffer (pH adjusted to 7.4 at 4°C) containing
   0.1 mg/ml bovine serum albumin
A filter manifold (e.g., model FH 225V; Hoefer, San Francisco, CA)
Whatman (Clifton, NJ) GF/F glass fiber filters
Borosilicate glass tubes (e.g., Kimble disposable culture tubes, 12 × 75
   mm, No. 73500 Kimble Glass Inc., Vineland, NJ)
Scintillation vials; scintillation cocktail (e.g., Aquasol; Du Pont-New
   England Nuclear, Wilmington, DE); a liquid scintillation counter

Procedure

1. To a borosilicate glass tube add in the following order: 100 μl of assay
buffer, 50 μl of assay buffer containing 10 mg/ml bovine serum albumin with/
without nonradioactive RTX, [^{3}H]RTX in a 50-μl volume of assay buffer
containing 10 mg/ml bovine serum albumin, and 50 μl of membrane suspension containing 25–30 μg of membrane protein. Membranes are thawed in an
ice/water mixture just prior to use. Both radioactive and nonradioactive RTX
stock solutions are made up in ethanol and added to the assay buffer at a
concentration such that the solvent concentration does not exceed 0.1% in
the final incubation mixture. Tubes are kept on ice while the additions are
made.

2. The tubes are thoroughly vortexed and then incubated in a shaking water
bath at 37°C. A 10-min incubation time is routinely used. The tubes are then
cooled on ice. The length of time for cooling is not critical: aliquots of the
same assay mixture filtered immediately after a 10-min incubation at 37°C or
filtered after keeping on ice over a period of 5–60 min gave similar bound
values.

3. After the tubes are cooled, a 50-μl aliquot of the assay mixture is
removed to determine total radioactivity. An additional 150 μl of the assay
mixture is pipetted onto a Whatman GF/F glass fiber filter presoaked with
10 mg/ml bovine serum albumin in 20 mM Tris-HCl (pH 7.4) and filtered
immediately. The filter is washed with at least 40 ml of ice-cold 20 mM Tris-
HCl (pH 7.4) containing 0.1 mg/ml bovine serum albumin, and the bound
radioactivity is determined by scintillation counting. To obtain consistent
measurements, we equilibrate the filters in scintillation cocktail for at least
10 hr before counting.

Notes and Suggestions

When capsaicin and other lipophilic and low-affinity ligands are assayed,
dimethyl sulfoxide (DMSO) may be included in the assay mixture at a final
concentration of 1% to enhance solubility.

We found that the pore size of the glass fiber filter is a critical factor: the Whatman GF/F filters (0.7 μm) are more effective in retaining the specific [^{3}H]RTX-binding activity than are the GF/C filters (1.2 μm). Some lots of Whatman GF/F filters gave markedly more scatter in replicate assays than did other lots. High, nonspecific radioligand binding by both GF/C and GF/F filters can be reduced by presoaking the filters with 10 mg/ml bovine serum albumin in 20 mM Tris-HCl (pH adjusted to 7.4 at 4°C). A number of other solutions sometimes used to minimize filter binding, such as 0.1% (w/v) polyethyleneimine, did not work for [^{3}H]RTX.

Nonspecific binding should be determined in the presence of 100–1000 nM nonradioactive RTX; concentrations of nonradioactive RTX higher than 1 μM should be avoided because in some experiments we observed increased nonspecific binding at high RTX concentrations. Under our usual binding conditions, specific binding at the K_d represented approximately 50% of the total in rat or pig DRG membranes. Approximately 30% of the nonspecific binding was due to sticking of [^{3}H]RTX to the filters. The remainder presumably reflects partitioning of RTX into the lipid phase of the membranes, as had been observed previously for typical phorbol esters. An advantage of using particulate preparations from pig dorsal horn is a more favorable ratio of specific to nonspecific [^{3}H]RTX binding: by using 40 μg of membrane protein specific binding comprised 90% of the total binding.

Although this filtration assay is rapid, convenient, and reliable it does not permit direct measurement of free [^{3}H]RTX concentrations. We have therefore also established conditions for a centrifugation assay. After chilling the samples at the end of the incubation, the membranes are pelleted by centrifugation for 15 min at maximum speed in a Beckman microfuge Model 12. An aliquot of the supernatant is removed to determine free [^{3}H]RTX concentration. The remainder of the supernatant is removed by aspiration, leaving perhaps 1–2 mm of liquid above the pellet. The pellet is dried with the tip of a rolled Kimwipe (Kimberley-Clark Corp., Roswell, GA), being careful not to disturb the surface of the pellet. The tip of the microcentrifuge tube, which contains the pellet, is cut off with a razor blade and transferred directly to a scintillation vial. For both safety and leverage, we normally use a razorblade holder.

For assays at [^{3}H]RTX concentrations below the K_d and at 20–30 μg of membrane protein, a significant proportion (20–30%) of the total [^{3}H]RTX added to the 250-μl assay mixture may be partitioning into the membranes, decreasing the actual free [^{3}H]RTX concentration below that calculated in the filtration assay. This effect can be minimized by increasing the assay volume to 2.5 ml to achieve a 10-fold receptor dilution. Under these assay conditions no more than 1% of the total added [³H]RTX is bound nonspecifically.

Comments on Buffers, pH, and Ions

In pig DRG or pig dorsal horn membranes specific [³H]RTX binding can readily be measured in a 10 mM HEPES (pH 7.4) buffer or a 20 mM Tris-HCl (pH 7.4) buffer. Although it appears that the pH optimum of the binding is below pH 7.0, we decided to carry out the binding experiments using a physiological pH (7.4). In pig DRG membranes none of the monovalent (Na$^+$, K$^+$) and divalent (Ca^{2+}, Mg^{2+}, Mn^{2+}) cations tested affected binding; neither did adenyl (ATP) or guanyl nucleotides (GTPγS). In contrast, in rat DRG membranes specific [³H]RTX binding cannot be measured unless K$^+$, Na$^+$, Mg^{2+}, and Ca^{2+} are present in the assay mixture; none of these cations alone can restore specific [³H]RTX binding by more than 50%. The ionic dependence for [³H]RTX binding of membrane preparations from other species has not been determined, nor is the basis of this difference known.

Comments on Choice between [³H]Resiniferatoxin-Binding Assays

We have established and described three binding assays using [³H]RTX: the assay using rat DRG membranes, the assay utilizing pig DRG membranes, and the assay employing a crude synaptic membrane/microsomal fraction obtained from the dorsal half of pig dorsal horn. Given the fact that vanilloids show striking species differences (1), rat DRG membranes are the choice when binding affinities are to be compared to biological effects determined in the rat. A disadvantage of this assay, however, is the small amount of material obtainable per rat. Pig DRG is a considerably more abundant source of tissue. Although our limited analysis did not reveal major differences in structure–activity relations for the vanilloid receptor in rat and pig DRG membranes (11), the different ion dependence, the approximately 10-fold lower affinity in pig DRG membranes, and the lack of information on *in vivo* vanilloid actions in the pig limit the use of pig DRG membranes in the [³H]RTX-binding assay. An advantage of the pig dorsal horn preparation for analysis of [³H]RTX binding is its physiological relevance: spinal vanilloid receptors are thought to play a central role in the antinociceptive activity of vanilloids (1). In addition, at the methodological level, the [³H]RTX-binding assay utilizing dorsal horn preparations represents a marked improvement compared to the binding assays using sensory ganglion membranes. The dorsal horn preparation provides a more favorable proportion of specific to total binding at the K_d; dorsal horn is an abundant source of material (approximately 1 mg of membrane protein/2-cm long portion of the spinal cord versus 200–300 μg of protein/rat for DRG membranes); and the dissection of the preparation is easier.

Analysis of Binding Data

We analyze our binding data using the collection of computer programs described by McPherson (13). Scatchard and Hill transformations are performed by the equilibrium binding data analysis program referred to as EBDA. Data are further analyzed by the curvilinear regression program LIGAND.

Binding Properties of the Vanilloid Receptor

Saturation of Specific [³H]Resiniferatoxin Binding

³H-Labeled RTX displays specific, saturable binding both to membranes from sensory ganglia and dorsal horn. Nonspecific binding, which is defined as that occurring in the presence of 100–1000 nM nonradioactive RTX, is not saturable and increases linearly with increasing concentration of the labeled compound. Scatchard analysis of the data cumulated from filtration assays using rat DRG membranes is consistent with a single component possessing a K_d of 300 pM and a B_{max} of 150 fmol/mg protein. The Hill coefficient was 0.96, suggesting that the binding sites are not cooperative. The curvilinear analysis of the data by the LIGAND program confirms the one-site model suggested by the Scatchard plot. Nonradioactive RTX displaced specific [³H]RTX binding with a K_i of 110 ± 40 pM (mean ± SEM, three determinations), in fair agreement with the K_d value. Scatchard analysis of the data obtained in the centrifugation assay, allowing us to measure the free [³H]RTX concentration directly, gave binding parameters of K_d = 100 pM and B_{max} = 180 fmol/mg protein, respectively.

The proportion of specific to total binding is somewhat lower in the pig DRG than is the case in the rat. Nonetheless, nonradioactive RTX displaced specific [³H]RTX binding with a K_i of 2.4 ± 0.3 nM (mean ± SEM, four determinations), significantly higher than that obtained in the rat. The values obtained by competition were confirmed by Scatchard analysis of direct binding (K_d = 1.7 nM, B_{max} = 700 fmol/mg protein; data from two separate determinations).

Scatchard analysis of direct [³H]RTX binding to particulate preparations from pig dorsal horn revealed a K_d value of 270 ± 30 pM and a B_{max} of 370 ± 40 fmol/mg protein (mean ± SEM, three determinations). The Hill coefficient was 0.95. The curvilinear analysis of the data again confirmed the one-site model suggested by the Scatchard plot. The values are in excellent agreement with the K_i and B_{max} values determined in the competition experiments, 260 ± 80 pM and 380 ± 25 fmol/mg protein, respectively.

Kinetics of Specific [³H]Resiniferatoxin Binding

At 37°C, specific [³H]RTX binding is a time-dependent process attaining half-maximal binding within 2 min, reaching a plateau by 10 min, and maintaining this level for at least 60 min. By contrast, nonspecific binding attains maximal values by 1 min. In addition, similar K_d values were measured for 10- and 60-min incubations at 37°C. Based on these results, binding is routinely measured following a 10-min incubation at 37°C. The association data appear to be consistent with a simple bimolecular reaction. In contrast, dissociation seems to be a complex process in which the dissociation rate is changing as a function of the time of incubation in the presence of [³]RTX. Following a 2-min incubation with [³H]RTX, displacement by nonradioactive RTX appears to be complete within 10 min. Following a 10-min incubation with [³H]RTX, however, nonradioactive RTX displaced only 20% of the labeled ligand during an additional 10 min of incubation. All of the remaining binding can be extracted by a chloroform : methanol mixture (3 : 1), indicating that the ligand is not covalently bound.

Although the biological significance of this phenomenon remains to be determined, an important practical implication is that membranes should be preincubated with highly lipophilic, slowly equilibrating ligands before [³H]RTX is added to the assay mixture.

Tissue Linearity, Thermal Stability of [³H]Resiniferatoxin Binding, and Additional Comments

Specific [³H]RTX binding increases linearly with increasing tissue concentration; specific binding is linear up to 0.25 mg/ml membrane protein using pig dorsal horn particulate preparations.

The thermal stability of specific [³H]RTX-binding sites has been examined by incubating membrane preparations at various temperatures for 10 min prior to the standard binding assay. In pig DRG membranes specific binding was completely abolished by heating to 55°C; in pig dorsal horn membranes specific binding sites were significantly reduced by a similar heat treatment. Complete inactivation, however, required either longer heating or higher (65°C) temperature.

Experiments have been carried out to determine whether [³H]RTX is metabolized during the binding process. Bound [³H]RTX extracted from dorsal horn membranes by a chloroform : methanol (3 : 1) mixture and free [³H]RTX recovered from the lyophilized supernatant of the assay mixture were subjected to normal-phase thin-layer chromatography (TLC; precoated TLC sheets, silica gel 60 F-254 (E. Merck, Darmstadt, Germany) developed in ethyl acetate]; both bound and unbound [³H]RTX migrated identically to authentic [³H]RTX. In addition, unbound [³H]RTX recovered and added to a second binding assay gave bound [³H]RTX values similar to those of authentic [³H]RTX.

Evidence that Specific [³H]Resiniferatoxin Binding Represents Vanilloid Receptor

Based on the *in vivo* effects of capsaicin, specific ligand binding must fulfill well-defined criteria, including pharmacological, tissue, and species specificity, to represent the postulated capsaicin receptor. Specific [³H]RTX binding fits all of these criteria.

Pharmacological Specificity

The pharmacological specificity of [³H]RTX binding was examined for three classes of compounds: vanilloids of the capsaicin and RTX types, phorbol-related activators of protein kinase C, and unrelated compounds sharing some homology to the homovanillyl moiety in vanilloids.

It is clear that the specific binding sites for [³H]RTX are distinct from protein kinase C, the receptor for typical phorbol esters. Specific [³H]RTX binding was inhibited neither by phorbol 12,13-dibutyrate (PDBu), the typical ligand used for analysis of binding to protein kinase C, nor by resiniferonol 9,13,14-ortho-phenylacetate, the C-20 deesterified parent compound of RTX. Conversely, RTX inhibited specific [³H]PDBu binding to protein kinase C only at concentrations higher than 100 nM. Capsaicin and RTX structural analogs (dihydrocapsaicin, nonanoylvanillylamide, piperine, zingerone, homovanilloyldecylamide, homovanilloyldodecylamide, homovanilloylcyclododecylamide, homovanilloylhexadecylamide/tinyatoxin, 12-deoxyphorbol 13-phenylacetate 20-homovanillate) inhibited specific [³H]RTX binding both to sensory ganglion and dorsal horn membranes in accord with their *in vivo* potencies. Catecholamines possess some homology to the 3-methoxy 4-hydroxyphenyl moiety in vanilloids; however, they did not compete for

[³H]RTX-binding sites. Neither did bryostatin 26-homovanillate, indicating that protein kinase C and the vanilloid receptor recognize different aspects of the diterpene moiety.

Tissue and Species Specificity

No specific [³H]RTX binding was observed for rat cerebellum or for pig ventral horn, neural tissues reported not to be affected by capsaicin (11). [We were also unable to detect [³H]RTX binding in areas of the central nervous system implicated in capsaicin actions, such as the preoptic area (11). Perhaps these negative results reflect the detection limit of the current binding methodology.] No binding was measured in DRG from chicken, in agreement with birds being unresponsive to the pungent activity of capsaicin (1). In rats treated with RTX as neonates, the reduction in specific [³H]RTX-binding sites in DRG membranes correlated with the loss of small DRG neurons (14).

Practical Applications of [³H]Resiniferatoxin

This binding assay is in use for the direct analysis of the pharmacology of vanilloid receptors. In addition, it has been utilized for estimation of the molecular weight (radiation inactivation size) of the receptor both in pig DRG and dorsal horn membranes; the apparent molecular size of 270 kDa suggests a receptor complex. Other applications include the isolation of the solubilized receptor, the detection of putative endogenous analogs, and autoradiographic mapping of possible vanilloid-sensitive structures in the central nervous system.

References

1. S. H. Buck and T. F. Burks, *Pharmacol. Rev.* **38,** 179 (1986).
2. S. Bevan and J. Szolcsanyi, *Trends Pharmacol. Sci.* **11,** 330 (1990).
3. R. W. Fuller, *Arch. Int. Pharmacodyn.* **303,** 147 (1990).
4. D. J. de Vries and P. M. Blumberg, *Life Sci.* **44,** 711 (1989).
5. A. Szallasi and P. M. Blumberg, *Neuroscience* **39,** 515 (1989).
6. A. Szallasi, F. Joo, and P. M. Blumberg, *Brain Res.* **503,** 68 (1989).
7. A. Szallasi, N. A. Sharkey, and P. M. Blumberg, *Phytother. Res.* **3,** 253 (1989).
8. A. Szallasi and P. M. Blumberg, *Life Sci.* **47,** 1399 (1990).
9. C. A. Maggi, R. Patacchini, M. Tramontana, R. Amann, S. Giuliani, and S. Santicioli, *Neuroscience* **37,** 531 (1990).

10. J. Szolcsanyi, A. Szallasi, Z. Szallasi, F. Joo, and P. M. Blumberg, *J. Pharmacol. Exp. Ther.* **255,** 923 (1990).
11. A. Szallasi and P. M. Blumberg, *Brain Res.* **524,** 106 (1990).
12. H. I. Yamamura (ed.), ''Methods in Neurotransmitter Receptor Analysis,'' Raven, New York, 1990.
13. G. A. McPherson, *J. Pharmacol. Methods* **14,** 213 (1985).
14. A. Szallasi, Z. Szallasi, and P. M. Blumberg, *Brain Res.* **537,** 182 (1990).

[28]   Scorpion Toxins Affecting Insects

Erwann P. Loret, François Sampieri, Claude Granier,
Françis Miranda, and Hervé Rochat

Introduction

The venom of North African scorpions shows toxicity both to mammals and to insects. This toxicity is due to small proteins (1), 60 to 70 amino acid residues long, cross-linked by 4 disulfide bridges, which exhibit a strong affinity for excitable cells (for a review, see Ref. 2). In the North African scorpion venoms, the proteins toxic to mammals differ from those toxic to insects (3). Electrophysiological and binding studies revealed that the target of most of the scorpion toxins was the voltage-dependent sodium channel of excitable cells (4). In the case of scorpion toxins acting on mammals, two types (α and β) have been described according to their pharmacological and electrophysiological effects (5, 6). The binding of α-type toxins on the sodium channel leads to a prolongation of the opening phase of the channel while the binding of β-type toxins brings out repetitive opening and closing phases of the channel. There is no competition between α- and β-type toxins in binding experiments, which probably means that there is a specific binding site for each type of toxin.

Depending on their mode of action, the scorpion toxins specific for insects were divided into two different categories: contraction-inducing toxins, which caused rapid excitatory contraction paralysis in *Sarcophaga argyrostoma* fly larvae, and depressant toxins, which induced a slow depressant flaccid paralysis (7). Each type showed distinct electrophysiological effects when tested in current- and voltage-clamp conditions on an isolated axonal preparation of *Periplaneta americana*, but both were capable of binding to a common site on the sodium channel of insects (8). The contraction-inducing toxins showed electrophysiological effects in insects that were similar to those observed in the case of β-type toxins acting on mammals, i.e., repetitive firing of the nerve. Recently, a new type of anti-insect toxin was described, which was shown to bind to a different site on the sodium channel of insects (9). This toxin showed electrophysiological effects comparable to those described for α-type toxins acting on mammals. Thus, it appeared that the sodium channels of insects and mammals may possess similar structures, leading to the division of the scorpion toxins acting either on insects or on mammal into two types, α and β, according to their specific pharmacological and electrophysiological effects.

Methods in Neurosciences, Volume 8

Due to their high toxicity toward insects and their absence of toxicity toward mammals, the contraction-inducing toxins have been the most studied in the last 10 years. Their primary structure presents two peculiarities: their peptidic chain is composed of 70 amino acids, while the average is 60 to 65 for the other scorpion toxins, and there is a shift in the position of one half-cystine residue whereas the position of the eight half-cystines was strictly conserved in the other scorpion toxins (10–12).

This chapter will focus on techniques applied to such contraction-inducing toxins isolated from venoms of North African scorpions, although toxins from other scorpion venoms have been described as active on insects. β-Type mammal toxins isolated from American scorpion venoms were found to exhibit a low toxicity in insects (13–15). Finally, short peptides called "insectotoxins," I5A and I2 (35 and 62 amino acid residues, respectively) from scorpions collected in the Caucasus area (Soviet Union) were described as being specifically but weakly toxic to insects (16). We will describe recent improvement in three areas: toxicity tests that can be used on insects, purification procedures for scorpion toxins active in insects, and a pharmacological assay, including insect dissection, membrane preparation, purification of a monoiodo derivative of a scorpion toxin active on insect, and binding test.

Toxicity Tests

Qualitative and Quantitative Toxicity Test

The toxicity of a scorpion venom or of scorpion toxins toward insects can be measured according to different criteria. The most obvious is the death of the insect, which makes it possible to determine the lethal dose corresponding to the amount of material able to kill the insect. However, the most convenient criterion for measuring the toxicity remains the paralysis of the insect, in that it is rapidly observable. Moreover, lower amounts of toxic material are needed to paralyze an insect than to kill it.

In some instances, a simple qualitative test allows one to know whether a venom or a fraction of the venom is toxic to insects or not, but this information is not sufficient in most cases. A quantitative statistical assay should be done that permits characterization of a sample and determination that the material producing any toxic effect is specific to the sample. Since all doses above a certain point will kill essentially 100% of insects treated, it is more convenient to determine a half-effect dose, that is, the amount of material that induces 50% of positive responses. Depending on toxicity test, a positive response can be either the death or paralysis of the insect.

Examples of Toxicity Tests Using Insects

The following animals, six insect species belonging to four different orders, are tested (17): male *Blattella germanica* and *Periplaneta americana*, *Dictyoptera*; male or female *Gryllus domesticus*, Orthoptera; L_4 larval instar *Spodoptera littoralis*, Lepidoptera; female *Musca domestica* and male and female *Sarcophaga argyrostoma*, Diptera.

Injections to insects can be performed with a metallic or glass microneedle (according to the size of the animal) joined by a flexible tube attached to a 25- or 50-μl Hamilton syringe delivering aliquots of 0.5 to 1 μl. The point of injection depends on the species used: (1) intersegmental membranes of the ventral (*B. germanica*, *P. americana*) or lateral side (*M. domestica*) of the abdomen or of the ventral side of the animal, (2) dorsolateral side of the thorax (*S. argyrostoma*) or lateral side of the posterior part of the body (*S. littoralis*), and (3) articular membranes of the legs (*G. domesticus*). It is more convenient to make the injections of *G. domesticus* under a binocular microscope. *Musca domestica*, *S. argyrostoma*, and *S. littoralis* must be anesthetized with ether before injection. Volumes injected vary from 1 to 8 μl or from 5 to 20 μl for the species whose weight is, respectively, less or more than 560 mg. The solvent used is 0.15 M NaCl containing 1 mg bovine serum albumin/ml. For each series of assays, control animals must be injected with solvent alone.

The following symptoms are chosen as criteria of toxicity: paralysis and mortality. In paralysis, the animal is unable to walk, loses its balance, and often lies on its dorsal side; it still moves, but with irregular movements of the limbs and the body. The paralyzing unit chosen is the Pu_{50} (paralyzing unit 50%), which is the dose required to get 50% of the insects paralyzed 1 hr after the injection. Mortality is often first noted 24 hr after the injection but it is finally expressed by the LD_{50} (lethal dose 50%) only after intervals of different times according to the species used. Thus mortality is determined after 24 hr for *S. argyrostoma*; 48 hr for *M. domestica*; 72 hr for *B. germanica* and the crustaceans; and 96 hr for *G. domesticus* and *P. americana*. As regards *S. littoralis*, mortality can be determined by counting larvae that did not reach the well-formed nymphal instar. Therefore, it can be noted only 15 days after the injection time. It is usual to express doses injected in nanograms or micrograms per 100 mg of body weight of insects.

Effect of Scorpion Toxins on Different Insect Species

The effect of the anti-insect toxin (AaH IT) from the scorpion *Androctonus australis Hector* on insects can be different according to the species tested

(17). AaH IT injection induces variable symptoms depending on the species and the dose injected. Observations of *G. domesticus, B. germanica,* and *P. americana* can be summarized as follows: (1) for *G. domesticus* and *B. germanica,* after a few seconds of uncoordinated motion, the animal falls on its dorsal side after the injection of a paralyzing dose. It manifests violent trembling of the body and the legs, attesting an excitatory effect. This phase is interrupted by periods of relaxation. This state can last several days depending on the injected dose. (2) For *P. americana,* a few seconds after the injection the insect is unable to move, but is still remaining on its legs. After a few minutes, the animal is indifferent to any stimulus (pinching of the legs, the antennae, or the cerci). After a delay ranging from a few minutes to several tens of minutes, the intoxicated animal occasionally loses its balance and falls on its dorsal side.

The paralyzing and lethal doses of a toxin change markedly depending on the species injected. The LD_{50} varies by a ratio of about 700 between *M. domestica* (LD_{50} 2 ng) and *S. littoralis* (LD_{50} 1310 ng). The intraspecies sensitivity to scorpion toxins seems to be more constant: for the *Orthoptera,* the PU_{50} on *G. domesticus* (240–290 ng) is comparable with the PU_{50} on *Locusta migratoria* (300 ng). For the coleopteron species *Tenebrio molitor,* the LD_{50} on larva and the PU_{50} on adult are about 50 and 90 ng, respectively. Doses are expressed in nanograms or micrograms per 100 mg of body weight of insects.

The paralysis induced by AaH IT does not necessarily lead to the death of the animal. The effect can be reversible depending on the dose injected. For *B. germanica, P. americana,* and *G. domesticus* (female), in particular, PU_{100} corresponds to the LD_{50}. For all three species, the order of magnitude of PU_{50}, PU_{100}, and LD_{50} is the same.

Mode of Application

The level of the toxicity can change with the mode of application. Various methods employed to evaluate the toxicity of synthetic insecticides have been used with AaH IT (18). In a solvent composed of 80% acetone and 20% water or in a solvent of 50% acetone and 50% dimethyl sulfoxide, AaH IT is toxic to the fly *M. domestica* just by topical application. However, no activity is observed against *Aphis craccivora* in surface-contact tests on glass, or against *Culex pipiens pipiens* larvae in water. On *M. domestica,* AaH IT, in weight, is only 1.5 times more active than propoxur or DDT and 10 times more active than malathion by topical application but apparently 2500 times more active than propoxur or DDT and 1000 times more active than malathion by injection, which is the method most closely resembling the natural stinging activity of a scorpion.

Determination of the Contraction Paralysis Unit (CPU)

In order to compare results from different laboratories, the same toxicity test should be used. For historical and practical reasons, the so-called contraction paralysis unit (CPU) described by Zlotkin *et al.* (3) can be considered as a reference test.

It is rather easy to obtain fly larvae and to maintain a breeding. The fly commonly used is *S. argyrostoma,* characterized by a black body with white lines on the posterior face of the thorax and red eyes. This fly has the habit of laying its eggs on meat and provides larvae of convenient size that are easy to inject. Thus a simple way to get such fly larvae is to leave a piece of meat outside and wait for a couple of days. This method provides, usually, larvae of different fly species at the first generation. These larvae must be isolated at 25°C in a box until all are transformed into pupae. Then the pupae are stored at 4°C for at least 1 week but not more than 2 months. The storage at 4°C allows synchronization of the metamorphosis cycle of the larvae for each species. The metamorphosis of an *S. argyrostoma* pupa into a fly is of 10 ± 1 days at 25°C, while the metamorphosis of the other fly species is typically more rapid. Providing water and food (powdered milk and sugar) only after the tenth day makes it possible to select the *S. argyrostoma* flies. After 10 more days at 25°C, the flies are in turn able to lay eggs on a piece of meat (bovine liver is the more appropriate). This piece of meat is removed from the box after 5 or 6 hr and stored in the dark at 25°C for 5 to 6 days before larvae may be used for the test.

Quantitative estimation of toxicity on fly larvae (5–6 days old, 100–120 mg body weight) is based on the determination of the contraction paralysis unit (CPU). In the CPU assay, aliquots (5 μl) of four solutions of increasing concentration are injected in the terminal segment of fly larvae (Fig. 1). It is also possible to use the same concentration and to vary the injected volume. A positive response is an immobility for at least 5 sec due to the spastic contraction of the larvae. The CPU is the amount of toxic material that induces 50% of positive responses. Figure 1A shows a fly larva before injection. The larva is fixed on a needle and spontaneously moves circularly around the tip of the needle. Short contractions often occur when the larva is fixed on the needle, so it is necessary to wait for injection until it moves circularly. The injection of a scorpion toxin rapidly induces immobility and contraction of the larva body, which reduces its size as shown in Fig. 1A. Any liquid injected in a fly larva can also induce short contractions by itself,

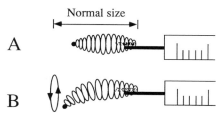

Fig. 1   Contraction paralysis assay on blowfly larvae. An *S. argyrostoma* larva is placed on a needle connected to a micrometric syringe. The needle is inserted into the ventral side of the last abdominal segment. (A) Contraction of the larva accompanied by complete immobility. (B) The larva on the needle prior to injection showing twisting movements.

and the 5-sec delay is necessary before a contraction can be considered as a positive response to scorpion toxin.

Purification

General Principles

Proteins active on insects have been purified from scorpion venoms collected in North Africa and the Middle East (3, 7, 11, 19–22), and also in China (23). Different methods can be used to purify toxic proteins from a crude scorpion venom. The different purification steps must be monitored by a quantitative toxicity test. Scorpion toxins can be purified according to three properties: the molecular weight, the electrical charge, and the hydrophobicity. The hydrophobicity is the most efficient property to exploit in the purification of scorpion toxins, but, due to the high number of proteins present in a scorpion venom, it is generally required to use all three characteristics. The complexity of a scorpion venom is increased when it is collected after electrical stimulation. Manual stimulation is the closest to natural excretion condition and provides a venom enriched in toxins when compared to ''electrical'' venom, which possesses many inactive proteins.

Purification of Toxins Active on Insects: AaH IT1 and AaH IT2 from the Venom of Scorpion Androctonus australis Hector

The venom of *Androctonus australis Hector,* collected in the area of Tozeur (Tunisia), contains different groups of proteins that are specifically toxic to mammals or insects. Among the various venom components obtained by electrical stimulation of this scorpion, the toxins correspond to only 3% of the protein in the venom, with 0.5 to 0.3% corresponding to the toxins specific to insects (Table I). The first purification step is a dialysis (membrane molecular weight cutoff of 3500) against water at 4°C. The dialyzed and lyophilized water extract of the venom is then twice subjected to low-pressure chromatography. The first is a Sephadex G-50 fine gel-filtration chromatography carried out on four columns (5 × 100 cm) in series, equilibrated and eluted with 0.1 M ammonium acetate buffer (pH 8.5, flow rate, 80 ml/hr). The second step is a DEAE-Sephadex anion-exchange chromatography carried out on a 2 × 200 cm column with 0.1 M ammonium acetate buffer (pH 8.5; flow rate, 20 ml/hr). Each chromatographic step is performed at 25°C. The fourth and fifth purification steps are carried out by semipreparative high-performance liquid chromatography (HPLC) with a C_8 column (C_8 HPLC). Semipreparative C_8 HPLC is carried out on a 10 × 250 mm column prepacked with Ultrasphere octyl, 5 μm (Beckman, Fullerton, CA). Column temperature is regulated at 25°C. The aqueous elution solvent (A) is 0.15 M ammonium formate (pH 2.75, conductivity 12 mS at 25°C) and the organic elution solvent (B) is pure acetonitrile (Carlo Erba) according to Bougis et al. (24). Flow rate is 4 ml/min.

Figures 2 and 3 show the elution profile of the different steps of purification. The gel filtration on Sephadex G-50 carried out on four columns in series makes it possible to perform two cycles. After the first cycle, the inactive fractions F1 and F2 are removed and the remaining fractions are recycled for another turn that makes it possible to separate the toxins active on insects (fraction IT) from the toxins active on mammals (fraction R1 and R2). Further separation by DEAE-Sephadex chromatography of fraction IT leads to four main fractions. The main toxicity (95%) is found in fraction B while only 5% is associated with other fractions. In the third purification step, fraction B is subjected to C_8 HPLC with elution by a gradient of 0.3% acetonitrile/min. All the toxicity on fly larvae is associated with fraction B', eluting between 47 and 52 min. In order to obtain pure proteins from fraction B', a last purification step is performed as before but with a less steep gradient (0.1% acetonitrile/min). Three proteins (AaH IT1, B50, and AaH IT2) are recovered. AaH IT1 and AaH IT2 are antiinsect toxins while B50 is devoid of toxicity on fly larvae.

Yields in terms of proteins and toxicity recovery are indicated in Table I for a purification of 7.4 g of crude venom. The content in protein material is measured from the specific ultraviolet absorbance of proteins at 280 nm and the yield in protein material is given, as is the amount of CPU in one absorbance unit, and the total CPU content. The yield in toxicity is also presented. The yield in protein material decreases with the purification but the

TABLE I Purification of AaH IT1 and AaH IT2 from *Androctonus australis Hector* Venom

Purification steps	Fraction subjected to purification	Fraction toxic to insects ($A_{280\ nm}$)	Yield in absorbance (%)	Specific toxicity (CPU/$A_{280\ nm}$)	Total Toxicity (CPU $\times$ 10^{-6})	Yield in toxicity (%)
—	Crude venom	7150	100	2,769 (±191)	19.8 (±1.4)	100
Sephadex G-50	Dialyzed water extract	750	10.5	16,600 (±1,145)	12.0 (±0.82)	61
DEAE-Sephadex	Fraction IT	105	1.5	100,000 (±6,900)	10.0 (±0.7)	50
C$_8$ HPLC (0.3% acetonitrile/min)	Fraction B	74	1.0	200,000 (±13,800)	14.7 (±1.0)	74
C$_8$ HPLC (0.1% acetonitrile/min)	Fraction B′	37 (AaH IT1)	0.5	240,000 (±16,560)	8.8 (±0.6)	44
		23 (AaH IT2)	0.3	255,000 (±17,600)	5.9 (±0.4)	29

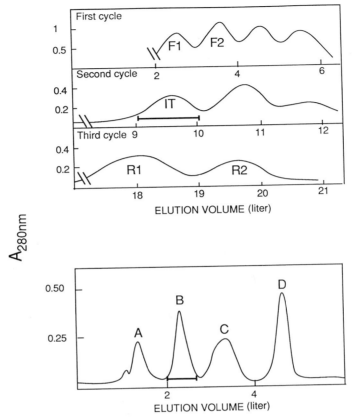

FIG. 2   Elution profiles of low-pressure liquid chromatographic steps. *Top:* Recycling gel filtration on Sephadex G-50 carried out on four columns (5 × 100 cm) in series (Marie-France Martin-Eauclaire, personal communication). The buffer is ammonium acetate, pH 8.5, and the flow rate is 80 ml/hr. IT is the fraction toxic to fly larvae, while R1 and R2 are the fractions toxic to mammals. F1 and F2 are nontoxic fractions removed after the first cycle. *Bottom:* DEAE chromatography of the fraction toxic to insects obtained from gel filtration on Sephadex G-50. The column (2 × 200 cm) is equilibrated, then eluted at a flow rate of 20 ml/hr with 0.1 *M* ammonium acetate, pH 8.5. The main toxicity is found in fraction B. The horizontal bar indicates the pooled fraction.

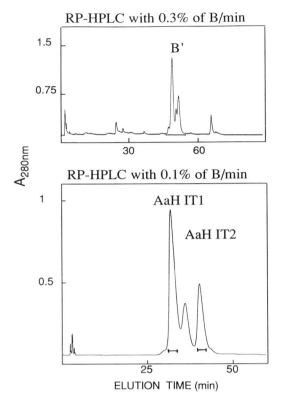

FIG. 3   Elution profiles of high-performance liquid chromatographic steps. *Top:* C_8 HPLC of fraction B on a semipreparative Ultrasphere reversed-phase C_8 column eluted by a linear gradient (from 15 to 40% acetonitrile) over 80 min (slope, 0.3% acetonitrile/min). Solvent A, 0.15 M ammonium formiate, pH 2.75; solvent B, acetonitrile; flow rate: 4 ml/min, at 25°C. Main toxicity is found between 47 and 55 min (fraction B'). *Bottom:* C_8 HPLC of fraction B' collected in the preceding step. Conditions are the same as those above, except that the gradient is 20 to 25% acetonitrile over 5 min and 25 to 35% acetonitrile over 100 min (slope, 0.1% acetonitrile/min). Horizontal bars indicate the pooled fractions.

yield in toxicity must remain close to 100%. The yield in toxicity increases after the purification step using C_8 HPLC (0.3% acetonitrile/min). This fact may be due to the presence of an antagonist of AaH IT1 and AaH IT2 in the whole venom. A protein able to bind to the sodium channel with low toxicity has been described recently (25).

Characterization

Electrophoresis must show that both toxins possess an identical mobility at pH 4.5 while AaH IT2 is more acidic than AaH IT1 at pH 9.5. AaH IT1 and AaH IT2 are closely related proteins of 70 amino acid residues with calculated molecular weights of 7830 and 7870, respectively. The experimental molar absorbance coefficients (277 nm) are 9.5 mM^{-1} and 11.7 mM^{-1}, respectively, for AaH IT1 and AaH IT2, similar to theoretical molar absorbance coefficients of 9.34 and 11.04 (taking into account only the contribution at 277 nm of tyrosines, phenylalanine, and disulfide bridges). Paralyzing contraction tests on fly larvae must give a CPU close to 1 ng for AaH IT1 and AaH IT2. In competition for the binding of the mono[^{125}I]iodo derivative of AaH IT1 to cockroach nerve cord synaptosomes (see Binding Test), AaH IT1 and AaH IT2 must display half-effects ($K_{0.5}$) close to 0.5 and 0.25 nM, respectively.

Binding Test

Purpose of Test

Besides the paralyzing or lethal effects that can be assessed for scorpion toxins, it is necessary to quantify the ability of the sample to bind to the same binding site as a reference scorpion toxin on the sodium channel of insects. Increasing concentrations of the sample are incubated with a given amount of radiolabeled scorpion toxin and insect nervous tissue membranes. After 2 hr at 20°C, the preparations are filtered on a filter retaining only the membranes and the sample or the radiolabeled scorpion toxin bound to the membranes, and the radioactivity retained on the filters is counted. It is the competition between the sample and one scorpion toxin, on the sodium channel of insects, that is measured in this assay. If the sample has a high affinity for the scorpion toxin binding site on the sodium channel, a low level of radioactivity will be observed at high concentration of the sample due to residual nonspecific binding of the radiolabeled scorpion toxins. On the other hand, a high level of radioactivity will be observed at low concentrations of the sample. If the sample has no affinity for the site of scorpion toxins a high level of radioactivity will be observed whatever the concentration of the sample. As a toxicity test the concentration of the sample corresponding to the half-effect ($K_{0.5}$), i.e., inhibition by 50% of the maximum binding observed in the absence of competitor, is used as a pharmacological characterization of the sample.

Radioiodination of Toxin AaH IT1 and Purification of Derivatives

Six tyrosine residues in AaH IT1 are available for radioiodination (the purification of this protein is described above). However, a careful purification of the radiolabeled derivatives is necessary since diiodinated derivatives possess a modified affinity for the sodium channel and therefore must be discarded. Only mono[^{125}I]iodo derivatives of AaH IT1 can be used for the binding assay. The use of C_8 HPLC makes it possible to eliminate free iodide, which elutes at the beginning of the gradient, and to separate the monoiodo derivatives from the native protein and from the diiodo derivatives.

The radioiodination and the purification of the radiolabeled derivatives are done as follows: 0.66 nmol AaH IT1 in 5 μl of water, 0.5 nmol Na^{125}I in 10 μl, 10 μl of lactoperoxidase (the stock solution of lactoperoxidase is at 250 mg/ml and the coefficient of molar absorbance at 412 nm is 114), and H_2O_2 diluted 1/50,000 in 10 μl are allowed to react for 2 min with 30 μl of a 50 mM phosphate buffer, pH 7.4. Then the volume is increased to 200 μl with 50 mM phosphate buffer containing 1 mg/ml bovine serum albumin (BSA), and the solution is injected in an HPLC column (4.6 × 250 mm 100 CH, 8/II, 5 mm, prepacked with Lichrospher; Hibar Merck, Darmstadt, Germany). This operation can be scaled up when necessary, but reagent ratios must remain unchanged. This ratio makes it possible to obtain roughly 40% monoiodo derivatives and 60% diiodo derivatives.

The mobile phase used for C_8 HPLC is a mixture of 0.15 M ammonium formate, pH 2.75, 12 mS (solvent A), and acetonitrile (solvent B). Elution is performed at 20°C with a linear gradient from 20 to 25% solvent B in solvent A for 5 min, followed by another linear gradient from 25 to 33% solvent B in solvent A for 80 min with a flow rate of 1.5 ml/min. These conditions are similar to those described in the preceding chapter for the last step of purification of AaH IT1. The eluant is collected in plastic tubes every minute and the measure of the radioactivity allows one to identify the fractions where the monoiodo derivatives and diiodo derivatives are localized. The observed elution times are usually 35 min for the native AaH IT1, 41 min for the monoiodo derivatives, and 45 min for the diiodo derivatives. The order of elution is always the same.

Dissection of Male Cockroaches Periplaneta americana

The cockroach *P. americana* is very useful for electrophysiological and pharmacological studies of insects. This animal possesses at the rear two appendices called cerci that are sensitive to vibrations. The mere opening of a door is picked up by the cerci and induces a flight reflex in the cockroach.

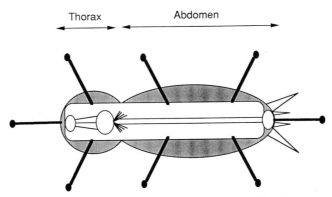

FIG. 4   Dissection of male cockroaches (*P. americana*). The diagram represents a posterior view of the insects after the cuticule and organs are removed. The nerve chord is represented in the middle, starting from the rear of the abdomen, with the abdominal ganglion located beside the cerci. At the other end the abdominal nerve chord is terminated by the thoracic ganglion. Two nerves starting from this ganglion run from the superior part of the thorax into the smallest ganglion. The muscular chiasma that must be cut with the cartilage to remove the thoracic ganglion is represented at the junction of the abdomen and the thorax.

This reflex of survival seems to be the cause of the developed abdominal nerve cord of this insect. This nerve chord is used for studies of the electrophysiology of insects and provides a high quantity of insect nervous tissues for synaptosomal preparations.

Male cockroaches are preferentially used due to their low content in fat tissues, which facilitates the dissection. An easy way to distinguish a male *P. americana* from a female is to compare the cerci, which are thinner in a male cockroach. For the dissection steps, the legs, the wings, and the head must first be removed. Although the insects are *prochordae,* and therefore their nervous system is located in the anterior part of the body, the dissection must nevertheless occur by the posterior face. The body of the animal is fixed by a pin at each extremity and three pins on each side, the cuticule is cut and stripped from the rear of the abdomen to the thorax (Fig. 4), and the different organs are removed until the cuticule of the anterior face is reached. At that point, a slim, white, almost translucent tissue that is the abdominal nerve chord becomes visible. This nervous chain is ended by one ganglion at the rear of the abdomen and one in the thorax. Physiological liquid must be added to the preparation during the dissection. The thoracic ganglion must be taken off first. It is located on the middle of the inferior part of the thorax. Two nerves start from this ganglion and run to the smallest ganglion, which is rather difficult to get to, located as it is in the superior part of the thorax. Before removal of the thoracic ganglion, the cartilage making the junction between thorax and abdomen must be cut. This is the most delicate part of the dissection because the nerve chord passes through the cartilage and can be torn out. Figure 4 shows the muscular chiasma that must be cut to reach the cartilage. When the thoracic ganglion is removed, the nerve chord is taken from the preparation, put in physiological liquid, and then stored in liquid nitrogen. On average, 50 to 100 nerve chords are necessary to start a synaptosome preparation. Fifty nerve chords correspond roughly to 600 mg of wet tissue.

Cockroach Nerve Chord Synaptosomal Preparation

A crude synaptosomal fraction is prepared according to the method of Lima *et al.* (26), from the thoracic and abdominal nerve cords of male cockroaches (*P. americana*). The nerve chords, at 10% (w/v) in an ice-cold buffer (10 mM glucose, 140 mM choline chloride, 5.4 mM KCl, 0.8 mM $MgSO_4$, 25 mM HEPES, adjusted to pH 7.4 with Tris) and a mixture of protease inhibitors [0.1 mM phenylmethylsulfonyl fluoride (PMSF), 1 mM iodacetamide, 1 mM 1,10-phenanthroline, 0.001 mM pepstatin A, and 1 mM EDTA], are homogenized with a Potter-Elvejhem apparatus (800 rpm, 15 strokes with a 1-min interval every 5 strokes to avoid heating). The homogenate is centrifuged at 1000 g for 10 min at 4°C and the pellet discarded. The supernatant is centrifuged at 30,000 g for 30 min and the pellet resuspended in the same buffer (1 ml/g nerve chords). The protein content is determined according to the method of Peterson (27) with BSA as a standard. Samples (50–100 μl) are stored in liquid nitrogen until use. They can be stored without loss of binding properties for at least 6 months.

Binding Assays

Binding and wash buffers are the homogenization buffer supplemented with 1.8 mM $CaCl_2$ and BSA (0.2% in binding buffer and 0.5% in wash buffer) in the absence of the protease inhibitors. The binding studies with the nerve chord synaptosomal fraction of cockroach (5 μg/ml) are carried out in 0.5 ml buffer, incubated at 20°C. The free ligand is separated from the bound by rapid filtration over BSA (2%, w/v)-pretreated GFB glass fiber filters. After washing twice with 4 ml ice-cold wash buffer, the radioactivity bound to the filters is measured. Filtration and washing take 12–15 sec.

References

1. F. Miranda and S. Lissitzky, *Nature (London)* **190**, 443 (1961).
2. H. Rochat, P. Bernard, and F. Couraud, *Adv. Cytopharmacol.* **3**, 325 (1979).
3. E. Zlotkin, H. Rochat, C. Kopeyan, F. Miranda, and S. Lissitzky, *Biochimie* **53**, 1073 (1970).
4. W. A. Catterall, *Annu. Rev. Pharmacol. Toxicol.* **20**, 15 (1980).
5. E. Jover, F. Couraud, and H. Rochat, *Biochem. Biophys. Res. Commun.* **95**, 1607 (1980).
6. F. Couraud, E. Jover, J.-M. Dubois, and H. Rochat, *Toxicon* **20**, 9 (1982).
7. E. Zlotkin, D. Kadouri, D. Gordon, M. Pelhate, M. F. Martin, and H. Rochat, *Arch. Biochem. Biophys.* **240**, 877 (1985).
8. D. Gordon, E. Jover, F. Couraud, and E. Zlotkin, *Biochim. Biophys. Acta* **778**, 349 (1984).
9. M. Eitan, E. Fowler, R. Herrmann, A. Duval, M. Pelhate, and E. Zlotkin, *Biochemistry* **29**, 5941 (1990).
10. H. Darbon, E. Zlotkin, C. Kopeyan, J. Van Rietschoten, and H. Rochat, *Int. J. Pept. Protein Res.* **20**, 320 (1982).
11. E. P. Loret, P. Mansuelle, H. Rochat, and C. Granier, *Biochemistry* **29**, 1492 (1990).
12. C. Kopeyan, P. Mansuelle, F. Sampieri, T. Brando, E. M. Bahraoui, H. Rochat, and C. Granier, *FEBS Lett.* **261**, 423 (1990).
13. D. D. Watt and J. M. Simard, *J. Toxicol.* **3**, 181 (1984).
14. M. E. Lima, M. F. Martin, C. R. Diniz, and H. Rochat, *Biochem. Biophys. Res. Commun.* **139**, 296 (1986).
15. A. C. Alagon, H. S. Guzman, B. M. Martin, A. N. Ramirez, E. Carbone, and L. D. Possani, *Comp. Biochem. Physiol.* **1**, 153 (1988).
16. E. V. Grishin, *Int. J. Quant. Chem.* **19**, 291 (1981).
17. S. De Dianous, F. Hoaro, and H. Rochat, *Toxicon* **25**, 411 (1987).
18. S. De Dianous, P. Carle, and H. Rochat, *Pestic. Sci.* **23**, 35 (1988).
19. E. Zlotkin, Z. Teitelbaum, H. Rochat, and F. Miranda, *Insect Biochem.* **9**, 347 (1979).
20. P. Lazarovici and E. Zlotkin, *J. Biol. Chem.* **257**, 8397 (1982).
21. D. Lester, P. Lazarovici, M. Pelhate, and E. Zlotkin, *Biochim. Biophys. Acta* **701**, 370 (1982).
22. S. De Dianous, C. Kopeyan, E. M. Bahraoui, and H. Rochat, *Toxicon* **25**, 731 (1987b).
23. J. Yong-Hua, Y. Kimura, K. Hsu, and S. Terakawa, *Comp. Biochem. Physiol. C* **90C**, 237 (1988).
24. P. E. Bougis, P. Marchot, and H. Rochat, *Biochemistry* **25**, 7235 (1986).
25. E. P. Loret, M. F. Martin-Eauclaire, P. Mansuelle, F. Sampieri, C. Granier, and H. Rochat, *Biochemistry* **30**, 633–640 (1991).
26. M. E. Lima, M. F. Martin, B. Hue, E. P. Loret, C. R. Dinitz, and H. Rochat, *Insect Biochem.* **19**, 413 (1989).
27. G. Peterson, *in* "Methods in Enzymology" (C. H. W. Hirs and S. N. Timasheff, eds.), Vol. 91, p. 95. Academic Press, New York, 1983.

[29] Potassium Channel-Blocking Toxins from Snake Venoms and Neuromuscular Transmission

A. L. Harvey, A. J. Anderson, and E. G. Rowan

Introduction

Many snake toxins affect the release of acetylcholine at the neuromuscular junction (1). The phospholipase toxins, which include β-bungarotoxin, crotoxin, notexin, and taipoxin, cause an irreversible block of acetylcholine release after a period in which release is augmented. The dendrotoxins from African mamba snakes do not block release or affect spontaneous release of acetylcholine, but only facilitate release in response to nerve action potentials.

The dendrotoxins (2–4) and at least some of the phospholipase toxins (5, 6) block certain K^+ currents in neurons. As a consequence, both types of toxins can facilitate the evoked release of acetylcholine from mammalian motor nerves, although probably by blocking different subtypes of K^+ channels (7, 8).

The toxins also act on central neurons following intracerebroventricular injection. They can be radiolabeled and shown to bind to specific high affinity sites on neuronal membranes (9–11). Consequently, the toxins have been used to probe the distribution of K^+ channels in the central nervous system (CNS) (12, 13) and to isolate putative K^+ channel proteins (14, 15). This is discussed elsewhere in this volume. In this chapter, we will concentrate on methods used to study the effects of such toxins on neuromuscular transmission and on the excitability of motor nerve endings.

Twitch Tension Recording Methods

Many isolated nerve–muscle preparations have been used for studying the effects of drugs and toxins on neuromuscular transmission. We routinely use two preparations for such functional studies: the chick biventer cervicis preparation and the mouse phrenic nerve–hemidiaphragm preparation. Both can be set up in small tissue baths (5 ml or less), and both are robust and stable over several hours *in vitro*. These features make them suitable for

Methods in Neurosciences, Volume 8

studying the effects of toxins, which are often available in only small quantities, and which are often slow in action. Because the chick biventer cervicis muscle contains both focally innervated twitch fibers and multiply innervated contracture-producing fibers, it can be stimulated by exogenously applied cholinomimetic agonists, as well as by stimulation of its motor nerve. This enables prejunctional effects to be distinguished from postjunctional effects.

Chick Biventer Cervicis Nerve–Muscle Preparation

Reagents

> Krebs–Henseleit solution (mM): NaCl, 118.4; KCl, 4.7; MgSO$_4$, 1.2; KH$_2$PO$_4$, 1.2; CaCl$_2$, 2.5; NaHCO$_3$, 25; and glucose, 11.1
> Acetylcholine chloride: 10^{-1} M
> Carbachol chloride: 10^{-3} M
> KCl: 1 M

Procedure

A chick (4–14 days) is killed by exposure to anesthetic ether. The down and feathers are plucked from the back of the head and neck to the middle of the back. The chick is pinned through its beak to a cork dissection board and its neck is supported by a 2-cm diameter cylinder. A central incision is made through the skin on the back of the neck and a cut is made in the skin from the middle of the back to the base of the skull. The two biventer cervicis muscles (16) will be seen on either side of the midline, lying on top of groups of other muscles. Throughout the dissection, the muscles should be kept moist with Krebs–Henseleit solution. Sharp-tipped scissors are used to pierce the connective tissue sheaths surrounding the muscles and their tendons, and then to cut the connective tissue along the length of the biventers. By gently raising each muscle in turn with forceps, the muscles can be freed from the underlying connective tissue and blood vessels. Care should be taken to avoid crushing parts of the long tendons, because the motor nerves run within them. A long thread is tied around the tops of the long tendons, and a thread is tied in a small loop at the bottom of each muscle. Both muscles are now removed to a beaker of Krebs–Henseleit solution.

Pairs of muscles and associated nerves are mounted in 2 ml, 5 ml, or 10-ml tissue baths containing Krebs–Henseleit solution (pH 7.3) continuously bubbled with oxygen containing 5% CO_2. The solution is maintained at a fixed temperature (either 37°C, or 32–33°C for more stable responses over a longer period).

A ring electrode is placed around the tendons and the long threads are connected to a force-displacement transducer. Twitches are evoked by stimulating the motor nerve at the desired frequency (routinely 0.1 Hz) with pulses of 0.2-msec duration and a voltage greater than that which produces a maximal twitch. The resting tension is set initially at 1 g, but it should be adjusted for each preparation so that nerve stimulation produces the maximum force from the muscle. In the absence of nerve stimulation, contractions to submaximal concentrations of exogenously applied acetylcholine ($1–3 \times 10^{-3} M$), carbachol ($1–4 \times 10^{-5} M$), and KCl ($1–4 \times 10^{-2} M$) are obtained prior to the addition of the toxin and at the end of the experiment. Acetylcholine and KCl are allowed to remain in contact with the preparations for 30 sec and carbachol for 60 sec. The preparations are then washed by overflow for 15 sec at between 5 and 10 ml/sec. After obtaining control responses to agonists, preparations are allowed to stabilize for about 30 min with continuous nerve stimulation (0.1 Hz) before the addition of toxin.

If required, preparations can be stimulated directly. Neuromuscular transmission is first abolished by, e.g., tubocurarine (10–20 μM), and the electrodes are placed around the belly of the muscle. Direct muscle stimulation can be evoked by increasing the pulse duration to 1–2 msec and by increasing the strength of the stimulus. As the multiply innervated fibers can give a slowly developing contracture during direct stimulation it is difficult to achieve a maximal twitch. Twitches and contractures are recorded isometrically on suitable ink-writing polygraphs.

Mouse Phrenic Nerve–Hemidiaphragm Preparation

Reagents

Krebs–Henseleit solution, as above

Procedure

The mouse phrenic nerve–hemidiaphragm preparation is dissected in the same way as the well-known rat diaphragm preparation (17).

The preparations are mounted in tissue baths under the same conditions as described above for the chick biventer cervicis preparations. The hemidiaphragm can be trimmed if necessary to fit in a small tissue bath. It should be noted that effects of dendrotoxins on mouse diaphragm preparations are not seen at room temperature or 30°C, but are clearly observed at 36–37°C.

For indirect stimulation, the phrenic nerve is stimulated (via a Burn and Rand electrode) at 0.1 Hz with pulses of 0.2-msec duration and of sufficient strength to produce a maximal twitch. For direct muscle stimulation, two silver electrodes are hooked onto either side of the rib; pulses of 2 msec are applied at 0.1 Hz with sufficient strength to produce a maximal twitch. Tubocurarine (10–20 μM) is used to prevent neuromuscular transmission.

Preparations can also be stimulated alternately indirectly via the phrenic nerve and directly via the hook electrodes at a frequency of 0.05 Hz. Under these conditions, tubocurarine is always added prior to the start of the experiment to ensure that activation of nerve endings by the field stimulation does not significantly contribute to the overall tension recorded in response to the direct stimulation. If there is more than a 10% decrease in responses to "direct" stimulation in the presence of tubocurarine, the hook electrodes are repositioned to avoid this artefact. After washout of the tubocurarine, preparations are allowed 30–60 min to stabilize prior to the addition of toxin.

Electrophysiological Methods

For electrophysiological studies on neuromuscular transmission, it is best to have a thin muscle so that end-plate regions can be located by visual identification. Additionally, fibers that are large enough to allow stable impalements for at least 1 hr are necessary for experiments with snake toxins because effects are often slow in onset.

Several preparations have been used: for example, frog sartorius and frog cutaneous pectoris (18), mouse or rat diaphragms, mouse triangularis sterni (19), and mouse levator auris longus (20). We will describe one mammalian (triangularis sterni of the mouse) and one amphibian (frog cutaneous pectoris) preparation.

Mouse Triangularis Sterni Nerve–Muscle Preparation

Reagents

Krebs–Henseleit solution, as above
HEPES physiological salt solution (mM): NaCl, 154; KCl, 5.0; MgCl$_2$, 1.2; CaCl$_2$, 2.5; glucose, 11.1; and Na-HEPES, 5.0 (pH 7.4)

Procedures

Dissection
Experiments are performed on the left triangularis sterni (TS) nerve–muscle preparation (19) isolated as described below from mice weighing about 20–25 g. As different strains of mice from different suppliers seem to vary in the

pattern of innervation of the TS, it may be necessary to select a strain that provides convenient access to the three nerves innervating the TS. The complete dissection of the muscle with its three nerves is performed under continuous perfusion at a rate of 15–20 ml/min with Krebs–Henseleit solution (aerated with oxygen containing 5% carbon dioxide). A dissecting microscope with transillumination is used to aid dissection.

The TS muscle is located on the inner surface of the rib cage. It is a trapezoidal sheet originating at the sternum and inserting at the intercalations of the ribs. The muscle is bounded by the second and seventh intercostal spaces, which form its inner and outer limits.

The entire rib cage is removed from mice killed by cervical dislocation and exsanguination. The rib cage is then pinned, with the inner ribs uppermost, to a Sylgard-lined (Dow Corning, Midland, MI) Petri dish. The inner area of rib is carefully cleared of all excess tissue, ensuring that the exposed TS is not damaged. The rib cage is now turned over and pinned to the Sylgard base with the outer ribs uppermost. To ease the dissection, the ribs are fanned out and secured with pins. At this point, two preparations can be made by carefully dividing the preparation longitudinally at the sternum, although we do not normally do this. The muscles at each intercostal space (starting at the abdominal end) are carefully removed in layers until the TS (or usually the nerve branch innervating the muscle) is visible. The remaining overlying muscle is removed a few millimeters proximal to the nerve branch; this is repeated at each intercostal space. The ribs are cut free of the sternum and cut a few millimeters proximal to the nerve branch and lifted free of the preparation. The surface of the TS can be cleaned of any remaining tissue that may cause obstructions. The separate nerve trunks running parallel to the rib are also isolated; at least 1 cm of nerve can be dissected out.

For experiments, the TS nerve–muscle preparation is pinned thoracic side downward to the base of a 2- to 3-ml Sylgard-lined tissue bath, and perfused at a rate of 5–10 ml/min with Krebs–Henseleit solution or HEPES-buffered solution. Twitching is abolished by addition of tubocurarine, α-bungarotoxin, or by using a high Mg^{2+}/low Ca^{2+} physiological salt solution, as appropriate for the particular experiment.

Electrophysiological Recording

Intact nerve–muscle preparations are observed using a binocular compound microscope with a movable stage. To assist the localization of superficial motor nerve endings for electrode placement, preparations are observed at a magnification of $\times 400$–600 using a high-magnification ($\times 40$), long working distance objective (Zeiss or Olympus).

Microelectrodes used for intracellular and extracellular recording are prepared from 1.2-mm (external diameter) borosilicate glass capillaries containing internal glass filaments (Clark Electromedical Instruments, Pang-bourne, UK; type GC120f). The microelectrodes are pulled on an electrode puller and filled with 2 M NaCl (resistance 5–15 MΩ) for extracellular recording, and 3 M KCl (resistance 10–20 MΩ) for intracellular recording.

The potential difference between a silver/silver chloride reference electrode (pellet type) in the bath and the recording electrode is measured by a high-impedance unity gain electrometer, displayed and amplified on a dual-beam storage oscilloscope and simultaneously stored on FM tape or video-tape, as described below under Data Analysis.

For extracellular recording of nerve terminal action potentials, the intercostal nerves are stimulated via a suction electrode every 2 sec with pulses of 50-μsec duration and supramaximal voltage. Recording electrodes are placed inside the perineural sheath (near end-plate areas) of one of the branches of an intercostal nerve (see Refs. 21–23). Usually 20–25 waveforms are recorded at each time period. As the shape of the waveform recorded is directly dependent on the electrode position, waveforms are monitored for 20 min prior to the start of the experiment and continuously from the same site throughout application of toxins and drugs. If the waveform changes by more than 10% during the initial 20-min monitoring period, the electrode position is adjusted or a new site is tried. The microelectrode should be as close as possible to the preterminal branching of the motor nerve. In general, the second negative waveform should be as large as possible (see Fig. 1). The first negative deflection is caused by the Na$^+$ current and the second negative deflection reflects the K$^+$ current at the terminals.

As shown in Fig. 1, the extracellular waveform in the TS preparation has different appearances at different recording positions. This is due to the asymmetrical distribution of Na$^+$ and K$^+$ channels in the mammalian motor nerve (see Refs. 21–23). Sodium ion channels are not present at high density in the nonmyelinated terminal regions; hence, the active depolarization at the last nodes of Ranvier and the heminodal region caused by the inward Na$^+$ current of the action potential gives rise to a local circuit current that appears to be outward at the terminal regions. Conversely, K$^+$ channels are found at the terminals, but not at the nodes of Ranvier. The active, outward K$^+$ current at the terminals creates a local circuit current that is inward at the heminode and final nodes of Ranvier.

We routinely use perineural recording in preference to focal recording from the terminals because the signal is larger, has a better signal-to-noise ratio, and is more stable. This last point is important when working with toxins that have a slow and progressive action on acetylcholine release.

Figure 2 shows typical effects of the phospholipase toxins β-bungarotoxin, crotoxin, notexin, and taipoxin on perineural waveforms. It can be seen that the toxins produce a significant reduction in the second negative deflection

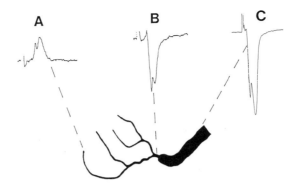

Fig. 1   Schematic diagram of a neuromuscular region in the mouse triangularis sterni preparation. The shape of the waveform associated with an action potential depends on the position of the extracellular recording electrode: (A) terminal region, (B) preterminal or heminodal region, and (C) perineural.

(associated with K^+ currents) with little effect on the first negative deflection (related to the Na^+ current).

Although a stable Na^+ spike is necessary in order to be confident about changes in the second negative deflection being caused by the toxin rather than change in electrode position, there are other problems of interpretation. For example, low concentrations of tetrodotoxin or μ-conotoxin can cause an apparently selective block of terminal ''K^+ currents'' (24). Higher concentrations reveal the expected block of the main Na^+ spike. The explanation is presumably because of a loss of some of the driving force for nerve terminal depolarization.

For intracellular recording, the microelectrode is inserted into a muscle fiber at an end-plate region. Cells are rejected if the initial membrane potential is less than -70 mV, if the membrane potential is not stable, or if the rise time of the end-plate potential (EPP) or miniature EPP is greater than 1 msec (see Fig. 4). Recordings are made continuously from one end plate before and during application of toxins.

Physiological solution (10–20 ml) containing the toxin at the desired concentration is perfused onto the preparation and recycled after aeration.

Most experiments are performed at room temperature, although it should be remembered that dendrotoxins have greater effects in mammalian preparations at body temperature (7), and the phospholipase toxins act more rapidly at higher temperatures. Figure 3 shows that the perineural waveform becomes much faster as temperature is increased. However, the phospholipase toxins still produce their characteristic block of a fraction of the K^+-related waveform (Fig. 4).

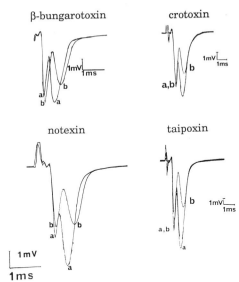

FIG. 2   Effects of four presynaptically active phospholipase A_2 neurotoxins on perineural waveforms from mouse TS preparations. a, Control waveform; b, waveform after a 60-min exposure to toxin.

For experiments performed at 30 or 37°C the perfusing solution is passed through a constant-temperature hot water jacket before entering the tissue bath. To reduce the temperature drop across the preparation the tissue bath is fitted into a water jacket mounted on the microscope stage. Hot water at the required temperature is pumped through the water jacket in the direction opposite to the flow of the physiological salt solution. This procedure allows countercurrent heat exchange to take place and thus prevent a temperature gradient in the tissue bath.

We have found that nerve terminal function is not well maintained in mouse TS preparations at 37°C in Krebs–Henseleit solution unless flow rate is rapid. Consequently, we often use a HEPES-buffered solution.

Frog Cutaneous Pectoris Nerve–Muscle Preparation

Reagents

Ringer's solution (mM): NaCl, 111; KCl, 2; NaHCO$_3$, 2; CaCl$_2$, 1.8 (pH 7.2)

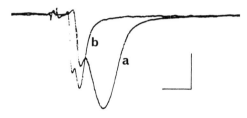

Fig. 3   Effect of temperature on perineural waveforms from a mouse TS preparation. a, Recorded at 20°C; b, recorded from the same site at 37°C. Calibration: 1 mV and 1 msec.

Procedures

Dissection

Left cutaneous pectoris preparations (18) are dissected from small frogs (*Rana pipiens* or *Rana temporaria*). The complete dissection of the muscle and nerve is performed in the presence of Ringer's solution, which is changed frequently during the dissection.

The cutaneous pectoris muscle is located just under the skin on the ventral side of the frog. It is a transparent rectangular sheet of muscle some three to six fibers thick. A branch of the ulnaris nerve, the pectoralis proprius, innervates the muscle.

A pithed frog is firmly pinned ventral side uppermost to a cork board viewed through a dissecting microscope. The skin overlying the cutaneous pectoris muscle, the ulnaris nerve, and pectoralis proprius nerve are carefully dissected free. It is important to ensure that the upper tendon attaching the muscle to the skin is not cut, as this piece of skin is used to manipulate the muscle during the dissection. A 2-cm long piece of ulnaris nerve is cut free from its surrounding tissue before being cut. This piece of ulnaris nerve is used to aid the dissection of the pectoralis proprius nerve from the surrounding tissue and up to the muscle. The strip of skin with the muscle attached is then dissected free of the surrounding tissue, and it, along with a portion of the lower tendon attachment of the muscle, is lifted free and pinned ventral side down to a Sylgard-lined Petri dish. By pinning the muscle by the attached piece of skin and the rectus abdominis muscle, the remnants of the deltoids and pectoralis muscle can be removed, leaving the pectoralis proprius nerve intact. The pectoralis proprius nerve runs on top of the muscle, crossing the muscle fibers in the middle. The muscle can now be transferred to the tissue bath used experimentally, while ensuring the muscle is kept in the same orientation as before.

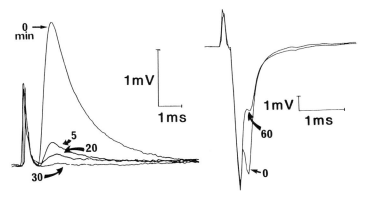

FIG. 4   Effect of crotoxin at 30°C on end-plate potentials (left) and perineural wave-forms (right) from mouse TS preparations. Note the rapid reduction in end-plate potential amplitude (over 30 min), although the perineural recording reveals that only the K^+-related waveform is affected.

For experiments, the cutaneous pectoris muscle preparation is pinned ventral side downward to the base of a 2- to 3-ml Sylgard-lined tissue bath. The Ringer's solution is changed several times before the start of the experiment, but thereafter the same solution can be used throughout. Toxins can be added directly to the bath solution, or in a perfusate.

Electrophysiological Recording

The procedures described above for recording from the triangularis sterni preparation can be followed. It should be remembered that the separation between Na^+ and K^+ channels is less in amphibian motor nerves than in mammalian ones. Therefore, the perineural waveform shows less distinction between Na^+- and K^+-dependent components.

Data Analysis

All signals collected on the FM or video tape recorder are amplified to approximately 4 V and then digitized by an analog-to-digital converter (CED 502, Cambridge Electronic Designs, Cambridge, UK). Each digitized event consists of 512 points collected every 40 μsec. These events are then analyzed by an IBM PC computer. The analysis program (SCAN or CDR, written by John Dempster, Department of Physiology and Pharmacology, University of Strathclyde and available on request) is used to visualize the digitized event and either accept it for further analysis or reject it. The accepted events are used by the computer to generate histograms and averaged records.

For intracellular records, the analysis program determines the amplitude, rise time, and decay time constant of the digitized signals. It can also determine quantal content by three methods (the direct method, by failures, or by analysis of variance).

The amplitude of an event is measured as the difference between 1 msec of preceding baseline and the point of greatest amplitude during the event. The rise time is calculated as the time between points at 10 and 90% of the peak amplitude derived from a straight line fitted to the points between 10 and 90% of the peak. The decay time constant is estimated as the inverse of the slope of a single exponential fitted to the points between 95 and 5% of the peak amplitude on the decay phase of the event.

References

1. A. L. Harvey, editor, "Snake Toxins." Pergamon, New York, 1991.
2. E. Benoit and J.-M. Dubois, *Brain Res.* **377**, 373 (1986).
3. J. V. Halliwell, I. B. Othman, A. Pelchen-Matthews, and J. O. Dolly, *Proc. Natl. Acad. Sci. U.S.A.* **83**, 493 (1986).
4. C. Stansfeld and A. Feltz, *Neurosci. Lett.* **93**, 49 (1988).
5. M. Petersen, R. Penner, F.-K. Pierau, and F. Dreyer, *Neurosci. Lett.* **68**, 141 (1986).
6. F. Dreyer and R. Penner, *J. Physiol. (London)* **386**, 455 (1987).
7. A. J. Anderson and A. L. Harvey, *Br. J. Pharmacol.* **93**, 215 (1988).
8. E. G. Rowan and A. L. Harvey, *Br. J. Pharmacol.* **94**, 839 (1988).
9. A. R. Black and J. O. Dolly, *Eur. J. Biochem.* **156**, 609 (1986).
10. H. Rehm, J.-N. Bidard, H. Schweitz, and M. Lazdunski, *Biochemistry* **27**, 1827 (1988).
11. A. L. Harvey, D. L. Marshall, F. A. De-Allie, and P. N. Strong, *Biochem. Biophys. Res. Commun.* **163**, 394 (1989).
12. J.-N. Bidard, C. Mourre, G. Gandolfo, H. Schweitz, C. Widmann, C. Gottesman, and M. Lazdunski, *Brain Res.* **495**, 45 (1989).
13. A. Pelchen-Matthews and J. O. Dolly, *Neuroscience* **29**, 347 (1989).
14. A. R. Black, C. M. Donegan, B. J. Denny, and J. O. Dolly, *Biochemistry* **27**, 6814 (1988).
15. H. Rehm and M. Lazdunski, *Proc. Natl. Acad. Sci. U.S.A.* **85**, 4949 (1988).
16. B. L. Ginsborg and J. Warriner, *Br. J. Pharmacol.* **15**, 410 (1960).
17. E. Bülbring, *Br. J. Pharmacol.* **1**, 38 (1946).
18. F. Dreyer and K. Peper, *Pfluegers Arch.* **348**, 257 (1974).
19. J. J. McArdle, D. Angaut-Petit, A. Mallart, R. Bournaud, L. Faille, and J. L. Brigant, *J. Neurosci. Methods* **4**, 109 (1981).

20. D. Angaut-Petit, J. Molgo, A. L. Connold, and L. Faille, *Neurosci. Lett.* **82,** 83 (1987).
21. A. Mallart, *J. Physiol. (London)* **368,** 565 (1985).
22. R. Penner and F. Dreyer, *Pfluegers Arch.* **406,** 190 (1986).
23. A. J. Anderson, A. L. Harvey, E. G. Rowan, and P. N. Strong, *Br. J. Pharmacol.* **95,** 1329 (1988).
24. A. J. Anderson, M. F. M. Braga, A. L. Harvey, and E. G. Rowan, *Br. J. Pharmacol.,* in press (1991).

Index